The Complete

ARTHRITIS

HEALTH, DIET GUIDE
& COOKBOOK

• SECOND EDITION •

The Complete
ARTHRITIS
HEALTH, DIET GUIDE
& COOKBOOK

• SECOND EDITION •

Includes 125 recipes for managing inflammation & arthritis pain

KIM ARREY, BSc, RD
with DR. MICHAEL R. STARR, MD, FRCPC

Robert
ROSE

The Complete Arthritis Health, Diet Guide & Cookbook, Second Edition

For complete cataloguing information, see page 337.

Disclaimer

This book is a general guide only and should never be a substitute for the skill, knowledge, and experience of a qualified medical professional dealing with the facts, circumstances, and symptoms of a particular case.

The nutritional, medical, and health information presented in this book is based on the research, training, and professional experience of the authors, and is true and complete to the best of their knowledge. However, this book is intended only as an informative guide for those wishing to know more about health, nutrition, and medicine; it is not intended to replace or countermand the advice given by the reader's personal physician. Because each person and situation is unique, the authors and the publisher urge the reader to check with a qualified health-care professional before using any procedure where there is a question as to its appropriateness. A physician should be consulted before beginning any exercise program. The authors and the publisher are not responsible for any adverse effects or consequences resulting from the use of the information in this book. It is the responsibility of the reader to consult a physician or other qualified health-care professional regarding his or her personal care.

This book contains references to products that may not be available everywhere. The intent of the information provided is to be helpful; however, there is no guarantee of results associated with the information provided. Use of brand names is for educational purposes only and does not imply endorsement.

The recipes in this book have been carefully tested by our kitchen and our tasters. To the best of our knowledge, they are safe and nutritious for ordinary use and users. For those people with food or other allergies, or who have special food requirements or health issues, please read the suggested contents of each recipe carefully and determine whether or not they may create a problem for you. All recipes are used at the risk of the consumer. We cannot be responsible for any hazards, loss, or damage that may occur as a result of any recipe use. For those with special needs, allergies, requirements, or health problems, in the event of any doubt, please contact your medical adviser prior to the use of any recipe.

At the time of publication, all URLs linked to existing websites. Robert Rose Inc. is not responsible for maintaining, and does not endorse the content of, any website or content not created by Robert Rose Inc.

Design and Production: Daniella Zanchetta/PageWave Graphics Inc.
Editor: Sue Sumeraj
Proofreader: Kelly Jones
Indexer: Gillian Watts
Illustrations (p.16, 20, 21, 68-73): Kveta (Three in a Box)
Illustration (p.144): hands © iStockphoto.com/Kharlamova
Cover image: Healthy indredients with plate © iStockphoto.com/Foxys_forest_manufacture
Back cover image: Healthy spring salmon salad © iStockphoto.com/Foxys_forest_manufacture

The publisher gratefully acknowledges the financial support of our publishing program by the Government of Canada through the Canada Book Fund.

Canadä

Published by Robert Rose Inc.
120 Eglinton Avenue East, Suite 800, Toronto, Ontario, Canada M4P 1E2
Tel: (416) 322-6552 Fax: (416) 322-6936
www.robertrose.ca

Printed and bound in USA

1 2 3 4 5 6 7 8 9 LSC 27 26 25 24 23 22 21 20 19

Contents

Foreword

Arthritis is a very common condition that affects adults the world over. In North America, it is estimated that one in five adults has some type of arthritis. This means that about 55 million North American adults currently suffer from arthritis, and this figure is expected to rise to 75 million courtesy of the baby boomers. Arthritis comes with a large price tag, not only in terms of the costs for medical care, but also in terms of quality of life. Approximately one in three people with arthritis has limitations on physical activity.

Referring to arthritis as though it is one disease is misleading. There are actually more than 100 different types of arthritis. We have decided to devote this book to osteoarthritis and rheumatoid arthritis because they are the types of arthritis we see most often in our practices, which are a reflection of the arthritis population in North America. We have many years of experience in treating patients with arthritis, as a medical doctor and as a registered dietitian, and we bring to this task the most recent clinical studies of arthritis.

> No matter what type of arthritis you have, the treatment goals are the same: to reduce pain, to control inflammation, to maintain or increase your ability to function, and to improve your quality of life.

The treatments for the different types of arthritis can vary greatly. We have made every effort to state clearly which treatments are applicable to patients with rheumatoid arthritis (RA), which are applicable to osteoarthritis (OA), and which could be used by people suffering from either OA or RA. Make sure that you are looking at the correct section and are reading the information that will be useful to you.

No matter what type of arthritis you have, the treatment goals are the same: to reduce pain, to control inflammation, to maintain or increase your ability to function, and to improve your quality of life. This book will help you achieve these goals. It will also help you manage conditions often associated with arthritis, such as obesity, heart disease, and diabetes. We made every attempt to keep these conditions in mind when developing management recommendations.

Recent advances, especially in the development of new drugs, have made the medical management of arthritis more successful in meeting the treatment goals. Therefore, you are encouraged to consult with your medical doctor to determine if there are any arthritis medications that might be appropriate for you. Optimal arthritis management involves more than drug treatments, however. A comprehensive approach also includes lifestyle changes and dietary therapy, and may even include surgery.

The focus of much of this book is on the role nutrition can play in managing arthritis. Although there is no diet or nutritional supplement that is proven to cure arthritis, we review the foods that can have an impact on arthritis management, as well as nutritional and herbal supplements that may be helpful in some cases. An effective diet is presented in a 28-day menu plan, and we've included more than 125 recipes chosen specifically for people managing arthritis. You will also find some helpful hints on how to make grocery shopping and cooking easier for you and your family.

We hope this book provides you with the information you need about the medical management of arthritis, and at the same time inspires you to add a nutrition component to your comprehensive arthritis management program.

Kim Arrey, BSc, RD
Dr. Michael R. Starr, MD, FRCPC

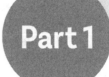

Part 1

UNDERSTANDING ARTHRITIS

CHAPTER 1

Who Gets Arthritis?

CASE HISTORY
Family Affair

George and Gladys came to the clinic complaining of pain in their joints. They had been married for 35 years and tended to do things together, including visiting their doctor. George, a 65-year-old retired carpenter, was experiencing pain in the knee and could feel something crunching and grinding when he walked. The pain was sufficiently severe that he avoided walking whenever possible and, as a result, had gained more than 10 pounds during the past year. George had previously enjoyed an active life, working hard at his job, but had begun to experience some general wear and tear as he grew older. He had looked forward to retirement to take a load off his back. Instead, his general quality of life had deteriorated and he was feeling somewhat depressed. The over-the-counter pain medications he was using didn't offer much relief.

Gladys, an active, 60-year-old real estate agent, was suffering from pain, swelling, and stiffness in her hands and wrists, especially first thing in the morning. At times, she found it impossible to grasp her knife and fork while eating. At work, she found it hard to complete legal forms, whether using a pen or a keyboard. Gladys suspected she had arthritis but wasn't sure of this self-diagnosis.

After completing a thorough physical examination and taking a family history (both sets of their parents had similar complaints later in life), they were directed to a laboratory for various tests. George's knee was X-rayed, and he underwent a local procedure known as joint aspiration to test the fluid in his knees. Gladys's painful joints were examined by X-ray and in an MRI machine, and her blood was tested for various factors and markers, including sedimentation rate, C-reactive protein (CRP), and rheumatoid factor. Her suspicions were correct. Gladys was diagnosed with rheumatoid arthritis, and George was diagnosed with osteoarthritis. What a pair!

They found some comfort in knowing their diagnoses, and we sat down with them to explain more about the causes of these conditions and the range of treatments available to them. They left the office joking with one another about who had the worst condition — and vowing to stick to their treatment plans, which included taking arthritis medications, making lifestyle modifications, and adopting an anti-arthritis diet plan.

Almost everyone we know complains occasionally about aches and pains in the joints, most often in the knees and the hands. These aches become especially prevalent as we get older, and most people think that arthritis is a disease that strikes only in older individuals as a result of wear and tear. But this condition can also occur in younger individuals.

Did You Know?

Two Basic Types of Arthritis

There are many different types of arthritis, but they are usually grouped into two broad categories: degenerative disorders, like osteoarthritis (OA), and autoimmune and inflammatory disorders, like rheumatoid arthritis (RA). Approximately 100 different types of arthritis fall into the autoimmune group.

Prevalence and Incidence

Osteoarthritis (OA) is the most common form of arthritis. It affects millions of people around the world. When a group of older adults gets together, it is quite common for some of them to have osteoarthritis. In fact, osteoarthritis is often called a disease of wear and tear because it is so common in older people.

- OA is the most commonly diagnosed form of arthritis. It is no longer considered only a disease of wear and tear, but a condition that results when the body cannot repair damaged joint tissues.

- OA can be the result of injury or can occur at any age. However, it is most frequently diagnosed in people over the age of 50.

- Rheumatoid arthritis (RA) is different in that it not only affects the joints, but it can also affect the whole body, and it usually strikes in the prime of life, between the ages of 30 and 60.

- Three times more women than men get RA. However, the men who do get RA often have a more severe type of the disease.

Signs and Symptoms

Arthritis is not usually a sudden-onset condition. The signs and symptoms are often slow to show, but when they become pronounced, they are easy to diagnose as osteoarthritis or rheumatoid arthritis.

Joint Pain

In both categories of arthritis, the major symptom that most people mention is joint pain. The pain may be in one particular joint (in OA) or in multiple joints in a symmetric pattern (in RA). In OA, the pain can be mild. It is often first noticed after exercise or when you put weight or pressure on the joint in question. As the bone starts to rub on the bone, the pain can become constant and even wake you up at night. In RA, the pain is very different. It can be sharp and intense, almost

Quick Guide to the Kinds of Arthritis

Kind	Common Location	Signs & Symptoms
Osteoarthritis	Weight-bearing joints such as hips and knees Also hands, feet, spine and neck	• Onset at approximately 50 years of age • Pain on movement • Joint stiffness • Loss of motion • Grinding and crunching in joints • Swelling of joints may occur
Autoimmune Conditions		
Rheumatoid arthritis	Hands and feet	• Onset between 30 and 60 years of age • Multiple joints • Joint swelling • Morning stiffness
Ankylosing spondylitis (AS), part of spondylo-arthritis	Lower back and buttocks	• Onset before the age of 40 to 45 • Back pain lasting at least 3 months • Back pain relieved by exercise • Can affect eyes, lungs, kidneys, bowels
Psoriatic arthritis	Finger joints, toe joints, pain in tendons and ligaments that attach to the bone	• Develops in up to 20% of patients with psoriasis • Generally appears between the ages of 20 and 50 • May mimic OA, RA or AS • Redness and swelling in end of finger or toe joints ("sausage digits") • Pain in fingers, back, feet, heels
Systemic lupus erythematosus (SLE)	Can involve the joints, heart, lungs, kidney, and nervous system	• Most lupus patients experience arthritis • Fever, fatigue, depression • Rashes are common especially with sun exposure
Crystal arthritis (gout)	Big toe, ankle, knee	• Occurs in men over 30, women over 50 years of age • Acute hot, painful swelling in big toe • Can occur in knee, ankle or foot • Often associated with red wine, red meat, seafood
Reactive arthritis	Joints in lower limbs; can affect eyes, skin, muscles or tendons, urethra	• Occurs in younger individuals, 18 to 40 years of age • Acute painful swelling of one or more joints • Recent infection, including from food
Septic arthritis	Joints	• Acute, hot, red, very painful swelling in one joint • Fever, chills • Caused by bacterial or fungal infection • Recent surgical procedure

as if someone is stabbing you. It can continue constantly for long periods at a time or be of a short duration, and it can affect many joints at the same time.

Joint Stiffness

In both types of arthritis, many people complain of stiffness in their joints. This is usually most pronounced in the morning, upon rising. In people with RA, the stiffness often lasts for at least 45 minutes to 1 hour but can last for up to 4 hours. In OA, morning stiffness usually lasts for less than 30 minutes. In both types of arthritis, there can also be pain after a long car ride or even sitting for too long.

Muscle Weakness

Muscle weakness can occur in both types of arthritis. In OA, muscle weakness occurs primarily as a result of lack of use. Often the pain of OA will reduce the amount of your physical activity. This will cause a loss of muscle strength.

Swelling of the Joint

People with RA will notice that their joints may become swollen. They can also become warm and painful. People with OA are more likely to complain of swollen joints after participating in an activity that stresses the joint.

Deformation of the Joint

In OA, the joints lose the cartilage that provides a cushion between the bones. This usually takes a long time to occur, so the deformations of the joints are often not noticed until years after the initial diagnosis. This can result in the bone resting on bone, which can lead to the formation of bone spurs. Deformation of the joints is most obvious in the joints of the fingers.

In RA, the joint deformation is more common and obvious. It can be caused by the eroding of cartilage or by damage to tendons or ligaments. When the tendons and ligaments no longer function properly, they no longer hold the joint in place. This will ultimately lead to deformation of the joints. People with RA often notice that their joints have become deformed soon after their diagnosis.

Reduced Range of Motion

In both OA and RA, the changes that occur in the joints can limit the range of motion. Muscle weakness also contributes to this problem.

CHAPTER 2

What Causes Arthritis?

Osteoarthritis (OA) is a degenerative joint disease, while rheumatoid arthritis (RA) is an autoimmune disorder. Both conditions can inflame the joints, which can cause chronic pain and reduce joint mobility. Recent research suggests that inflammation may be the common denominator in OA and RA.

Joint Anatomy and Pathophysiology

A healthy joint has many different components, each of which has a specific job. Any of the different parts of a joint can be injured, worn down, or inflamed. Some can even break. Each of these components can play a role in the development of arthritis.

Muscles

Muscles do many jobs, including giving the body its structure by supporting the bones.

Strong muscles can help reduce the strain on your weight-bearing bones. The muscles surrounding the joints are called skeletal muscles. They only contract when they get a signal from the brain. The signal passes down the nerve and is then transmitted to the muscle cells. Different types of fibers in the muscles then contract. Muscles can become bigger and stronger the more that you use them. When they are not used very often, as can be the case when you have OA or RA, the muscles become weaker and weaker and are eventually invaded by fat cells, which cause them to atrophy and break down.

> A healthy joint has many different components, each of which has a specific job. Any of the different parts of a joint can be injured, worn down, or inflamed. Some can even break.

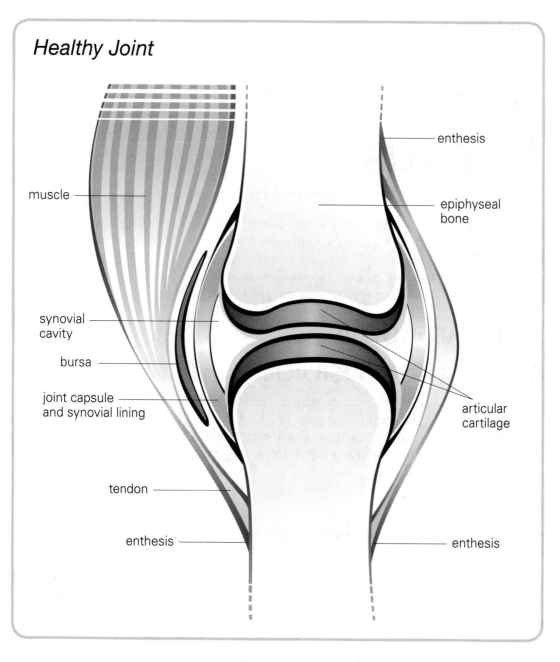

Healthy Joint

muscle

synovial
cavity

bursa

joint capsule
and synovial lining

tendon

enthesis

enthesis

epiphyseal
bone

articular
cartilage

enthesis

Tendons

Tendons attach the muscles to the bone. The tendons are
workhorses. They act like a pulley, taking the force of the
muscle contraction and transferring it to the bone so the body
moves the way you want it to. In OA, as the muscles get weaker,
the tendons have to work harder and may become irritated and
start to break down. In RA, the tendons can rupture or they
can be moved into new positions because of the swelling that
occurs in the joints.

Muscle Size

Recent studies suggest that there are differences in the muscle size (length and strength) in patients with OA as compared with patients who do not suffer from arthritis. The results of this study have led to more questions because it is not known if the changes in the muscles are a result or a cause of the disease. When RA is active, patients seems to burn calories at a faster rate, so they lose weight even if they eat as much as they usually eat. In people with RA, this is most likely to result in a loss of muscle mass, which leads to loss of muscle strength. Studies have shown that resistance training can help to maintain muscle mass, which in turn leads to being able to stand for longer periods of time and a feeling of well-being. Keeping active and participating in a specially designed exercise program that includes stretching, cardiovascular exercise, and resistance training is one of the best ways to reduce the damage to your muscles that may occur.

Ligaments

Ligaments are used to connect the bones to the bones. They are made of collagen, which is a bit elastic. Ligaments help to keep the joint strong and add stability to the joint. OA causes a bit of a dilemma for scientists. It is believed that suffering an injury to the ligaments might be a cause of arthritis, but it is also believed that the changes in the structure of the joint might lead to injuries of the ligament. In RA, as the disease attacks that joint, it is possible that toxic chemicals are released and these chemicals can cause inflammation and damage to the ligaments.

Synovial Cavity and Fluid

This cavity is filled with synovial fluid, which is like the stuffing in a pillow. When the synovial fluid is healthy and present in a good quantity, the bones of the joint are well cushioned and don't rub together. Another job the synovium performs is to bring nourishment to the cartilage. In OA, the synovial fluid becomes filled with substances that are fighting inflammation. This will eventually cause the cartilage to break down, leading to the development of pain and reduced mobility. In RA, the fluid becomes filled with chemicals that are toxic to the joint. There is a buildup of antibodies and other immune cells, blood vessels, and fibrous cells in the synovial cavity, which can form a pannus. This pannus grows very quickly and soon runs out of

Did You Know?

Bursa Cushion

The bursa is like a little pillow between the two bones of a joint, the bones and the tendon, and the bones and the ligaments. It acts like a cushion between all of these different parts. A healthy bursa keeps the bones from touching and allows for smooth movement. In both types of arthritis, the bursa may be damaged and become irritated and inflamed. This will cause even more pain.

space, causing it to wear away the cartilage and the bone that is near it. The warmth that you feel in your joint, along with the swelling and pain associated with RA, are caused by the inflammation and formation of the pannus.

Cartilage

Cartilage is also present in most joints. It is made up of collagen, water, and proteoglycans. Its role is to make sure that there is no friction between the two bones of a joint. This means that the bone will slide easily and not get stuck. Cartilage plays a key role in the development of OA. Cartilage starts to break down, but it is not repaired as quickly as it is broken down. Over time, the cartilage becomes brittle and eventually starts to wear away. This will result in bone rubbing on bone. In RA, the cartilage is broken down through a different mechanism. The toxic chemicals that are produced by the cells in the lining of the synovial cavity can damage the cartilage and the bone, eventually causing the cartilage to wear away and bone to rub on bone.

Did You Know?

Many Collagens

Collagen is a protein that is part of the structure of the different connective tissues — including tendons, ligaments, and cartilage — and is produced by chondrocytes, the cells in cartilage. Scientists have discovered up to 27 different types of collagen that seem to be variably affected in the different types of arthritis. In RA, it is believed that some changes to collagen can cause the body's defense system to go into high gear, causing the formation of an antibody to the collagen. This starts the cascade of inflammation. In osteoarthritis, the different types of collagen that make up the articular cartilage can malfunction, which plays a role in the development and progression of the disease.

Proteoglycans

Proteoglycans are one type of molecule that contribute to the formation of cartilage. They attach to water molecules, and this liquid occupies the spaces between the cells. This allows the cartilage to act like a pillow, cushioning the ends of the bones. One of the major proteoglycans that is found in the knee is chondroitin sulfate. In the beginning stages of OA, the cartilage will lose proteoglycans and, as a consequence, water. As the cartilage dries out, it will no longer be able to act like a cushion, which can lead to pain and inflammation in the joint.

In RA, a slightly different process seems to take place. As a result of the toxic chemicals and antibodies produced in the joint that is attacked by RA, the proteoglycans are torn away from the water molecules that they usually hold on to. This generally causes the cartilage to dry up and become brittle. As the cartilage breaks down, the bone rubs on bone, which can contribute to pain and inflammation.

Enthesis

The ligaments and tendons attach to the bone at the enthesis. Generally speaking, this area does not become diseased in OA or RA. However, it has been known to become inflamed in other types of inflammatory arthritis, such as septic arthritis, ankylosing spondylitis, and psoriatic arthritis. It is often the site affected in juvenile arthritis.

Epiphyseal Bone

Epiphyseal bone refers to the rounded end of a long bone. It is covered in cartilage. In OA, as the cartilage wears away, the body tries to repair it. Unfortunately, instead of repairing the cartilage, the bone starts to change. This can lead to the formation of odd-shaped bones. In RA, the cartilage and the bone are both attacked by toxic chemicals. As the body tries to repair the damage caused by the toxins, the bone can actually become misshapen. Misshapen bones often lead to pain and instability in the joint.

> **As the body tries to repair the damage caused by the toxins, the bone can actually become misshapen. Misshapen bones often lead to pain and instability in the joint.**

Anatomy of Osteoarthritis

Osteoarthritis (OA) affects all of the tissues in the joints. It does not seem to affect the rest of the body directly. In OA, the cartilage between the joints wears away or becomes damaged so that the bones rub against one another. People generally feel pain because bone is touching bone without any cushioning from the bursa or synovial fluid. Sometimes pieces of the bone (bone spurs) break off and float around in the joint, causing additional pain and discomfort.

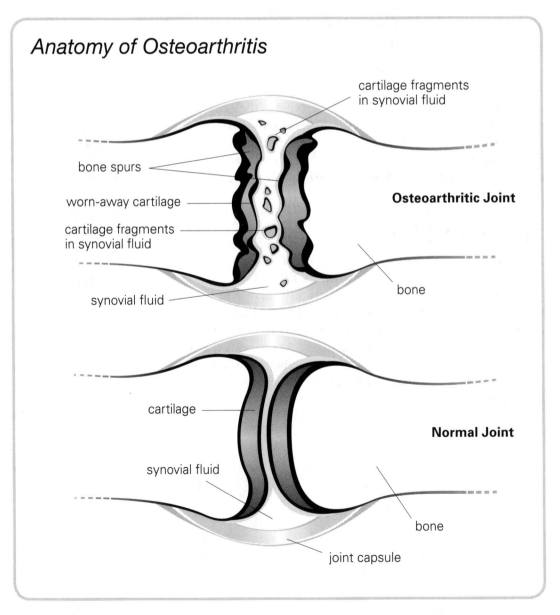

Anatomy of Osteoarthritis

cartilage fragments in synovial fluid

bone spurs

worn-away cartilage

cartilage fragments in synovial fluid

synovial fluid

Osteoarthritic Joint

bone

cartilage

synovial fluid

Normal Joint

bone

joint capsule

Anatomy of Rheumatoid Arthritis

Rheumatoid arthritis (RA) can affect the small joints in the hands and feet, as well as larger joints in the wrist, knee, shoulder, and neck. Typically, the joints are affected in a symmetrical pattern. For example, a person with RA is likely to have swelling and joint pain in both hands. RA is not usually found in only one side of the body. In RA, there is bone erosion and cartilage loss resulting from inflammation in the synovium and joint capsule. Because RA affects the whole body, it is a systemic condition. People with RA are often fatigued and lack energy.

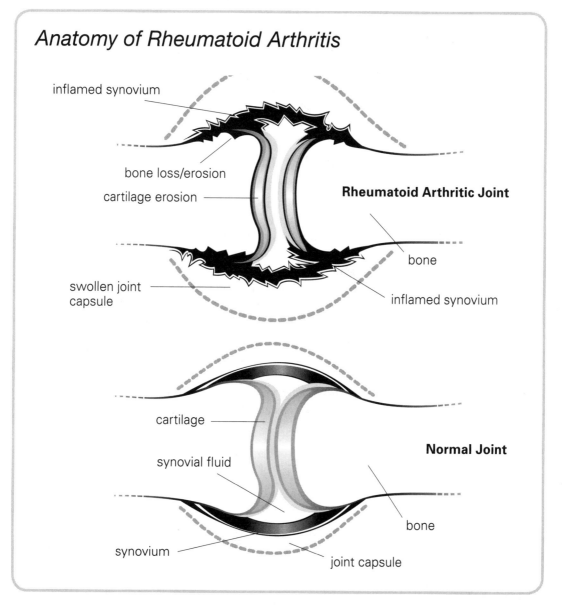

Anatomy of Rheumatoid Arthritis

inflamed synovium

bone loss/erosion

cartilage erosion

Rheumatoid Arthritic Joint

bone

inflamed synovium

swollen joint capsule

cartilage

Normal Joint

synovial fluid

bone

synovium

joint capsule

Immunity

The immune system is the body's defense against harmful invading organisms, such as bacteria, viruses, fungi, and parasites, collectively known as pathogens. Much as our armed forces are made up of different types of soldiers who have different duties, our immune system is made up of cells, proteins, tissues, and organs that work together as a network to protect the body. However, in some forms of arthritis, such as RA, these soldiers of good health have trouble resisting attack — in fact, in a peculiar physiological reaction, they can turn on themselves.

> **Much as our armed forces are made up of different types of soldiers who have different duties, our immune system is made up of cells, proteins, tissues, and organs that work together as a network to protect the body.**

White Blood Cells

White blood cells, or more specifically leukocytes, seek and destroy disease-causing substances, such as bacteria, parasites, or any other substance that does not seem to belong in the body. These cells travel throughout the body in blood and lymph circulation systems. Leukocytes are manufactured and stored in various locations of the body, including the thymus gland, spleen, lymph nodes, and bone marrow.

Phagocytes and Lymphocytes

There are two forms of leukocyte cells: phagocytes and lymphocytes. Phagocytes engulf, or "eat," the substance that is invading the body. There are many types of phagocytes, but the most common one is the neutrophil, whose primary job is to fight bacteria.

Lymphocytes are the memory of the immune system. Their job is to remember and recognize previous invaders. There are two types of lymphocytes: B lymphocytes and T lymphocytes. They are produced in the bone marrow. Some lymphocytes mature into B-cells in the bone marrow and become the body's military intelligence system, seeking out targets and sending out the troops to defend against them. Other lymphocytes leave the marrow and go to the thymus gland, where they mature into T-cells. T-cells are the troops that are sent out to destroy the enemy.

Antibodies

When foreign substances, called antigens, invade the body, the B lymphocytes spring into action and start to produce antibodies, special proteins that tag onto specific antigens. If the same antigen ever reenters the body, the antibodies are able to recognize it and act more efficiently in protecting the body against the harmful substance.

Antibodies are able to recognize and tag an antigen, but they are not able to destroy it. This is the job of the T-cells, which destroy the antigens that have been tagged by the antibodies, as well as other mutated cells.

Antibodies have other roles in the body. They can aid in the neutralization of toxins or poisonous substances in the body, and they can activate a group of proteins called complements, which also assist in the destruction of harmful substances.

Types of Immunity

Human beings have three types of immunity: innate, adaptive, and passive.

Innate Immunity
Humans are all born with innate immunity, also called natural immunity, which serves as the body's first line of defense against microbes, such as viruses, bacteria, fungi, and parasites. Innate immunity provides us with protection from viruses that can affect other animals. Innate immunity also includes our physical barriers to the external environment, chiefly our skin, hair, sweat, saliva, and tears. Not many microorganisms can penetrate intact skin. In addition, various skin and tear glands produce antimicrobial chemicals. All these products can inhibit or destroy the progression of pathogens into our bodies.

Adaptive Immunity
Adaptive immunity is the body's second line of defense. It is developed throughout life as we are exposed to diseases and immunized through vaccination. The adaptive immune system enhances some of the effects of the innate immune system by further protecting the body from invading pathogens.

Passive Immunity
Passive immunity is "borrowed" from another source and only lasts for a short time. For example, a baby receives antibodies through the mother's breast milk, which provides temporary immunity to diseases the mother has been exposed to. In the early years of childhood, this helps protect the baby against infection.

Disorders of the Immune System

Sometimes, the immune system fails to do its job and allows pathogens or foreign substances to harm the body. At other times, the body's immune system attacks its own tissues, acting as if its normal tissues were foreign or infected. This reversal is called autoimmunity — and this is what happens in rheumatoid arthritis.

Inflammation

> **Inflammation is the first response of the immune system to harmful stimuli, such as an infection, an irritant, a physical injury, or a foreign substance.**

Inflammation is the first response of the immune system to harmful stimuli, such as an infection, an irritant, a physical injury, or a foreign substance. The immune system is trying to protect the body by removing the harmful stimuli and initiating the healing process. The inflammatory response can be divided into three stages:

1. Vasodilation
2. Phagocytosis
3. Tissue repair

Stage 1: Vasodilation

When the body's tissues are damaged by harmful stimuli, the damaged cells release three key chemicals (histamine, bradykinin, and prostaglandin) into the blood or affected tissue. This serves as an alarm signal to the body to summon its forces to rid itself of foreign substances.

These chemicals initiate the inflammatory response and increase blood flow to the area. This causes dilation of the blood vessels, also known as vasodilation. During this process, more diffusion occurs as the blood vessels begin to leak fluid into the tissues, which allows the foreign substance to be isolated from further contact with the body's tissues.

Stage 2: Phagocytosis

As blood flow to the affected area increases, the plasma of the blood seeps toward the damaged tissues. The release of kinins and prostaglandins attract phagocytes and specific white blood cells (leukocytes) to the affected area. The leukocytes squeeze out of the blood vessels and approach the damaged tissues. This increase in blood flow, blood plasma, and leukocytes causes redness, heat, and swelling, which are common symptoms of inflammation.

Stage 3: Tissue Repair

Once the leukocytes reach the affected area, they engulf the bacteria and any dead body cells that remain. This may also lead to the death of the leukocytes, which, in turn, may also be digested. For this reason, pus, which is mainly composed of white blood cells and blood plasma, is usually but not always found at the site of infection.

Autoimmunity

An autoimmune disease occurs when the immune system gets confused. Instead of defending our bodies against invading bacteria or another irritant, or a type of infection, the immune system gets confused and attacks healthy cells. This leads to an inflammatory response that can be tracked through blood tests.

RA is the classic form of autoimmune arthritis. OA is not an autoimmune disease, so there are no signs of inflammation in the blood. There is some localized inflammation inside the joint itself, but it is less extensive than in RA.

Autoimmune Attack

In RA, the white blood cells charge to the joints and head for the synovium, the tissue that lines the joints. Once they are there, the white blood cells produce chemicals, such as cytokines and enzymes, that cause the tissues to become irritated, and that wear down the cartilage. These chemicals can also cause inflammation and swelling in the lining of the joint or synovium. This leads to more synovial fluid or joint fluid being manufactured and transported to the joint. This starts a chain reaction that can cause different types of damage to the joints.

- Immune cells, blood vessels, and fibrous cells join together to form a pannus, which causes the cartilage to wear away and the joints to become misshapen.

- Cartilage can be destroyed, causing bone to rub on bone.

- Synovium can eat its way into the bone, causing the joint to be painful, red, and swollen.

Inflammation is not limited to the joints in RA; it can also affect other parts of the body, including the eyes, heart, and lungs.

Inflammation is not limited to the joints in RA; it can also affect other parts of the body, including the eyes, heart, and lungs.

The Gut and a Healthy Immune System

To help our immune system to work effectively, we need to have a variety of different types of bacteria in the intestines. If our gut bacteria become imbalanced due to illness, stress or diet, that is likely to cause problems.

Scientists are now more convinced than ever that the immune system response may depend largely on how healthy your intestines are and on how your immune system reacts with the bacteria in your gut. The "control panel" of the immune system seems to be in the gut, where the immune system intercepts many of the pathogens coming into the body. The gut is also where the immune system learns to recognize something that is foreign but not harmful. For example, protein from food is not harmful, but it is a foreign substance that is entering our body.

Gut bacteria that do not cause us harm are present even before we are born. One of the reasons they are there is to teach our immune system not to overreact to every newcomer to our bodies. In fact, when babies are delivered by a caesarean, they usually have fewer bacteria in their intestines and often have more allergies and are more likely to develop an autoimmune disease.

To help our immune system to work effectively, we need to have a variety of different types of bacteria in the intestines. If our gut bacteria become imbalanced due to illness, stress or diet, that is likely to cause problems.

Some scientists also believe that if the cells in your intestines are unhealthy, this can lead to the development of small holes in the wall of the intestines. The intestinal wall is our body's first line of defense. It is part of the innate immune system, and it forms a barrier between the inside of the body and the outside world. If for some reason the cells in the intestinal wall are more fragile, it is possible for this barrier to become less resistant, which may allow for small molecules to seep into the body and potentially cause problems.

CHAPTER 3

What Is My Risk of Developing Arthritis?

....

In osteoarthritis, bone wear and tear, caused gradually by repetitive movement or instantly due to injury, is the precipitating cause of bone loss and pain. In rheumatoid arthritis, autoimmunity initiates factors that lead to bone loss and pain.

Osteoarthritis
Age

The number one factor that will predict your risk of developing OA is your age. The older we are, the greater the likelihood that our joints will be affected by OA. The disease typically shows up in the joints in our hands, especially the fingers, in our feet, and in our spine.

Genetics

Another risk factor is family history. If people in your immediate family (your mother, father, or siblings) have osteoarthritis, there is a greater chance that you will develop it. This seems to be particularly true for OA of the joints in the fingers and hands.

Currently, researchers are trying to determine which genes might be involved in the development of osteoarthritis that affects joints other than finger joints. It is possible that some inherited traits, such as being double-jointed or the way your joints fit together, may be factors that will increase your chances of developing arthritis.

> **Another risk factor is family history. If people in your immediate family (your mother, father, or siblings) have osteoarthritis, there is a greater chance that you will develop it.**

Q. What Is Collagen?

A. Collagen, produced by the cells in the cartilage, is a group of fibrous proteins that form a woven connective tissue. As we get older, our ability to make more collagen slows down, so our cartilage becomes weaker and weaker. This ultimately leads to a lack of cartilage in the joint and bone rubbing on bone. Sometimes, when a joint is injured, the body cannot replace the collagen, which leads to the cartilage breaking or wearing away. It is possible that our genes determine how much collagen we make and how easy it is for us to make it. Not being able to make enough collagen will ultimately lead to arthritis.

Recently, scientists have discovered that the process of wearing down collagen can be affected by different pro-inflammatory cytokines and enzymes that are present in the joint. We do not know what triggers this inflammatory process, but the result is that this breakdown and repair cycle gets shifted so that more collagen is broken down than is repaired. The pro-inflammatory cytokines and enzymes are present in the joint long before there is any pain in OA and before any OA joint damage can be seen in an X-ray.

> **The more weight you are carrying, the more stress you put on your joints. Studies have shown that for each pound you gain, your hips feel like you have gained six pounds, and it feels like a three-pound gain to your knees.**

Weight

Being overweight or obese will significantly increase your chances of having osteoarthritis in the hips, knees, and feet. The more weight you are carrying, the more stress you put on your joints. Studies have shown that for each pound you gain, your hips feel like you have gained six pounds, and it feels like a three-pound gain to your knees.

Losing weight will help reduce the pain and inflammation caused by the arthritis. A small amount of weight loss, perhaps 10% to 15 % of your current weight, can yield large gains in comfort and quality of life, so the effort is well worth it.

Gender

Women are more likely to develop OA, especially in the hands.

Injury

An injury to your joint or frequently performing the same repetitive movement can also lead to OA. Anyone who has broken a bone or torn the ligaments of a joint is more likely to have arthritis. OA might occur years after the initial injury, but it can occur. This is the type of arthritis that is often seen in athletes, musicians, and people who do jobs that require them to repeat the same movement over and over again.

Lifestyle

Lifestyle factors can influence your chances of developing arthritis, although we are not sure exactly what role they may play. Exercising regularly, consuming a varied and balanced diet, getting 8 hours of sleep every night, and not smoking have all been linked to a lower risk of developing OA. Scientists are not sure why this happens. These are all factors that decrease inflammation in the body, so it could be that OA is due to a systemic problem, not just wear and tear. Other scientists think it could simply be that people who have good lifestyle habits are more likely to be at a healthy weight and so less likely to have OA.

Rheumatoid Arthritis

Currently, there is no known cause for the autoimmunity that results in joint inflammation, but several genetic and environmental factors predispose individuals to develop RA.

Genetics

There do seem to be some genetic patterns involved in the onset of RA. For instance, it seems to run in families, with specific genes involved. So far, investigators have found at least six genes that play a role in the development of RA. Some researchers believe that even more genes are involved. Some of the genes involved include:

- **HLA:** These genes provide the recipe for making human leukocyte antigens. These antigens are the ones that decide which proteins belong to our bodies and which ones belong to foreign invaders like bacteria or viruses. The HLA-DRB1 gene will make you more inclined to develop anti-CCP antibodies, which are often found in the joints and blood of people with RA. Their presence seems to indicate that the body has started to attack some of the proteins that make up healthy cartilage. For some reason, smokers are more likely to have higher levels of anti-CCP antibodies.

For some reason, smokers are more likely to have higher levels of anti-CCP antibodies.

- **PTPN22:** This gene provides the recipe for making the enzyme LYP. This enzyme plays a critical role in our immune system because it helps wake up the different white blood cells, including the T-cells. People who test positive for anti-CCP antibodies are also more likely to have this gene. If you have this gene, your risk of developing RA may be doubled.

- **CTLA4:** This gene provides the recipe for making a chemical that is found on the outside of T-cells. This chemical is responsible for making sure that enough T-cells are made and for waking them up. People who test positive for anti-CCP are more likely to have this gene.

- **PADI4:** This gene provides the recipe to make peptidylarginine deiminase 4, an enzyme that plays a key role in the transformation of some very specific proteins. Although this gene is found in some North Americans, it is more commonly found in people of Asian descent.

- **STAT4:** This gene plays a role in the development of the different white blood cells. Someone who has two copies of this gene has a 60% higher risk of having RA.

- **TRAF1/C5:** These genes are located on the same chromosomes. They are associated with a 35% increase in the risk of developing RA. People who have these genes are more likely to make antibodies that get confused and attack the body — rather than a foreign invading substance.

As we become more familiar with, and more able to understand, all of the information available about our genes, we may learn that more genes are involved in RA.

Environment

Not everyone who has these genes gets RA. Scientists think that something in the environment may be the trigger that turns on the RA genes.

- **Smoking** has long been associated with an increased risk of RA. Scientists have established that individuals with the HLA-DRB1 gene who smoke have a 35% higher risk of developing RA, while those with two copies of this gene had a 55% higher risk of developing RA. Scientists are also looking at other ways that our genes can interact with some of the components in cigarette smoke.

However, smoking is a risk factor for developing RA regardless of your genetic makeup. A new study suggests that up to 1 out of 6 cases of RA may be caused by cigarette smoking. If you have stopped smoking for at least 10 years, the risk for developing RA becomes the same as it is for the general population. Being exposed to second-hand smoke does not seem to be a risk factor for developing RA.

- **Exposure to silica:** Silica is a mineral that is present in rocks. It can be inhaled by people who do foundry or quarry work, rock drilling, stone cutting, or tunneling. Studies show that people who are exposed to high amounts of silica are more likely to develop RA than people who do not have a high level of exposure to this mineral. And people who smoke and are exposed to silica have a much higher risk of developing RA, which suggests that there are some interactions between environmental triggers of RA.

- **Air pollution:** Inhaling more air pollution may be linked to an increase in the incidence of RA.

- **Geography:** In the U.S., studies have shown that women who live in the Northeast and Midwest have higher rates of developing RA than those who live in the West. Scientists are not sure what factor in the environment is responsible for this difference.

- **Socioeconomic factors:** These factors have recently been found to be a risk factor for developing RA. Some studies show that people who are born into a poorer family or who are born to young mothers are more likely to develop RA. Other studies show that people who have a university education are less likely to develop RA. The type of job that you do can also influence the likelihood that a person will develop RA. Doing manual labor may be associated with an increase in RA.

- **Infections:** Gum disease, in particular, is linked to the development of RA. More severe gum disease is linked to more severe RA. Studies are being done to determine if other bacteria or viruses could trigger RA.

> **A new study suggests that up to 1 out of 6 cases of RA may be caused by cigarette smoking.**

> **Some studies show that people who are born into a poorer family or who are born to young mothers are more likely to develop RA.**

Q. What role do hormones play in the development of RA?

A. Scientists are becoming more convinced that female hormones play a role in the development of RA. Since the amount of female and male hormones in a woman's body changes throughout her life cycle, the influence these hormones has can vary. However, scientists have noticed a few patterns:

1. Postmenopausal women are more likely to develop RA than younger women. The younger you become menopausal, the more the risk increases.

2. The period immediately after the birth of a child is often when RA is diagnosed. The risk is highest in the first 3 months after childbirth and decreases over the next 9 months.

3. Taking medications that block the effects of estrogen in the breast tissue, such as SERMs (selective estrogen receptor modulators), increases the likelihood of developing RA. Other medications that reduce the amount of estrogen that is produced, like aromatase inhibitors, also seem to be associated with increased risk. These medications can play a very important role in the treatment of some types of breast cancer, so it is important to weigh the small risk with the possible benefits.

The constant here is the rapid decrease in the production of estrogen. Maintaining normal estrogen levels by taking either birth control pills or hormone replacement therapy has so far provided mixed results; some studies say these treatments reduce the risk of developing RA, while others say they either have no effect or could even increase the risk. More research is clearly needed in this area.

Did You Know?

Food Preservatives

Although it is possible that there is some correlation between arthritis and food preservatives (because our immune system may not recognize some of the molecules that we are consuming), there does not seem to be a clear link between either RA or OA and any food preservatives.

Pro-Inflammatory Activities

Certain activities may be involved in initiating and sustaining the autoimmune reaction. This can have an impact on both RA and OA by causing the immune system to spring into action.

Smoking

Smokers seem to have higher levels of systemic inflammation. For years, it has been observed that people who smoke have higher levels of CRP (C-reactive protein), which is associated with higher levels of inflammation. They also have lower levels of vitamins A and C, which are powerful antioxidants in the bloodstream. Why does this happen? Every time a puff of smoke is inhaled, billions of molecules go into the system. These chemicals cause a huge amount of oxidative stress on the body, which leads to various chemical reactions in the different systems of the body.

Pro-Inflammatory Foods

A diet that is low in nutrients that reduce inflammation — like omega-3 fats and some vitamins and minerals — is likely to increase your level of inflammation. For some people, foods that contain gluten, a protein that is found in some grains, are also linked to increased levels of inflammation. Studies suggest that consuming a diet that is both vegan and gluten free can result in an improvement in RA symptoms in about 25% of the people affected by it. Many people hope that a specific allergic reaction is causing their RA, but this is rarely the case.

AGEs

Advanced glycation end products (AGEs) are formed in our food as a result of some naturally occurring chemical reactions. These chemical reactions are related to the browning of food. AGEs can be found in all food products but are most prevalent in animal protein foods. The AGEs seem to cause systemic inflammation, which can intensify symptoms of RA and OA.

Did You Know?

Spontaneous Remission

There have been occasional case reports of RA going into complete remission when an offending food has been removed from the diet, but all attempts to show that these foods may cause RA in a large group of people have failed. Although you might notice a slight difference in how you feel if you remove a food from your diet, most people will only see a difference if they change their whole diet.

CHAPTER 4

How Is Arthritis Diagnosed?

Did You Know?

Location of Pain

The joints that are most often affected by OA are the hips, knees, neck, and lower back. The joints of the hands and feet can frequently be affected as well. Usually OA will occur in the joint at the base of the thumb or at the base of the big toe. There are three joints in each finger, and OA typically occurs in the joint that is closest to the fingertip or in the middle joint.

If **you suspect** that you have arthritis, based on your symptoms, you should schedule an appointment with your family doctor. The first thing your doctor will do is take a family and medical history. After looking at the affected joints, your doctor may ask you to move around to see if your arthritis is affecting your range of motion or if moving causes you any pain. The next step in the process is to have some tests done. OA is often diagnosed after a physical exam and a thorough discussion of your family history and the type of pain you are experiencing.

Osteoarthritis Diagnosis
Laboratory Tests (OA)
Blood Tests

At this time, there are no specific blood tests that can detect OA. Your doctor may ask you to have other blood tests, however, to rule out any other causes of your pain. New research on how OA affects all of the tissues in the joint may eventually lead to the identification of some markers of OA in blood tests.

X-rays

Taking an X-ray of your joints is a good way to see what is happening to your bones and the tissues around them. An X-ray will allow your doctor to tell whether your cartilage has started to break down or if you have bone spurs, both of which are signs of arthritis. It will also allow your doctor to compare one joint to another — for example, your left knee with your right knee — which could help illustrate damage to the joint.

Remember that it is possible for your doctor to see signs of damage in your joint due to OA long before you start to have any symptoms. If this occurs, it is still important to learn about what you can do to protect the joint from deteriorating for as long as possible.

Magnetic Resonance Imaging (MRI)

MRIs allow your doctor to see a two-dimensional image of your joint, which enables a more precise diagnosis. However, MRIs are expensive. Many doctors will only do this test if an X-ray is not conclusive.

Rheumatoid Arthritis Diagnosis

Although some of the symptoms are similar to those of osteoarthritis, the causes and the tests to diagnose RA are very different, as are some of the treatments. Because your whole immune system is turned on, it is reasonable to expect that you might have some other symptoms. In fact, people with RA often mention that they have flu-like symptoms. They notice that they are tired and lethargic, and have less appetite, sore muscles, and even a slight fever.

Physical Examination

Much as with osteoarthritis, the first thing your doctor will do is ask you a number of questions about how you are feeling and conduct a physical examination to confirm your answers. Your doctor will want to determine:

- Whether you suffer from joint stiffness in the morning
- Whether you have swelling in your joints
- Whether your joints are painful
- Whether your joints are warm and red
- Whether your pain is the same on both sides of your body

Your doctor will also want to know whether anyone in your family has had RA. After learning about your medical history and doing a physical examination of your joints, your doctor may recommend a range of laboratory tests.

Did You Know?

Joint Aspiration

Another way for your doctor to determine whether you have osteoarthritis and not another form of arthritis is to perform a joint aspiration. This is a simple procedure. A needle is inserted into your joint and some of the synovial fluid is removed and then analyzed. This test is usually used to rule out other types of arthritis. New research on how OA affects all of the tissues in the joint may eventually lead to the identification of some markers of OA in the fluid that surrounds the joint or in the bloodstream. This could lead to earlier diagnosis of OA and new treatments.

Laboratory Tests (RA)
Blood Tests

Your doctor will request a number of specific blood tests.

- **Rheumatoid factor:** This type of antibody is present in about 80% of the people who have RA.
- **Anti-CCP blood test:** This test determines whether an antibody to a specific type of protein is in your bloodstream.
- **Erythrocyte sedimentation rate (ESR):** This test will tell your doctor whether there is any inflammation present in your body. When your blood is in a test tube, the red blood cells tend to fall to the bottom of the tube. If this happens quickly, there is some inflammation in your body.
- **C-reactive protein (CRP):** This is another test for inflammation in the body. It is usually elevated in patients with RA.

CHAPTER 5

What Other Conditions Are Associated with Arthritis?

Osteoarthritis and rheumatoid arthritis can contribute to the development of other medical conditions that are discomforting, if not life-threatening.

Bones

Both chronic inflammation and the use of corticosteroid drugs can lead to osteoporosis. Osteoporosis causes the bone to become thinner and more brittle, increasing the risk of fracture.

Skin Problems

People with RA often develop different skin problems. Some problems can be a reaction to the medications that are being taken to manage the RA. The most common skin effect is the formation of rheumatoid nodules, which are lumps of tissue usually found near the elbows, forearms, fingers, and heels. The formation of this type of nodule is tied to a higher level of RA activity. A condition called vasculitis that looks like skin ulcers can also develop as a result of the toll that inflammation is taking on the blood vessels.

Eyes

Inflammation can cause a few different problems in the eyes. Some can be serious and others are not, but they are very bothersome. The membrane that covers the white of the eye can become inflamed. This will cause redness and pain in the eye area, but it is not serious and not likely to lead to permanent damage to the eye. However, sometimes the white of the eye

> Inflammation can cause a few different problems in the eyes. Some can be serious and others are not, but they are very bothersome.

can become severely inflamed, and this may actually lead to blindness if left untreated.

Another problem that could occur as a complication of RA is the development of Sjögren's syndrome, where the immune system attacks the glands that produce tears. The result is eyes that are very dry. Tears play an important role in helping to keep the eyes free of bacteria. If we do not produce enough tears, we are more likely to develop eye infections. An eye infection could lead to scarring of the cornea and of the membrane that covers the eye. Ask your doctor to refer you to an ophthalmologist for an eye examination on a regular basis.

Did You Know?

Lung Disease

The membrane that lines the lungs can be attacked by inflammation (pleuritis). Fluid can also accumulate on the lungs, making breathing difficult. Methotrexate is an RA medication that modifies how the disease progresses. One of the side effects of taking methotrexate can be shortness of breath, a cough, and a fever, which will clear up soon after the methotrexate is stopped. Discuss any changes in your breathing with your doctor.

Heart and Blood Vessels

Different types of heart ailments may result from arthritis. The heart is surrounded by a membrane called the pericardium. This membrane can become inflamed as a result of RA. This could cause the membrane to become thicker, and that would affect how the heart pumps blood. The inflammation can also cause a buildup of fluid between the pericardium and the heart, which can become infected. This usually happens only when RA disease activity is high.

The risk of developing cardiovascular disease is higher when systemic inflammation is present. People with RA are at a higher risk of having a heart attack or a stroke. They are often found to have higher levels of cholesterol in their blood and higher blood pressure, both of which are risk factors for having a heart attack or a stroke. Your doctor will routinely perform blood tests to check your cholesterol and blood sugar levels, as well as suggest other tests that will help assess how fit your heart and blood vessels are. The great news is that exercising, following an anti-inflammatory diet, and managing stress, all of which can help your RA, will also reduce your risk of developing heart disease. Obesity, which is often linked to OA, is also a risk factor for the development of heart disease.

Diabetes

Some recent studies suggest that systemic inflammation also causes diabetes. Rates of diabetes seem to be higher in people with RA than they are in the rest of the population.

Fatigue

People with arthritis, particularly patients with RA, often complain of being fatigued. Certainly it is possible that pain may interrupt your sleep, but recent studies have found a higher incidence of sleep apnea in people with RA. One of the most important conditions that is linked to weight gain is lack of sleep. Some RA patients may struggle to maintain a healthy body weight, and many people with OA become overweight, and extra weight puts extra strain on already creaky joints. This is one of the reasons why it is important to tell your doctor about any changes in your sleep habits and to take charge of the situation.

Another reason people with RA often feel more fatigued is that they are more prone to developing anemia.

Recent studies have found a higher incidence of sleep apnea in people with RA.

Q. Does Arthritis Cause Depression?

A. Depression is common in people with RA and in people with some types of OA. It seems that the more pain a person is in, the more likely they are to be depressed. The other factor that seems to influence people's mood is the inability to partake in regular day-to-day activities. Discuss how you feel with your doctor, who may be able to put you in contact with a support group in your area or with a psychologist who is familiar with treating people who are coping with the limitations of arthritis. Diet, exercise, and stress management play a key role in the treatment of depression. A diet high in omega-3 fatty acids has been linked to a reduced risk of suffering from depression. Regular exercise has also been linked to a decrease in the incidence of depression. Your doctor may also prescribe medication to help with your depression. These medications may provide an added benefit, as some of them can help you to sleep.

Part 2

MANAGING ARTHRITIS

CHAPTER 6
Lifestyle Changes

CASE HISTORY
Turning Points

Derek was 62 years old when he was diagnosed with severe osteoarthritis of the knee. The bone was rubbing on bone. He decided on his own to take over-the-counter NSAIDs to relieve the pain. Forty-eight hours after he started taking the medication, Derek mentioned to his daughter that he had vomited, but that oddly it had looked like coffee grounds. He rushed to the hospital, where doctors found that the lining of his stomach had started bleeding because of the medication. He stayed in the hospital overnight.

When he was released the next day, Derek had a new medication to use, prescribed by his doctor: a cream containing NSAIDs, which would relieve his sore knees without harming his stomach. He also started to use a medication to protect his stomach.

After meeting with his family doctor, Derek added a number of tools to his osteoarthritis and pain management toolbox. He realized there were many approaches to managing his pain that did not involve taking medication. He visited a physiotherapist, who taught him some specific exercises to strengthen the muscles surrounding his knee and stressed the importance of using heat and ice after exercising, to help manage his pain. The physiotherapist also suggested that Derek use a knee brace to support his knee until his muscles got strong enough to help him. He started to go on walks, and learned the importance of pacing himself. He found that he could easily walk for 10 minutes, three times a day, but could not walk for 30 minutes at a time. He started using walking poles, which helped him with his balance and gave him confidence that if his knee gave out he would not fall. He planned his routes so that he could always find a park bench to sit down on if needed. After a while, Derek added tai chi to his exercise routine, having learned that it is very beneficial to people with both OA and RA.

But Derek knew he had to make more fundamental changes to his lifestyle to reduce his pain. On his first visit to our clinic, Derek mentioned that he was taking medication to control heartburn and reflux. We gave him a tip sheet on dietary and lifestyle changes he could make to manage these conditions. Derek also said he was ready to make a serious attempt to lose weight. We were thrilled by this decision, because Derek had a body mass index of 33.5, which is considered obese. He also had type 2 diabetes and a heart condition.

continued...

The goals we set were modest. On our advice, Derek made some simple changes to his eating habits. To start, he aimed to lose 10 pounds in 6 months. He joined a cardiac rehabilitation program, where his exercise sessions were modified by a kinesiologist to suit his various medical conditions. He used an elliptical machine to do cardiovascular exercise, and followed a strength training program with resistance bands, eventually moving on to weight machines. After about 4 months, Derek had lost 10 pounds. His blood sugar levels were now managed with much less medication. As an added bonus, Derek had less pain in his knees. His doctor decided to try a hyaluronic acid injection to see if that would act as a cushion between the bones of his knees. This helped Derek so much that he was able to go back to taking his dogs for long walks.

Following a suspected diagnosis of arthritis, your family doctor will likely refer you to a rheumatologist, who is a specialist in treating this type of disease. The rheumatologist will confirm your doctor's initial diagnosis and verify the type of arthritis you have. Sometimes your doctor will ask you to work with other health-care specialists. These specialists could include orthopedic surgeons to do various types of surgery on your joints, physical therapists to improve your mobility, occupational therapists to help you keep up with your daily activities, and dietitians to help you manage your diet. In many cases, managing your arthritis will involve significant changes to your lifestyle. With the support of your health-care team, these often difficult changes can be made.

Lifestyle Factors in Arthritis

Maintaining a healthy lifestyle can play a central role in the management of the disease. Look at your exercise, sleeping, and eating habits with a critical eye to see how they may contribute to the progress of your arthritis and make your inflammation worse.

There are many practical things you can do to help manage your pain and your disease. Some you can do at home on your own, though it is always best to discuss using these treatments with your physician or the other members of your health-care team. These simple techniques can be added to your treatment toolbox. In your kitchen or workshop, it is best to have a wide range of tools so you can choose the best one to do the job. In your arthritis toolbox, it is best to have a variety of tools to use in conjunction with the treatment your doctor prescribes for you.

Treatments for Arthritis

There are several accepted treatments for arthritis. They are not exclusive and can be complementary or synergistic.

- Lifestyle changes
- Medication
- Surgery
- Dietary therapy
- Complementary and alternative medicine
- Nutritional and herbal supplements

Each treatment intervention can play a role in how well you feel. And each type of intervention can have an impact on the other. If you have osteoarthritis, for instance, doing regular exercise can maintain your range of motion, keep your muscles strong, and maintain a healthy weight. This may, in turn, play a role in how much pain you are in and how quickly your joints will deteriorate, which will ultimately play a role in helping your doctor to determine the best medicines for you and if and when you might need surgery. The same applies for RA.

Conversely, if you do not take enough pain medication, you may not be able to do your exercises — and you may stiffen up and have less range of motion. Moving less might lead to eating more. If you gain a lot of weight, this puts more stress on your joints, which, in turn, may cause more pain and reduce your range of motion even more.

Excessive Stress

Stress can cause many different reactions in the body, most notably the secretion of the hormone cortisol. Any type of stress causes the body to go into the "fight or flight" defense mode, which will cause the adrenal glands, located near the kidneys, to secrete cortisol. Cortisol then acts on all the systems in the body so that the maximum amount of energy and effort can go into fleeing or combating the source of stress. In response to stress, cortisol actually reduces inflammation in the body; in fact, corticosteroid medications have been developed to simulate this response.

If we feel stressed excessively and continuously, our immune system is affected and we become vulnerable to inflammatory and autoimmune diseases, such as rheumatoid arthritis. In fact, high levels of emotional stress have been linked to elevated levels of many of the markers of inflammation, including IL-6 and TNF-α. Other consequences of producing too much cortisol include increased levels of body fat, in particular visceral fat in the abdomen, which is the type of fat most commonly associated with health problems such as diabetes and heart disease. This is the type of fat that secretes the most adipokines, chemicals that can lead to inflammation.

Did You Know?

Stop Smoking

If you smoke, try to stop now. Smoking cigarettes has been found to increase inflammation. Blood levels of C-reactive protein (CRP) are higher in smokers than in non-smokers. Both cigarette smoke and cigarette tar contain chemicals that increase inflammation. This may be why smoking cigarettes causes heart disease. When people stop smoking, their CRP levels start to decrease; however, they may take 5 to 10 years to return to normal.

Lack of Sleep

One study of our sleep habits showed that people who got less than 7 to 9 hours of sleep a night have higher levels of C-reactive protein. Although scientists have not figured out exactly how this happens, they have suggested a few possibilities.

When we do not sleep enough, the body produces more pro-inflammatory cytokines, and cortisol levels may increase. People who do not get enough sleep tend to be more overweight, which is a separate risk factor for developing OA. When we are tired, the body makes more of the hormone ghrelin, which makes us feel hungry, so we eat more. Often, the foods that we tend to snack on are high in sugar and fat, which cause us to gain weight. Alone, these foods are also linked to higher levels of the markers of inflammation.

Sometimes when people are too tired, they also do not engage in as much physical activity, which is another factor that can reduce sleep. Recently, studies have confirmed that, in particular, women with RA may have more difficulty sleeping.

Good Sleep Hygiene

Sleeping well for an optimal time will help you reduce levels of inflammation, manage your weight and feel more able to cope with your arthritis. Here are some tips for getting a great sleep:

1. Stick to a sleep schedule.
2. Have a bedtime routine that calms you.
3. Create a great bedroom that is dark, quiet, and calming.
4. Decrease your intake of caffeine-containing foods, beverages and medications.
5. Decrease your intake of alcoholic beverages, cigarettes and vaping.
6. Turn off all screens 1 hour before your scheduled bedtime.
7. Increase your level of physical activity.
8. Meditate.

Weight Management

Being overweight or obese often increases the symptoms of arthritis because it raises the level of inflammatory markers. This is especially true of the fat that is stored in the belly area. In the past, it was thought that fat tissue (adipose tissue) was only used by the body to store fat. Now scientists know that it actually secretes so many different substances that it could be considered an endocrine gland. Some of the chemicals that are secreted can increase inflammation.

Losing weight will reduce stress on the joints. In addition, when weight is lost, levels of C-reactive protein go down. The more weight you lose, the more the CRP levels go down.

Body Mass Index

The body mass index (BMI) is a tool used by dietitians and medical professionals to assess, classify, and monitor changes in body weight. A BMI greater than 30.0 is considered obese.

BMI is calculated as follows:

International (metric) units: BMI = Weight (kg) $\div$ (Height (m))^2
Imperial units: BMI = Weight (lbs) x 703 $\div$ (Height (in))^2

For example, if you weigh 120 kg and are 165 cm tall, your BMI is 44.1.

BMI = 120 $\div$ (1.65 x 1.65) = 44.1

BMI ranges from underweight (less than 18.5) to obese (more than 30.0). Each classification is connected to a risk of developing health problems. The risk of developing arthritis increases as BMI increases.

BMI Classifications

BMI Category (kg $\div$ m2)	Classification	Risk of developing health problems
< 18.5	Underweight	Increased
18.5–24.9	Normal weight	Least
25.0–29.9	Overweight	Increased
30.0–34.9	Obese class I	High
35.0–39.9	Obese class II	Very high
≥ 40	Obese class III	Extremely high

Waist Measurement

Fat that is located in the abdominal area produces chemicals that increase inflammation. Measuring your waist can help determine your health risk.

Men
Waist measurement ≥ 94 cm (37 inches) = increased health risk
> 102 cm (40 inches) = even greater increase in health risk

Women
Waist measurement ≥ 80 cm (31.5 inches) = increased health risk
> 88 cm (35 inches) = even greater increase in health risk

BMI	19	20	21	22	23	24	25	26	27	28	29	30	31	32	33	34	35	36
Height (inches)	Body Weight (pounds)																	
	NORMAL						OVERWEIGHT					OBESE						
58	91	96	100	105	110	115	119	124	129	134	138	143	148	153	158	162	167	172
59	94	99	104	109	114	119	124	128	133	138	143	148	153	158	163	168	173	178
60	97	102	107	112	118	123	128	133	138	143	148	153	158	163	168	174	179	184
61	100	106	111	116	122	127	132	137	143	148	153	158	164	169	174	180	185	190
62	104	109	115	120	126	131	136	142	147	153	158	164	169	175	180	186	191	196
63	107	113	118	124	130	135	141	146	152	158	163	169	175	180	186	191	197	203
64	110	116	122	128	134	140	145	151	157	163	169	174	180	186	192	197	204	209
65	114	120	126	132	138	144	150	156	162	168	174	180	186	192	198	204	210	216
66	118	124	130	136	142	148	155	161	167	173	179	186	192	198	204	210	216	223
67	121	127	134	140	146	153	159	166	172	178	185	191	198	204	211	217	223	230
68	125	131	138	144	151	158	164	171	177	184	190	197	203	210	216	223	230	236
69	128	135	142	149	155	162	169	176	182	189	196	203	209	216	223	230	236	243
70	132	139	146	153	160	167	174	181	188	195	202	209	216	222	229	236	243	250
71	136	143	150	157	165	172	179	186	193	200	208	215	222	229	236	243	250	257
72	140	147	154	162	169	177	184	191	199	206	213	221	228	235	242	250	258	265
73	144	151	159	166	174	182	189	197	204	212	219	227	235	242	250	257	265	272
74	148	155	163	171	179	186	194	202	210	218	225	233	241	249	256	264	272	280
75	152	160	168	176	184	192	200	208	216	224	232	240	248	256	264	272	279	287
76	156	164	172	180	189	197	205	213	221	230	238	246	254	263	271	279	287	295

Source: Adapted with permission from *Clinical Guidelines on the Identification, Evaluation, and Treatment of Overweight and Obesity in Adults: The Evidence Report.*

THE FIRST STEP:
Stop Gaining Weight

1. Balance your meals. A balanced meal should contain a plate that is one-half vegetables, one-quarter meat and alternatives, and one-quarter grains and grain products, along with a glass of water and some healthy fats.
2. Choose fish, legumes, nuts, and seeds as alternatives to meat more often.
3. Select lower-fat dairy products, such as skim, 1%, or 2% milk, low-fat yogurt (less than 2% milk fat, or M.F.) and cheeses that have less than 20% M.F.
4. Eat raw vegetables, fruit, and low-fat yogurt as snacks instead of baked goods or other high-calorie snacks.
5. Try eating more slowly, ideally taking at least 20 minutes to finish your meal.

BODY MASS INDEX TABLE

BMI	37	38	39	40	41	42	43	44	45	46	47	48	49	50	51	52	53	54
Height (inches)	Body Weight (pounds)																	
	OBESE			EXTREME OBESITY														
58	177	181	186	191	196	201	205	210	215	220	224	229	234	239	244	248	253	258
59	183	188	193	198	203	208	212	217	222	227	232	237	242	247	252	257	262	267
60	189	194	199	204	209	215	220	225	230	235	240	245	250	255	261	266	271	276
61	195	201	206	211	217	222	227	232	238	243	248	254	259	264	269	275	280	285
62	202	207	213	218	224	229	235	240	246	251	256	262	267	273	278	284	289	295
63	208	214	220	225	231	237	242	248	254	259	265	270	278	282	287	293	299	304
64	215	221	227	232	238	244	250	256	262	267	273	279	285	291	296	302	308	314
65	222	228	234	240	246	252	258	264	270	276	282	288	294	300	306	312	318	324
66	229	235	241	247	253	260	266	272	278	284	291	297	303	309	315	322	328	334
67	236	242	249	255	261	268	274	280	287	293	299	306	312	319	325	331	338	344
68	243	249	256	262	269	276	282	289	295	302	308	315	322	328	335	341	348	354
69	250	257	263	270	277	284	291	297	304	311	318	324	331	338	345	351	358	365
70	257	264	271	278	285	292	299	306	313	320	327	334	341	348	355	362	369	376
71	265	272	279	286	293	301	308	315	322	329	338	343	351	358	365	372	379	386
72	272	279	287	294	302	309	316	324	331	338	346	353	361	368	375	383	390	397
73	280	288	295	302	310	318	325	333	340	348	355	363	371	378	386	393	401	408
74	287	295	303	311	319	326	334	342	350	358	365	373	381	389	396	404	412	420
75	295	303	311	319	327	335	343	351	359	367	375	383	391	399	407	415	423	431
76	304	312	320	328	336	344	353	361	369	377	385	394	402	410	418	426	435	443

6. Include high-fiber foods to help you feel full for longer.

7. Choose water instead of high-calorie drinks. Drinking a large glass of water 30 minutes before eating will lead to consuming a smaller meal.

8. Eat three meals daily. Even if you get up late, plan to eat three meals. You may wish to start with a smaller breakfast, a regular-sized lunch, and a regular-sized dinner. Some people prefer to eat a larger breakfast with a late lunch and a light supper. People who eat meals regularly tend to be thinner.

9. Eat with friends and family, and enjoy your meals!

10. Be more physically active, if approved by your doctor.

Physical Activity

Stay as physically active as possible. Ask your physical therapist what types of activities are best for you. Physical activity will have many benefits. Aside from helping your body cope with arthritis, participating in regular physical activity will help you sleep better, maintain your weight, and stave off depression. Choose the type of activity that suits your needs and preferences best, make sure you have comfortable shoes and clothes to wear, and learn to pace yourself. Trying to do too much too soon can bring to an abrupt end any attempt to increase your level of fitness and to alleviate your arthritis symptoms.

Improving Muscle Strength

Strong muscles will help to support the joints and keep them stable. And this will result in less damage to your joints and less pain.

The saying "use it or lose it" applies to muscles and muscle strength. The less you use your muscles, the weaker they become. The best way to strengthen muscles is to make them work a bit harder every time you use them. You can add a resistance to the exercise in the form of weights or resistance bands. It is typically recommended that strength training be done three times weekly, but sometimes a physiotherapist will suggest that specific exercises be done daily.

Tips for Improving Muscle Strength

1. Consult with your doctor, physiotherapist or kinesiologist before starting an exercise program. Some exercises can put too much stress on your joints and cause additional damage. Ask your physiotherapist to give you some safe strength training exercises.

2. Find out whether your local arthritis support group offers strength training classes adapted for people with arthritis.

3. Use soup cans, bottles of water, and even a pair of pantyhose instead of weights and resistance bands. You don't need any special expensive equipment and you don't need to go to a gym.

4. Try a Pilates class. This will help build muscles, especially the core muscles in the trunk. Ask your physiotherapist to tell you which exercises you might want to either avoid or to modify.

5. Try a program that is done in the water. Water adds resistance but takes some of the stress off the knees, hips, and spine.

Maintaining Range of Motion and Flexibility

Do specific exercises that will help you stretch out and relax your muscles and tendons. These exercises also take away stiffness. Range of motion and stretching exercises will help reduce the risk of injury to your joints. They also help you relax tense muscles. Some people do a few quick stretches in the morning before they get out of bed to help relieve morning stiffness. This type of exercise can be done on a daily basis. Start slowly with one or two exercises and gradually work your way up to doing 15 to 20 minutes of exercise. Once you can do this, you are ready to move on to more strenuous exercises.

Supporting Heart and Lungs

Aerobic conditioning exercises your heart and lungs while "burning" more calories and helping maintain your weight. Aerobic activities also help produce endorphins that have a positive impact on your mood. They will help you sleep better as well.

Choose low-impact aerobic activities, such as walking, cycling, and swimming. Use an elliptical trainer or join a water aerobics program. Remember that some household chores, such as raking leaves, cutting the grass, or even vacuuming, are good aerobic exercises.

> **Start slowly with one or two exercises and gradually work your way up to doing 15 to 20 minutes of exercise. Once you can do this, you are ready to move on to more strenuous exercises.**

Tips for Improving Range of Motion

1. Join a tai chi or yoga class. Choose your classes carefully and make sure you go slowly. Do not try to compete with the other members of your class. Not every yoga or tai chi class is adapted to people with arthritis, so choose an appropriate class.

2. Ask your local arthritis support group to start a specially adapted stretching program.

3. Ask your physiotherapist to develop a special stretching program just for you or for help choosing appropriate yoga or tai chi exercises.

4. Search the Internet for interesting classes and exercises you can do at home (with the approval of your physiotherapist).

The goals are simple. Start doing more than what you're doing now. The American guidelines for physical activity suggest that the first goal is to do 2 hours and 30 minutes of aerobic activity a week and then to progress to 5 hours a week. Rather than exercise for 1 hour at one time, consider breaking up the session into 10-minute intervals.

Home Remedies for Managing Pain

Applications of heat or cold to the affected joint can help you deal with the pain. Some treatments you can do at home on your own, but it is always best to discuss how you are using these treatments with your physician or the other members of your health-care team.

Heat and Cold

Heat can work wonders for osteoarthritis and rheumatoid arthritis — and it feels sooo good. Heat can help alleviate your pain, soothe tense muscles, and increase your range of motion. There are a few different approaches to using heat, but always keep in mind that if your joints are very swollen and inflamed, heat may not help — it might actually make you feel more pain.

Hot Baths or Hot Tub

Relax tense muscles with a soak in a warm bath or hot tub. A soak can also help you sleep. Make sure that the water is not too hot. Very hot water is not recommended for people over the age of 70, people with heart conditions, or people with chronic respiratory problems. Always consult with your doctor or other member of your health-care team to make sure that taking warm baths is appropriate for you.

Did You Know?

Hot Caution
Heating pads, hot water bottles, and hot packs are great ways to apply heat to a specific area. Just be careful. Every year, thousands of people burn themselves with these devices. Continuous low-level heat wraps are another way of delivering heat to specific joints. They provide up to 8 hours of heat, and you are not likely to burn yourself with these products.

Paraffin Wax

Applying paraffin wax to your hands or feet does feel amazing! Check the temperature of the wax before applying it to make sure you don't burn yourself.

Hot/Cold

Alternate placing a heating pad and an ice pack on the affected area. The heat may be recommended before exercise and cold afterwards.

Cold

Cold can also be used to provide relief from pain. Applying cold will also decrease swelling and reduce inflammation. Commercially available cold packs, water bottles filled with ice, or even a plastic bag filled with ice cubes will do the trick. Put the pack on a towel or thin sheet of fabric so it does not lie directly on the skin.

Did You Know?

Pacing

Learning to pace yourself can be one of the most effective strategies you can use for reducing pain. You can rest a joint by relaxing, by alternating different activities, or by wearing a splint or support bandage. These strategies can help you feel less pain and be more energetic.

CHAPTER 7

Medications for Arthritis

....

CASE HISTORY
Coping with Medications

Jennifer was diagnosed with RA about 10 years ago, just after the birth of her first child. She had X-rays and many blood tests before her doctor was able to make a final diagnosis. Her family doctor prescribed NSAIDs for the pain, but these medications upset her stomach. She found that eating small meals often helped her stomach.

Once Jennifer met with her rheumatologist, he added cortisone to her treatments. When her diagnosis was confirmed, she started to take methotrexate. This medication helped her to manage her pain. However, she could not take it during her next pregnancy. Although her rheumatologist told her about several medications that can be safely taken during pregnancy, Jennifer chose to follow a non-drug approach.

At that time, with the help of her dietitian, she began to follow an anti-inflammatory diet. She started taking some omega-3 fatty acid supplements. Jennifer also added a gentle stretching yoga program to her daily routine. All this helped her to take only small amounts of Tylenol during her pregnancy.

One of the first things your doctor will do once you are diagnosed with arthritis is to recommend or prescribe medication to manage your pain and inflammation. There is a wide array of arthritis medications to choose from. Some drugs are used to treat both OA and RA, and others are specific to one type of arthritis. Your doctor may need to prescribe several different drugs before you find relief from your pain. And, although these medications are helpful in managing pain, many of them come with unwanted side effects.

Over-the-Counter and Prescription Medications

Some arthritis medications are available over the counter at your local pharmacy, and others are medications prescribed by your doctor. Be sure to consult with your pharmacist before taking any over-the-counter drugs so you understand how much medication to take and how often to take it.

Over-the-counter medications may interact adversely with other medications you are taking or with food you may eat. Your dietitian and your pharmacist will be your best sources of information if you want to know which foods might interact with your medication. If the over-the-counter versions of these medicines are not effective, stronger versions or combinations may be prescribed by your doctor. Some prescription medicines have the potential to become habit forming, so your doctor will prescribe them with great caution.

Over-the-counter medications may interact adversely with other medications you are taking or with food you may eat. Your dietitian and your pharmacist will be your best sources of information if you want to know which foods might interact with your medication.

Categories of Analgesic and Anti-inflammatory Medications

- Analgesics and non-steroidal anti-inflammatory medications (NSAIDs), either pills or topical ointments
- Corticosteroids
- Disease-modifying anti-rheumatic drugs (DMARDs)
- Advanced therapies such as biologic drugs and *JAK* inhibitors
- Injected cortisone and hyaluronic acid

QUICK REFERENCE GUIDE

This chapter is intended to be a quick reference guide to medications for arthritis. For more complete information, consult with your health-care provider. Always tell your pharmacist about any medications and supplements you may be taking.

Analgesics and NSAIDs

Analgesics (pain killers) are sold over the counter under such generic and brand names as acetaminophen, Tylenol, and Atasol. NSAIDs are sold under the generic and brand names Aleve, Motrin, ibuprofen, Advil, and Aspirin. They are designed to decrease the amount of pain and swelling in your joints by reducing inflammation. Examples of prescription NSAIDs are Voltaren (XR), Lodine (XL), Oruvail, Mobicox, Celebrex, Relafen, Naprelan, Daypro, Feldene, Arthrotec, Ansaid, Indocid, and Orudis. Other analgesics include narcotics, chiefly codeine. They may be habit forming, so your doctor will be very cautious about prescribing these drugs.

Aspirin

Known generically as Aspirin, acetylsalicylic acid (ASA) and other medicines containing salicylates (and all NSAIDs) can be very hard on the stomach, particularly when taken at higher doses. If you have the tendency to have heartburn or acid reflux, mention this to your doctor before you start to take these medications. Another medication can be prescribed to help protect your stomach and avoid further discomfort. This medication is not usually recommended for pain management.

Did You Know?

Quick Start

When trying to manage your pain, remember to take your medicine when the pain starts rather than waiting until it is unbearable. Once the pain reaches that level, it is more difficult to make it go away.

Did You Know?

Heart Consequences

Recent studies suggest that taking a low dose of Aspirin may promote heart health, but taking NSAID medications can increase your risk of having a heart attack. Check with your doctor or pharmacist before taking these medications and do not exceed the recommended dosage.

Acetaminophen

Acetaminophen does not present the same gastrointestinal problems but can be problematic for people with liver disease. Be sure to tell your doctor or pharmacist if you have liver problems before you start to take acetaminophen.

COX-2 Inhibitors

These newer drugs reduce pain, swelling, and inflammation without common NSAID side effects (heartburn, stomach pain, and bleeding). However, some studies have linked these medications to an increased risk of having a heart attack. Some examples of COX-2 inhibitors are Celebrex and Arcoxia.

Be sure to tell your doctor or pharmacist if you have liver problems before you start to take acetaminophen.

Did You Know?

Anticoagulant Caution

NSAIDs can interact with medications, such as Coumadin and Warfarin, that thin your blood. They should not be taken if you are already taking anticoagulants. Some nutritional supplements and herbs can also act as blood thinners, so check with your pharmacist or dietitian to make sure you're not taking a supplement that might worsen this problem. Take only what you need, making sure you do not take more than the recommended dosage.

Corticosteroids

This group of medications is used to reduce and control inflammation. They work on the whole body, so they will reduce the inflammation in your joints and wherever else it may be in your body. These drugs are usually quite fast acting, quickly bringing relief from swelling, stiffness, pain, and fatigue. Prednisone is the most commonly prescribed corticosteroid. Once the Disease-Modifying Anti-Rheumatic Drugs (see page 54) take effect, your doctor will wean you off prednisone. Corticosteroids can be injected directly into the joints, which may be especially effective in patients with OA because the inflammation is localized.

Some of the side effects of taking corticosteroid pills are weight gain, increased appetite, insomnia, and osteoporosis. There are also other potential side effects of these medications, so consult your doctor and your pharmacist to make sure that you know exactly what to expect.

Did You Know?

Viscosupplementation

In a joint affected by OA, the natural lubricating agent, called hyaluronic acid, is deficient. It is now possible for your doctor to inject hyaluronic acid (hyaluronan) into the joint. This treatment is usually used in OA of the knees and hips. The medication seems to help the body produce more of its own lubricating fluid, and it may also act to help reduce inflammation. There are few reactions to this medication, and if there are any, they seem to be mostly related to the site of the injection. Occasionally, clients can have nausea and an irritated stomach. It can take 4 to 6 weeks to feel the benefits of this treatment. New, more effective formulations of the medication are being developed.

Creams and Ointments

There are a number of different types of creams and ointments to help you feel less pain. They have different active ingredients that work in different ways to help you feel better. Make sure that you wash your hands after using one of these creams and do not put your hands near your eyes after application. None of these creams should be used if your skin is irritated or broken from a cut or scrape.

These creams and ointments are the first treatments you should try if you have OA:

Salicylate Creams

These creams are similar to Aspirin and work by releasing a small amount of anti-inflammatory medicine that goes through the skin into the blood vessels. A salicylate cream is not as strong as a pill, but because you rub it right on the joint that hurts, a salicylate cream can be quite effective at reducing pain and inflammation locally. However, these ointments can cause the same side effects as the over-the-counter medications containing salicylates. These creams can also interact with blood-thinning medications (anticoagulants), so check with your doctor or pharmacist before using them.

NSAID Creams

These creams contain diclofenac, an anti-inflammatory medication, and usually do not present the same side effects as NSAIDs in pill form.

Capsaicin Creams

Capsaicin is found naturally in cayenne pepper and is the active ingredient in creams and liniments such as Capzasin-P, Zostrix, and Zostrix-HP. It works by causing your nerve cells to feel heat. When you do this repeatedly, there is a reduction in the amount of chemicals that are released to communicate pain to your brain, which reduces pain. These creams may take more than one application to work, and they need to be applied on a regular schedule. Use these creams on pain that is near the surface of the skin — for example, in your fingers, toes, and knees.

Counterirritants

This is another group of creams, liniments, and gels that work by tricking the brain. In this case, the active ingredients cause your brain to feel extreme heat or cold. While your brain is occupied with these feelings, it does not feel the pain from your arthritis. Some of the active ingredients in these products are wintergreen oil, eucalyptus oil, camphor, menthol, and turpentine oil. Some of the brand names of these products are Icy Hot, Eucalyptamint, ArthriCare, and Therapeutic Mineral Ice.

Disease-Modifying Anti-Rheumatic Drugs (DMARDs)

These medications are designed for patients with RA and work by modifying how the disease progresses. In RA, the immune system starts attacking healthy cells of the body as if they were invaders and were about to attack the body. DMARDs slow down this process.

There are many types of DMARD drugs, and each has a different way of reducing inflammation and slowing down the effect that RA has on the body. The most commonly used DMARD is methotrexate.

Treatment with this type of medication is started as soon as possible because early intervention with these drugs can reduce the damage that is done to your joints. It can take up to 6 weeks for the DMARD drugs to start working. During that time, patients are often asked to continue to take NSAIDs or corticosteroids to reduce pain and improve function and mobility.

These medications are quite strong. Make sure that your doctor knows about all the other medications and supplements that you may be taking. Also inform your doctor if you are planning to become pregnant or father a child — this may make a difference in the medication that you are prescribed. Because of the possibility of side effects with some of these medications, your doctor may ask you to go for blood tests on a regular basis to ensure that all systems are functioning normally.

Disease-Modifying Osteoarthritis Drugs (DMOADs)

Doctors, patients, and researchers all agree: it would be very helpful to be able to modify the progress of osteoarthritis or even find a medication that would stop it in its tracks. We are discovering more ways to identify OA in its early stages, and at the same time, we are learning exactly what is happening in the joint to cause the problem. Finding different markers of the disease will eventually allow doctors to prescribe medication that will slow down the progression of OA and keep joints from deteriorating. Although there are no DMOADs currently available to doctors, there is a lot of ongoing research, so look for these medications in the future.

Profiles of Commonly Used DMARDs

Methotrexate

Used to treat severe, active RA; it is usually the first DMARD tried.

How it works: Reduces cell growth and suppresses the actions of the immune system.

How to take it: Pill, once a week. Can be injected.

How long will it take to see results? 3–6 weeks; follow up with regular blood tests.

Possible side effects: Nausea, vomiting, malaise, mouth sores.

Caution: Cannot be used during pregnancy; do not take unless you are using a very reliable form of birth control. Do not consume alcoholic beverages. Have regular blood tests to monitor liver and bone marrow function.

Food interactions: Take with or without food, be consistent, may need folic acid supplementation, consume lots of fluids.

Contraindications: Check with your pharmacist.

Barictinib (Olumiant)

Used to treat moderate to severe RA.

How it works: Stops the production of enzymes that are essential for the pro-inflammatory cycle to begin.

How to take it: Pill, once a day.

Possible side effects: Upper respiratory tract infections and gastrointestinal symptoms like nausea and diarrhea. Before you start this medication, ask your doctor if you should have the shingles vaccine.

Interactions: Can be taken with methotrexate.

Hydroxychloroquine (e.g., Plaquenil)

Used to treat mild RA.

How it works: At this time, we do not know how it works in RA, but it does affect the immune system and calms RA.

How to take it: 1–2 pills daily.

How long will it take to see results? 2–4 months.

Possible side effects: Mild side effects include a skin rash and digestive difficulties. It can affect the eyes. Have eye exam before starting medication, and then on a yearly basis. Wear sunglasses, a sun hat and sunscreen to avoid exposure to bright sun and reduce the risk of eye problems.

Food interactions: Take with a meal or glass of milk.

continued...

JAK inhibitors (Janus kinase inhibitors)

This new class of medication, used to treat RA, has effects similar to biologics (see page 63). This type of medication works differently from other RA medications, disrupting the pro-inflammatory response from inside the cells.

Leflunomide (e.g., Arava)

Used to treat active RA.

How it works: Inhibits production of lymphocytes, a type of white blood cell that is involved in the autoimmune response.

How to take it: Pill form, usually start with a larger dose, then stabilize dose.

How long will it take to see results? Up to 2 months.

Possible side effects: Diarrhea, nausea and dizziness can occur.

Caution: Cannot be used during pregnancy; do not take unless you are using a very reliable form of birth control.

Food interactions: None.

Sulfasalazine

Used to treat RA in patients who did not do well on other NSAIDs.

How it works: May be anti-inflammatory, may regulate immune system.

How to take it: Pill form up to 2 times daily. Gradually increasing the dose may decrease side effects.

How long will it take to see results? Up to 3 months.

Possible side effects: Decreased appetite, nausea, diarrhea; have regular blood tests.

Food interactions: Take after meals or snacks, may decrease absorption of folate and folic acid; consume up to 8 cups (2 L) of fluids daily.

Contraindications: Do not take if you are allergic to sulfa or Aspirin.

Tofacitinib (Xeljanz, Xeljanz XR)

Used to treat moderate to severe RA.

How it works: Stops the production of enzymes that are essential for the pro-inflammatory cycle to begin.

How to take it: Pill, once or twice a day.

Possible side effects: Upper respiratory tract infections, headache, diarrhea, increased blood pressure and blood cholesterol levels. Before you start this medication, ask your doctor if you should have the shingles vaccine.

Interactions: Can be taken with methotrexate.

HOW TO
Cope with Nausea and Vomiting

A common side effect of drug therapy is nausea and vomiting. Your doctor may prescribe medication to counter this response, but you can also help the situation by following these guidelines:

1. Eat small, frequent meals throughout the day.
2. Eat slowly.
3. If the smells from cooking upset your stomach, ask somebody to help prepare your meals.
4. If the smells bother you at mealtime, try eating your foods cold or at room temperature. You can also open a window or use a fan to bring fresh air into the room.
5. Try nibbling on dry, bland food, such as crackers, toast, cereals, or bread, every few hours throughout the day.
6. Avoid foods with a pronounced taste (sweet, fried, or spicy) or smell.
7. Limit your intake of liquids with meals. Sip water and other liquids, such as flat ginger ale, sports drinks, broth, and herbal teas, between meals.
8. Keep your mouth clean by brushing your teeth at least twice daily. This will help reduce any unpleasant tastes in your mouth that may make you feel nauseated.
9. Wait 1 hour after eating before lying down.

Did You Know?

Folic Acid Supplement
When methotrexate is prescribed, your doctor will likely include a folic acid supplement. The addition of folic acid to the diet seems to reduce the likelihood that patients will have some of the common side effects that are associated with this medication, such as mouth ulcers, nausea, vomiting, diarrhea, or liver problems.

Biologic Response–Modifying Drugs

These medications are fast becoming a mainstay in the treatment of RA because they are so effective. Many studies have shown that these medications are able to slow the progress, reduce the symptoms, and prevent permanent damage to the joints caused by RA. Typically, these medications are added to your treatment if you have not received the desired results when you were treated with methotrexate or other DMARDs, if you have a condition that would be incompatible with the use of DMARDs, or if your RA is more active. They are often used in combination with methotrexate or other DMARDs.

These agents act on the immune system, although in a different way than the DMARDs do. They are called biologics because they are copies of parts of the immune system. Scientists have found a way to make in the laboratory some of the proteins that are important components of our immune system. There are several different biologic medications that act on different parts of the immune system — if one doesn't work, it is very possible that another one will.

In RA, the immune system is turned on, as though the body is defending against an invader. The body produces cytokines that send a message to turn on the production of interleukins and tumor necrosis factor (TNF). These substances are responsible for turning on the inflammation process. The inflammation then runs out of control. Biologics are made to intercept or attach to particular interleukins or the tumor necrosis factor, or to B-cells, which will effectively block their action.

At this time, the biologics are not available in pill form. Some are injected and others are given as part of an intravenous solution. You can learn to inject yourself, but you will have to visit a doctor or hospital to have the intravenous solution administered. These medications often take effect quite quickly; however, some patients will only see results after several weeks or months.

Side Effects

There may be some side effects associated with these medications. Most notably, the immune system is turned down to reduce inflammation and make it stop attacking the body. This means that the immune system will also be slower to attack any invaders or infections. All biologics may increase your risk of getting infections. Advise your doctor if you have any infections before starting treatment or during treatment with this type of medication. Your doctor will also want to test you for tuberculosis before you start and will probably ask you to have blood tests at regular intervals to monitor your condition. In addition, prior to starting biologics, patients should have all appropriate vaccinations updated.

Profiles of Biologic Agents

Abatacept (Orencia)

Used to treat moderate to severe RA.

How it works: Blocks signals that activate T-cells.

How to take it: Intravenous infusion on a monthly basis, or a weekly subcutaneous injection.

Possible side effects: Increased risk of infection, particularly a respiratory tract infection.

Contraindications: Can be taken with other RA medications, including DMARDs, but not with other biologics.

Adalimumab (Humira)

Used to treat moderate to severe RA.

How it works: Blocks tumor necrosis factor (TNF), which turns on inflammation.

How to take it: One subcutaneous injection every 2 weeks. Patients, their family, or caregivers can learn how to give the injections.

Possible side effects: Pain and redness at injection site, infections in the respiratory tract, headaches, and a rash.

Interactions/contraindications: Can be taken with other RA medications, including DMARDs, but not with other biologics. Biosimilars of Adalimumab are available.

continued...

Anakinra (Kineret)

Used to treat moderate to severe RA.

How it works: Blocks interleukin-1 (IL-1).

How to take it: One subcutaneous injection daily. Patients, their families, or caregivers can learn how to give the injections.

Possible side effects: Redness, swelling, and/or pain at the injection site. Increased risk of infections.

Interactions/contraindications: Can be taken with other RA medications, including methotrexate or other DMARDs, but do not use with other biologics.

Certolizumab (Cimzia)

Used to treat moderate to severe RA.

How it works: Blocks TNF, which turns on inflammation.

How to take it: One subcutaneous injection every 2 to 4 weeks. Patients, their families, or caregivers can learn how to give the injections.

Possible side effects: Pain where you had the injection. Increased risk of infections.

Interactions/contraindications: Can be taken with other medications, including methotrexate or other DMARDs, but not with other biologics.

Etanercept (Enbrel)

Used to treat moderate to severe RA.

How it works: Blocks TNF, which turns on inflammation.

How to take it: One subcutaneous injection once or twice a week. Patients, their families, or caregivers can learn how to give the injections.

Possible side effects: Pain where you had the injection. Increased risk of infections.

Interactions/contraindications: Can be used with methotrexate or other DMARDs. Do not use with other biologics. Biosimilars of Etanercept are now available.

Golimumab (Simponi)

Used to treat moderate to severe RA.

How it works: Blocks TNF, which turns on inflammation.

How to take it: One subcutaneous injection monthly (patients, their families, or caregivers can learn how to give the injections) or an intravenous infusion once every 12 months.

Possible side effects: Increased risk of infections.

Interactions/contraindications: Can be used with methotrexate and other DMARDs. Do not use with other biologics.

Infliximab (Remicade)

Used to treat moderate to severe RA.

How it works: Blocks TNF, which turns on inflammation.

How to take it: Intravenous infusions three times during the first 6 weeks of therapy, then every 8 weeks.

Possible side effects: Rarely, you can have an allergic reaction to the infusion, so it is important to be monitored while you are having it. Other side effects include upper respiratory infections, headache, and nausea.

Interactions: Taken with other RA medicines, usually with methotrexate, but not with other biologics. Biosimilars of Infliximab are now available.

Rituximab (Rituxan)

Used to treat moderate to severe RA.

How it works: Decreases the number of B-cells in the body. B-cells are a crucial part of the immune system.

How to take it: Intravenous infusion, initially two doses over 2 weeks, usually repeated every 6 to 12 months.

Possible side effects: Rarely, you can have an allergic reaction to the infusion; must be monitored during the process. Infusion reaction resembles the flu. Increased risk of infections.

Interactions/contraindications: Can be taken with methotrexate, but not with other biologics. Biosimilars of Rituximab are now available.

Sarilumab (Kevzara)

Used to treat moderate to severe RA.

How it works: Stops IL-6 receptor cells from receiving messages in the immune system.

How to take it: One subcutaneous injection every 2 weeks.

Possible side effects: Redness at the injection site, upper respiratory tract infection, urinary tract infection, sore throat, runny nose and nasal congestion, increased cholesterol levels.

Interactions: Can be taken with methotrexate or other biologic medications.

Tocilizumab (Actemra)

Used to treat moderate to severe RA.

How it works: Stops IL-6 from transferring messages in the immune system.

How to take it: Monthly intravenous infusions or subcutaneous injections once a week or once every 2 weeks.

Possible side effects: Respiratory tract infections, headache, can increase cholesterol levels.

Interactions: Can be taken with other RA medicines, with methotrexate, or alone, but not with other biologics.

CHAPTER 8

Surgery

CASE HISTORY
Successful Surgery

Louise is a healthy woman, who, at the age of 70, developed severe pain in her left knee. She had no other medical problems, and her BMI was 25, which is on the high side of normal. She tried to manage the pain with Advil. She also iced her knee on a regular basis. She had a regular visit with a physiotherapist and she did her exercises on a daily basis and used topical creams. However, the pain continued to get worse so her doctor sent her for an X-ray. Louise had severe osteoarthritis in her left knee; in fact, the bone was rubbing on the bone. Her doctor recommended she see an orthopedic surgeon.

The surgeon agreed with the diagnosis, and said that the best treatment would be to have a total knee replacement. The surgery was scheduled to take place in 2 months. During that 2-month period, Louise continued to work with her physiotherapist in order to maintain her muscle strength and her flexibility. She also took particular care of her diet. She made sure that she was eating a balanced diet that included enough protein.

Louise knew that once she came out of the hospital she would not be able to cook much, so she filled her freezer with meals for herself and her husband.

Louise had her surgery, and she was released from the hospital after 5 days. She was prescribed pain medication and an iron supplement because her iron levels were low, as well as a multivitamin and mineral supplement.

She went to her physiotherapist the next week, and started doing exercises to maintain the strength in her good leg and to start rebuilding strength in her new knee. She did the exercises she had to do at home on a regular basis. At first it was difficult because the temptation was to do too much, but Louise soon realized that she had to listen to her body. It was better to do less if she felt tired or pain. If she forced herself to do more, Louise quickly realized that the result was the opposite of what she desired. Doing too much resulted in more pain and ultimately less movement.

Initially, her appetite was quite small and she was frequently very tired. She ate small meals often. Louise made sure that she was eating some protein at every meal and at every snack. She also chose red meat more often than usual to help improve her iron levels. She took an iron pill in the morning and before bed. To make sure that the iron was absorbed, she did not consume any dairy products or tea or coffee with her breakfast, all of which reduce iron absorption. She took the pill with a glass of orange juice, a good source of vitamin C, which we think helps to increase iron absorption. Louise continued to eat more protein than usual, and a few extra calories to help the healing process, but she did not eat enough to gain weight.

After a few short months, Louise was back on her feet and doing most of her everyday activities. She continued to do special exercises for her knee, including water exercises, and gradually started to do her hikes again. A year later, she had resumed all her regular activities except those that required her to kneel. She continued to take a multivitamin supplement, but she no longer took her iron supplements.

Surgery is a viable option for people who suffer from either RA or OA. Almost any joint can be treated surgically to reduce pain or improve your ability to function. We have all heard of people with OA who have had their hips or knees replaced. However, surgery does not stop the inflammatory process that is ongoing in RA and possibly OA. Make sure that you understand exactly what to expect from the surgery, as well as how this might affect the rest of the treatment plan.

Make sure that you understand exactly what to expect from the surgery, as well as how this might affect the rest of the treatment plan.

Surgical Procedures

There are many different surgeries for arthritis. Some of the procedures can be quite simple, and others, such as joint replacement, are more complicated.

Arthroscopic Debridement (OA)

This surgery removes any bone chips and other debris, such as pieces of cartilage, that might be floating in the joint.

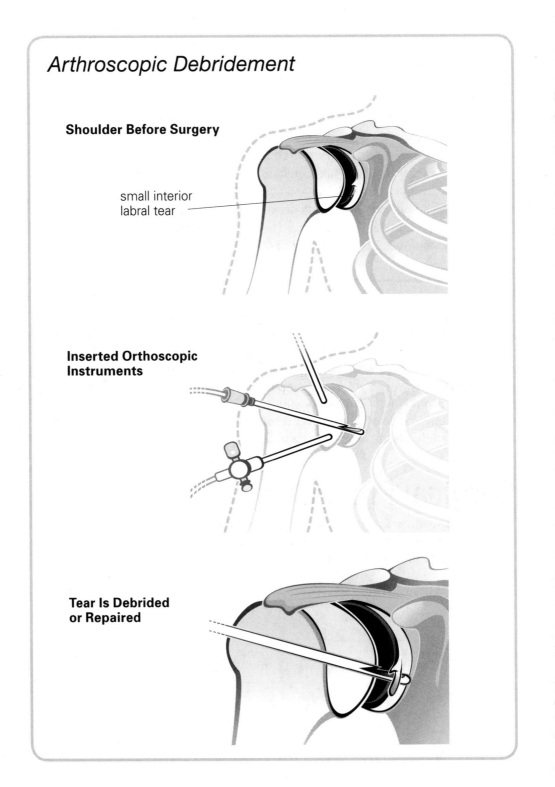

Arthroscopic Debridement

Shoulder Before Surgery

small interior labral tear

Inserted Orthoscopic Instruments

Tear Is Debrided or Repaired

Synovectomy (RA)

The goal of this procedure is to remove the synovial tissue in the joint, which decreases the amount of damage to the bone and cartilage and reduces pain and swelling.

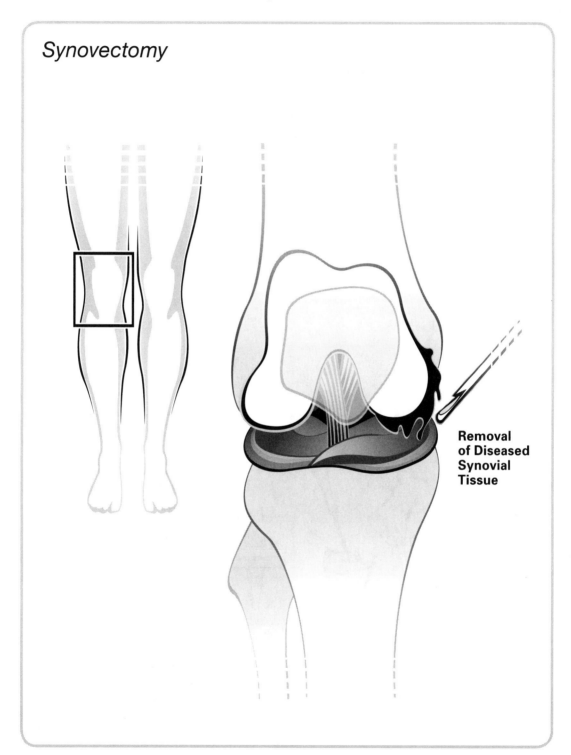

Synovectomy

Removal of Diseased Synovial Tissue

Resection (RA)

In this procedure, the bones and joints that have been damaged by RA are completely removed. This can be done in some of the smaller bones in the feet.

Resection Arthroplasty for Rheumatoid Forefoot Deformity

Removal of metatarsal heads of smaller toes, bases of toes left untouched. Removal of metatarsal head and base of proximal phalanx of great toe.

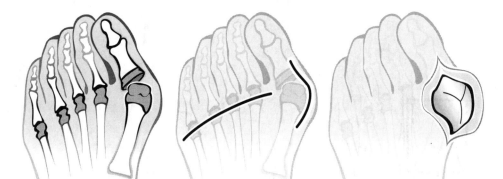

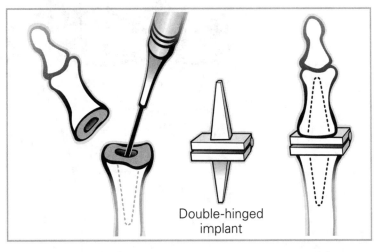

Double-hinged implant

Bone drilled to receive implant stems

Implant inserted and bones aligned

Joint Replacement (OA and RA)

This procedure is done when the joints become severely damaged. Usually, the joint is replaced with a plastic or steel joint called an implant. Most of us know someone who has had either a knee or a hip replaced — these are the joints that are most commonly replaced — but it is possible to replace other joints, including the elbow, knuckles, shoulders, and even ankles.

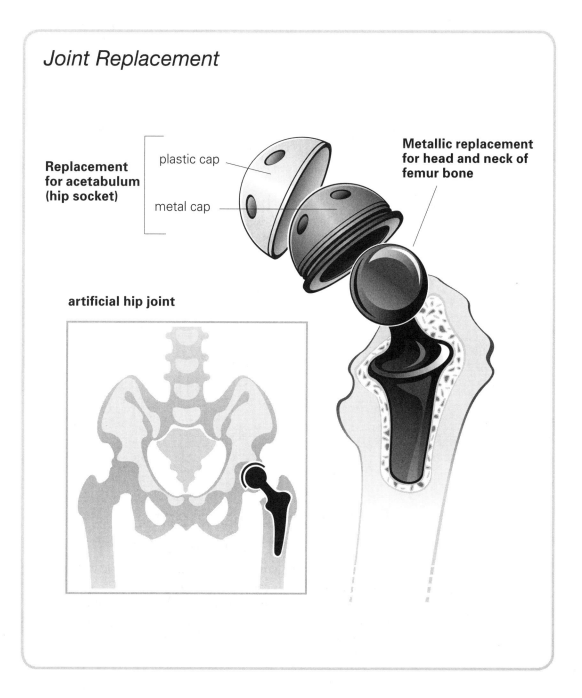

Joint Replacement

Replacement for acetabulum (hip socket)

plastic cap

metal cap

Metallic replacement for head and neck of femur bone

artificial hip joint

Joint Fusion (OA and RA)

This procedure involves joining two bones. After this procedure, the joint is no longer flexible but it will be able to bear weight. Joints in the spine, wrist, fingers, feet, and ankle can be treated with surgical fusion.

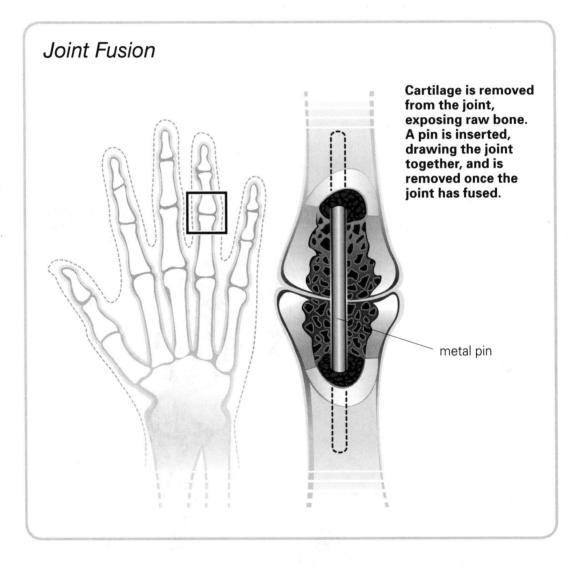

Joint Fusion

Cartilage is removed from the joint, exposing raw bone. A pin is inserted, drawing the joint together, and is removed once the joint has fused.

metal pin

Tendon and Ligament Adjustments (OA and RA)

Your tendons and ligaments play an important role in helping your joints remain anchored in position. If they are torn or stretched, the joint can become unstable, which can cause more pain and limit your mobility. Surgeons can realign, tighten, and adjust tendons and ligaments.

New Treatments for OA

Cartilage replacement is a relatively new category of treatments for osteoarthritis. The basic procedure involves removing a small amount of cartilage from a healthy joint, growing it in a test tube, and then implanting this cartilage into the joint affected by OA.

In an even newer type of treatment, stem cells are taken from the bone marrow and placed in the joint that is damaged by OA. This treatment shows promising results, but it is currently being performed only in certain specialized centers.

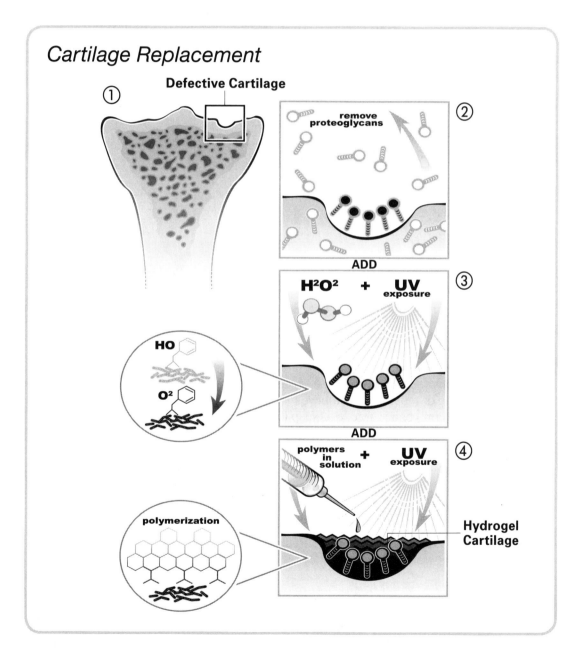

Cartilage Replacement

① Defective Cartilage

② remove proteoglycans

ADD

③ H^2O^2 + **UV** exposure

HO

O^2

ADD

④ polymers in solution + **UV** exposure

polymerization

Hydrogel Cartilage

Platelet-rich plasma (PRP), which is being used to treat both OA and ligament and tendon injuries, involves taking a small amount of blood from the patient, removing the growth factor–rich solution, and injecting it into the afflicted joint. The solution may help to decrease inflammation while helping to repair the tissue. This treatment is available, but may be quite expensive.

Recovery

Your surgeon and health-care team, from your dietitian to your physiotherapist, will help you recover from your surgery. There is much you can do yourself in advance of your surgery to ensure a speedy recovery.

HOW TO
Prepare for a Speedy Recovery

Everyone hopes to recover as quickly as possible after surgery. Try these strategies to get a head start on recovery:

1. Prior to surgery, try to achieve a healthy body weight. This will help you recover from your surgery.

2. Eat high-fiber foods, such as whole grains, fruits, vegetables, legumes, and nuts, before your surgery to prevent constipation. It is important to have regular bowel habits prior to surgery.

3. Drink at least 8 glasses of water throughout the day to prevent dehydration and constipation.

4. Try to eat at least 3 servings of meat and alternatives and 3 servings of milk and alternatives every day — protein promotes healing after surgery. One serving of meat and alternatives = 3 oz (90 g) meat/poultry/fish, 2 eggs, $\frac{3}{4}$ cup (175 mL) beans/tofu, or 2 tbsp (30 mL) peanut butter. One serving of milk and alternative = 1 cup (250 mL) milk/soy beverage, 2 oz (60 g) cheese, or $\frac{3}{4}$ cup (175 mL) yogurt.

5. Consider taking a multivitamin that includes vitamin B_{12} and iron to promote healing. B_{12} and iron can aid the bone marrow in forming new blood cells. Discuss this option with your doctor or your dietitian to make sure that you choose the correct multivitamin.

6. Participate in an exercise program before and after surgery to strengthen the muscles around the joint.

CHAPTER 9

Complementary and Alternative Medicine

CASE HISTORY
New Directions

Theresa started to look for new ways to deal with her RA after her last flare-up. Her use of a heating pad and her exercise program had helped her maintain her range of motion and gain some strength, but neither her exercise program nor her use of a DMARD had alleviated the pain in her foot or prevented flare-ups.

Theresa decided to look into some complementary and alternative ways of helping her manage her RA. She went to see her doctor and asked him if he had any recommendations. Based on his advice, she went to see an acupuncturist to see if traditional Chinese medicine could help the pain in her foot. She experienced some relief from these treatments. The acupuncturist suggested that meditation or relaxation exercises might help and explained that her bad posture was putting added strain on her shoulders.

Theresa also visited a clinic specializing in biofeedback and other complementary procedures. They designed a biofeedback program to help her become aware of her posture and to encourage good posture. They also recommended that Theresa should try a yoga routine.

These various complementary and alternative medicines helped Theresa to manage pain and to take some stress off her joints. She stayed on her DMARD, and she needed only a small amount of NSAIDs to feel better.

Popularity of CAM

In 2017, the Fraser Institute in Canada published a study showing that about 60% of individuals with some type of arthritis or rheumatism used complementary and alternative medicine. This percentage has stayed in the same range since 1997. The most commonly used treatments were massage therapy and relaxation techniques. In the United States, the National Center for Complementary and Integrative Health found that about 40% of the people with arthritis pain used some type of complementary health treatment. Another study suggests that up to 58% of patients with RA use complementary therapies. In these studies, most of the participants tried vitamins or supplements.

More and more people are turning to complementary and alternative medicine (CAM) for managing their arthritis. The National Center for Complementary and Integrative Health defines complementary medicine as a "group of diverse medical and health-care systems, practices, and products that are not generally considered part of conventional medicine." These treatments are used to supplement the treatments offered by doctors, dietitians, physical therapists, and other members of the conventional health-care team. These same practices are considered "alternative medicine" when they are used instead of conventional medicine; when they are used as part of conventional medicine, these practices are known as integrative medicine.

There are starting to be some studies that support integrating certain CAM practices into the conventional treatment of some conditions, including OA and RA.

Some studies have suggested that various CAM treatments may help to manage the symptoms of arthritis. Patients may report reduced morning stiffness, being better able to manage pain, or even reduced CRP levels. Even if you choose to add some of these treatments to your toolbox for managing your arthritis, you must also continue your traditional medical treatments. Make sure to discuss the use of CAM treatments with your doctor, physiotherapist, pharmacist, or dietitian.

CAM Practices

There are many practices, ranging from the scientific to the spiritual, categorized under the CAM title, including:

- Practices of traditional healers
- Mind-body work
- Natural products including herbs, vitamins, minerals and probiotics

The National Center for Complementary and Integrative Health (NCCIH) groups these treatments into two big categories: complementary health and integrative health. Complementary health approaches are not mainstream but are used at the same time as conventional medical treatment. Integrative health care meshes both conventional and complementary health care in a more coordinated way.

The NCCIH further classifies these treatments as natural products like dietary supplements, mind-body treatments like yoga and massage therapy, and finally practices of traditional healers.

Mind-Body Treatments

Numerous mind-body medicines have been used in the treatment of both OA and RA. To date, there have been no negative side effects reported in studies that have included patients with either OA or RA.

Tai Chi

Tai chi is a form of martial arts from China that can be traced back about 2,500 years. Most of us know it as a form of gentle exercise and even active meditation, but it is also part of Chinese medicine. It is now being studied by Western medicine and has been found to be helpful in managing many conditions.

When used in the treatment of both RA and OA, tai chi has been found to increase muscle function, improve self-efficacy, and reduce depression and pain. There was no change in disease activity, although some studies have shown a link between participating in tai chi and a decrease in inflammation.

So far, none of the studies show that arthritis was made worse by participating in a tai chi program. As always, discuss your participation in any type of exercise program with your doctor and physiotherapist to make sure the program is right for you.

Yoga

Yoga is an ancient Indian tradition that dates back 5,000 years. It encompasses movement, breathing techniques, and meditation. Studies have suggested that, like the practice of tai chi, participating in a yoga program can result in increased strength and flexibility, ease of movement, and pain reduction. Recent studies have shown that people who were experts in doing yoga had lower blood levels of the various markers of inflammation.

Arthritis is not a contraindication for taking part in a yoga program, but you may have to modify some of the exercises to safeguard your joints. Discuss undertaking this or any other exercise program with your doctor or physiotherapist. You may find yoga classes designed for people with arthritis.

Acupuncture

Acupuncture was introduced to Western medical practice in the 1970s and has grown in popularity year by year. Acupuncture is used to stimulate various points along the energy-carrying meridians, or pathways, to bring the body back into balance. During an acupuncture treatment, disposable sterilized needles are strategically placed in the body of the patient. This starts a string of events that involves the release of chemicals (neurotransmitters) secreted in the brain, which explains why acupuncture is often associated with managing pain.

Did You Know?

Promising Studies
Recent studies suggest that when placed at specific points, acupuncture will reduce pain. Some clinical trials have demonstrated that when acupuncture is added to conventional treatment for knee osteoarthritis, patients feel less pain and report improved levels of function. The effects of acupuncture on RA are still being explored. To date there have been no large clinical trials that have shown acupuncture to be effective in the treatment of RA.

Guided Imagery

Using your thoughts and imagination to help your body to feel less pain and heal itself is a technique that is gaining in popularity. A 2015 review of the scientific literature showed that guided imagery could be a helpful technique for people with arthritis. There seem to be no contraindications to this type of treatment.

Meditation

Meditation is becoming more popular. It involves relaxing your mind and learning to listen to your feelings regarding pain and any other difficulties you have encountered. A number of studies suggest that the use of mindful meditation can help to manage mood and also help the brain perceive pain differently. An added benefit is that there are no side effects.

Biofeedback

Biofeedback can assist you in developing new patterns of movement that will protect your joints from further damage. It can also be used to help you become more aware of your stress levels and teach you how to manage them. Less stress means your body will secrete less cortisol, which may lead to less inflammation.

This technique uses a device that measures muscle tension, the temperature of your skin, or your brain waves and then gives you immediate feedback on the results. For example, the device can measure whether you are performing your exercises correctly and strengthening the muscles you want. The immediate feedback will help you make any needed adjustments instantly as you continue the program. The same type of information can help you relax, manage pain, and avoid stress. There are no major contraindications to using biofeedback.

This technique uses a device that measures muscle tension, the temperature of your skin, or your brain waves and then gives you immediate feedback on the results.

Massage Therapy

Massage therapy has been considered an essential part of many healing systems for thousands of years. There are currently more than a hundred different techniques, ranging from traditional massage to reflexology to Watsu. The techniques that have been studied most in the treatment of arthritis include Swedish massage and shiatsu.

During a massage, the muscles, ligaments, synovial membranes, nerves, blood vessels, and other soft tissues are physically maneuvered, but we are not sure how massage actually works. Studies are now being performed to determine exactly what happens inside the body during a massage. We are learning that there are effects on the muscles, the way the blood circulates, the nervous system, and even the way waste products are eliminated from the body (the lymphatic system). Studies have suggested that, for those with arthritis, massage therapy may help reduce depression, reduce pain, and increase the range of motion and functionality.

Patients with RA who are having a flare-up should not use massage. If you have any other chronic medical conditions, please consult your doctor before having a massage. There are some contraindications. For example, if you are suffering from blood clots in the legs, infections — either on the skin or of the tissues (cellulitis) — or broken skin, it is important to avoid massage unless you have medical clearance.

If you are suffering from blood clots in the legs, infections — either on the skin or of the tissues (cellulitis) — or broken skin, it is important to avoid massage without medical clearance.

Chiropractic

Chiropractic was developed in the United States in the late 1800s using a philosophy that included a combination of both centuries-old and newer technologies. The premise of chiropractic is that the spine can become misaligned, causing the whole body to be out of whack and adversely affecting its natural ability to heal itself.

Patients with RA who are in a flare-up should avoid chiropractic treatments unless they receive permission or instructions from their doctor.

Q. **Is chiropractic effective for treating osteoarthritis?**

A. To date, there have been a few studies that suggest that people with either knee or hip osteoarthritis demonstrated less pain, more range of motion, and other benefits after chiropractic treatment. In one study, patients waiting for knee replacement surgery were more comfortable and had more range of movement following a specified regimen of chiropractic treatments, but they still needed the surgery.

Practices of Traditional Healers

These CAM treatments include traditional medicine philosophies from around the world, such as traditional Chinese medicine (TCM), Ayurvedic medicine, Native medicine, and naturopathic medicine.

Traditional Chinese Medicine (TCM)

This ancient medical practice is made up of various treatments, including acupuncture, herbal medicine, and tai chi. When combined, these treatments comprise the system called TCM. Despite some initial studies, there is no evidence to support the use of TCM in its entirety as a treatment for RA and OA; however, some studies suggest that tai chi (see page 77) and acupuncture (see page 78) in particular may be helpful in promoting pain management and well-being.

Ayurvedic Medicine

This healing system, based on the principle that the mind, body, and spirit must be integrated to prevent and treat disease, has been used in India for more than 2,000 years. In India, 80% of the population uses Ayurvedic medicine, either alone or in conjunction with Western medicine. The Indian government began studying the effectiveness of Ayurvedic medicine in the late 1960s.

Treatments are developed after a careful assessment of a person's constitution and life force has been completed, along with a study of their physical body and physical signs, such as their pulse. Ayurvedic medicine uses diet, mind-body techniques, and herbal medicine to relieve symptoms, cure disease, and prevent diseases from occurring.

Studies have shown conflicting results for the use of Ayurvedic medicine to treat OA and RA.

Native Medicine

Native medicine systems have been used among North American and other First Nations people from around the world to treat and prevent illness for thousands of years. Like Chinese and Ayurvedic practices, Native medicine takes a more comprehensive approach to healing. Native healers believe that illness is the result of imbalances between a person and society, and between a person and the surrounding natural environment. Illness is seen as an opportunity to look at lifestyle and make changes to improve life balance. Medicines are plant-based and nontoxic. In a database of traditional North American Native peoples' medicines, 76 different medicines for arthritis were found. There has been a growing interest in these treatments, but there has not been a systematic evaluation of their usefulness in OA or RA.

Native healers believe that illness is the result of imbalances between a person and the surrounding environment. Illness is seen as an opportunity to look at lifestyle and make changes to improve life balance.

Naturopathic Medicine

Naturopathic medicine is founded on the vitalistic principle of the *vis natura medicatrix*, or healing power of nature, which posits that the physician's job is to remove any impediment to this "nature cure." Naturopathic medicine is eclectic, encompassing clinical nutrition, botanical medicine, homeopathic medicine, traditional Chinese medicine, bodywork and mind-body strategies. There is little evidence to support the use of naturopathic medicine in the treatment of OA or RA.

CHAPTER 10

Nutritional and Herbal Supplements

CASE HISTORY
Nutrient Boost

Lilly was diagnosed with RA about 10 years ago. Over the years, she had taken many different medications to control her symptoms. After her most recent flare-up, her rheumatologist started her on a new medication. She was also very stiff in the morning and found it difficult to get her daughter ready for school. In addition, she was feeling very sluggish. Her doctor suggested that she see a dietitian.

After reviewing Lilly's diet, we realized that Lilly might not be consuming enough omega-3 fatty acids. Lilly and her daughter did not eat much fish and consumed only very small amounts of oils and other foods that contain omega-3 fatty acids. After a short discussion with Lilly, we decided that the best way to make sure she consumed enough omega-3 fats on a daily basis was to take a supplement. With the approval of her doctor, Lilly started taking 3 g of omega-3 fatty acid supplements. When she chooses her supplements, she makes sure they are purified, meaning that all the toxins had been removed from the fish oil. After a period of about 1 month, Lilly noticed that she was not taking as many NSAIDs and she was not as stiff in the morning.

At the same time, Lilly's doctor referred her for a blood test, and he shared these results with us. It turned out that Lilly's blood levels of vitamin D (25-hydroxy-vitamin D) were very low. Based on this information, as well as the information about Lilly's diet, it was decided that the best way to replace the vitamin D was to take a supplement. Initially, her doctor suggested a dose of 2000 IU (international units) daily and to repeat the blood test in 2 months. Two months later, the new blood test showed that although her levels of vitamin D had improved, Lilly still had low levels. This regime was maintained, and subsequent blood tests showed that Lilly's blood levels of vitamin D returned to normal.

At that time, the doctor reduced the dose of vitamin D to 1000 IU daily, which helped maintain her vitamin D levels in the normal range.

Because she had been taking cortisone on and off for a few years, Lilly's doctor suggested that she have a bone density test. It showed that her bone density was decreasing, so we decided to add a calcium supplement to the mix. We prescribed a liquid form of calcium supplement, which the body can absorb more easily. This arrested the loss of bone density and alleviated some of her arthritis symptoms. This regime should help Lilly maintain good bone health in the coming years.

The demand for complementary and alternative medical therapies in managing arthritis is growing, especially the demand for nutrients and herbs that can be used therapeutically or medicinally. Every day, it seems that a new supplement is heralded as an improved treatment for arthritis. This suggests that nutritional and herbal supplement research, much like research into medications, is in a state of flux. Exercise caution if you use supplements and consult with your doctor, pharmacist, or dietitian before starting these treatments to be sure there are no drug interactions or side effects that might affect your general health adversely. Just because most of these supplements are natural does not necessarily mean they are safe for you.

Did You Know?

Half the Population

A study by the National Health and Nutrition Examination Survey (NHANES) on the dietary habits of Americans, including the use of supplements, for the years 1999 to 2012 found that up to 50% were taking a nutritional supplement. In Canada, up to 70% of adults are taking some kind of natural health herbal product. Although the most popular form of nutritional supplement is a multivitamin, many people are now taking a wide array of nutritional and herbal products. For example, sales of omega-3 fatty acid and vitamin D supplements have increased significantly.

Did You Know?

Fortification

Supplementing the diet with nutrients is a preventive measure. White bread, for example, is fortified with thiamin, riboflavin, and niacin (vitamin B_1, B_2, and B_3, respectively), and dairy products are sometimes supplemented with vitamin D. Recently, nutrients have been used therapeutically in larger-than-preventive doses as medicine for treating illnesses, including arthritis.

Supplementation

Nutrients

Nutrients needed for good health are naturally derived from our food, but when our diet does not supply sufficient amounts, serious nutrient deficiency diseases can result. For example, scurvy can develop from a deficiency of vitamin C, pellagra can be caused by a deficiency of vitamin B_3, iron-deficient anemia can result from a shortage of iron in the food supply, and rickets is caused by a deficiency of vitamin D.

Herbal Medicines

Herbal, or botanical, medicines contain chemical substances that in some cases act as pharmaceutical medications. For a long time, Western medicine has focused on the use of pharmaceuticals to treat diseases. Some of these medicines are derived from plants or adapted from herbal remedies. Take, for example, digoxin, which is now used to treat congestive heart failure and abnormal heart rhythms. In the late eighteenth century, while treating a patient with heart problems, a physician in England noticed that the patient's health improved when she took a medicine recommended by a herbalist. The physician discovered that the active ingredient was derived from the otherwise poisonous foxglove plant (*Digitalis purpurea*). More and more study led to the development of a standard formula for the preparation of digoxin, now a common prescription medication.

Safety and Efficacy Standards

Not all nutrients and herbs have been studied as rigorously as digitalis, but several government health agencies in North America are starting to set standards for efficacy, safety, and dosage. The Federal Drug Agency (FDA) and Health Canada regulate the pharmaceutical industry in their respective countries. To be approved for use, a drug has to go through a rigorous process, which includes at least three stages of clinical trials where the drug is investigated for safety and effectiveness. Once the drug has been approved, it is continually re-evaluated. However, the rules that apply to the pharmaceutical industry do not apply to the nutritional and herbal supplement industry.

In the United States, the regulations state that it is the responsibility of the manufacturer of the supplement or of the individual ingredients to make sure that the products are safe and effective before they sell them. They do not have to register the product, although manufacturers must comply with the

Nutrient Classifications

There are many chemicals that we collectively call nutrients. In turn, these nutrients are commonly classified as vitamins, minerals, amino acids, essential fatty acids and enzymes. Probiotics are supplements, but they are not nutrients.

Vitamins: organic chemicals that the body requires to function properly. These substances cannot be made by the body or cannot be made in required amounts by the body, so must be obtained from food. This class of nutrients is further divided into water soluble vitamins, which cannot be stored in the body, and fat soluble vitamins, which are stored in the body.

Minerals: inorganic chemicals that the body requires to function properly. These substances are essential for the body to function, helping muscles, for example, to contract or in the formation of bone. Some minerals are needed in larger amounts and some are needed in very tiny or trace amounts.

Amino acids: the building blocks of protein molecules. Amino acids fall into three categories. Essential amino acids are necessary for the body to build up protein molecules, and must be obtained from the food we eat because they cannot be manufactured by the body. Nonessential amino acids can be made in adequate amounts by the body, and conditional amino acids are only essential when the body is under stress, for example during an illness.

Essential fatty acids: fats that we need for good health that cannot be made by our bodies and must come from our food or from supplements. These fats are called "essential." They are often referred to as fatty acids.

Enzymes: chemical structures that are made up of proteins. They are found in every cell of the body. They are a part of every chemical reaction that occurs in the body. Their role is to speed up these reactions so that the body runs smoothly.

Probiotics: healthy bacteria that live in the human intestines. Instead of harming humans, they actually provide us with health benefits. They can help to prevent colds and help to regulate the function of the immune system. (Technically, probiotics are bacteria, not nutrients).

recommendations in the FDA's Dietary Supplement Current Good Manufacturing Practices and the Interim Final Rule.

In Canada, supplements are regulated by the Natural and Non-prescription Health Products Directorate. All supplements and homeopathic products must be registered with this agency of Health Canada. The products are assigned a number, which is printed on their label. For nutritional supplements and herbal products, it is called a natural product number (NPN), and for homeopathic products, a drug identification number (DIN-HM) is assigned. The site that manufactures the supplements must also have a license.

Q. **How can I tell if I am getting accurate information on the use of supplements?**

A. Be wary of some of the information you find on the Internet and in pamphlets from health food stores. Some sites are designed to sell products, whereas others are there strictly to provide information. Verify who owns the site and who is providing the information. Look to see what type of credentials they have. Note whether scientific studies are quoted and references given. Ask your doctor or pharmacist whether the product could interact with any treatment that you are receiving, with any medicine that you are taking, or with any food that you eat.

Nutritional Supplements and Medicinal Herbs for Arthritis

Some nutritional and herbal supplements may be effective and safe for helping to manage arthritis symptoms. Your doctor, your dietitian, or your pharmacist may recommend them. Some supplements can be used exclusively to help in the management of RA, others only for OA, but some can be used to manage both. Do not start taking any supplement on your own without consulting with your doctor or other members of your health-care team. Results may vary from person to person.

Nutritional Supplements for OA

Glucosamine Sulfate and Chondroitin Sulfate

These are probably the most popular arthritis supplements. Many studies have been published suggesting that these products may help in the treatment of OA; however, the Osteoarthritis Research Society International (OARSI) states in its treatment guidelines that there is not enough evidence to support the efficacy of either of these supplements in maintaining cartilage or for pain management. Two recent review articles came to the same conclusion.

Recently, the American College of Rheumatology (ACR) and the American Association of Orthopaedic Surgeons (AAOS) recommended against using glucosamine sulfate and chondroitin sulfate, but the updated 2018 European League Against Rheumatism (EULAR) guidelines on the treatment of osteoarthritis recommend considering chondroitin sulfate to treat OA of the hand.

Here are some facts to keep in mind if you decide to take either of these supplements.

Therapeutic Dose

- Glucosamine sulfate: 1500 mg once daily or 500 mg three times daily.

- Chondroitin sulfate: 1000 to 1200 mg once daily or 400 mg three times daily.

Drug Interactions

- If you are taking blood thinners (such as warfarin): Glucosamine and chondroitin can impede clotting, which could lead to bruising or bleeding.

- If you are undergoing chemotherapy: Some medications that are used in chemotherapy cause the cancer cells to copy themselves more slowly. Glucosamine may get in the way of these medications and stop them from working, which would allow the cancer cells to keep copying themselves very quickly. If you are undergoing chemotherapy, check with your health-care team before taking glucosamine sulphate.

Possible Side Effects

- Mild side effects of these supplements include an upset stomach.

- If you have diabetes: Glucosamine might cause your blood sugar levels to go down. If you decide to take glucosamine sulphate, check your blood sugar levels more often, then check with your doctor or your dietitian to see if you need to adjust your diabetes medicine.

- If you have asthma: Some research suggests that glucosamine and chondroitin could make breathing more difficult. Discuss using these supplements with your health-care team.

- If you are pregnant or breastfeeding: Be cautious. There is not enough information available about these supplements to recommend them to women who are pregnant or breastfeeding.

> ## Did You Know?
>
> ### Exercise Caution
> One of the leading causes of liver injury in Canada and the United States is supplement use. This could be because of interactions between the supplements and other medications or conditions, or because the supplements do not contain the amounts of the ingredients they are supposed to. Always exercise caution when taking supplements.

- If you have a shellfish allergy: Avoid glucosamine sulfate. There is some evidence that you could have an allergic reaction.

- If you have or are at risk of getting prostate cancer: There is some evidence that this condition can be made worse by chondroitin, and research suggests that prostate cancer may recur even if it has been successfully treated. Although there is no proof that this type of supplement actually affects prostate cancer, it is better to be safe and avoid using it if you have a high risk of getting prostate cancer.

SAMe

SAMe (or S-adenosylmethionine) is another popular nutritional supplement. Although it is naturally produced in our livers, taking an additional supplement seems to help build and activate some very important chemicals. SAMe is found in the synovial fluid, where it seems to trigger the cartilage to grow and repair itself. It might also help protect the synovial cells from damage. In osteoarthritis, it helps reduce pain and acts as an anti-inflammatory. Some studies show that it is as effective as traditional pain medication.

Therapeutic Dose

400 mg up to three times daily. This medication will take up to 30 days to work, so be patient. Make sure that the major ingredient in this supplement is made of butanedisulfonate salt because it is the best-absorbed form of SAMe.

Drug Interactions

- If you are taking antidepressants: Like most anti-depressants, SAMe sometimes acts by increasing the amount of serotonin in the brain. If you take these medications together, discuss this combination with your health-care provider.

Side Effects

- This supplement is well tolerated, but it might cause some stomach upset, nausea, flatulence, headache or fatigue.

- If you are pregnant or breastfeeding: There is not enough information about this supplement to recommend its use if you are pregnant or breastfeeding.

- If you have bipolar disorder or Parkinson's disease: Do not use this supplement.

- If you are having surgery: Stop taking SAMe 2 weeks before you have any surgery.

Medications to Avoid Using with SAMe

- Antidepressants: such as Paxil, Elavil, Zoloft
- Monoamine oxidase inhibitors (MAOIs)
- Medicinal herbs: St. John's wort, L-tryptophan
- Dextromethorphan (ingredient in some cough medicines)
- Levodopa: SAMe breaks down this medication, used by people with Parkinson's disease
- Pethidine (e.g., Demerol)
- Tramadol (e.g., Ultram)
- Pentazocine (e.g., Talwin)

Q. **What is an enzyme?**

A. An enzyme is a protein that is used by every cell in the body to help speed up all the chemical reactions that have to take place to enable the cell to perform its role in the body. One of the jobs that enzymes do is to break down food into the nutrients that can be used by the body.

Collagen

Part of the bones, cartilage, and other tissues in humans and animals, the collagen from chickens has been used in supplements used to treat OA. Some studies show that taking it may help reduce pain and stiffness in knee OA.

Therapeutic Dose
Varies depending on the product.

Drug and Supplement Interactions
None are known.

Side Effects
- Some collagen supplements are made from chicken collagen, so if you have an allergy to chicken or eggs, you may have an allergic reaction to these products.
- If you are pregnant or breastfeeding: There is no information to show that this product is safe for you or your baby.

Medicinal Herbs for OA

Boswellia

Also known as frankincense, this herb has been used for generations to treat osteoarthritis and rheumatoid arthritis. Early research shows that boswellia could be effective in OA. It contains some chemicals that are anti-inflammatory, others that might stimulate cartilage repair, and still others that reduce the production of antibodies. Some preparations of boswellia reduced OA pain by 65% while improving mobility. The results of studies on RA are not as promising.

Therapeutic Dose
- OA: 100 to 1000 mg of a specific formulation of boswellia extract.
- RA: No recommendation at this time.

Drug Interactions
- This herb interacts with medications that are broken down in the liver. Ask your pharmacist if boswellia will interact with any medications you take.

Side Effects
- New research shows that boswellia might stimulate the immune system. It is not recommended for people with an autoimmune disease like RA. Frankincense is safe if used as a seasoning in food.

Devil's Claw

This plant is native to Africa and was introduced to Europe and North America around 1950. Scientists have found several different chemicals in devil's claw that help reduce pain and inflammation. Some studies show that devil's claw is only effective for pain that occurs during an activity but does not seem to help pain that occurs when resting.

Therapeutic Dose
The amount of devil's claw needed to effectively manage pain will depend on which chemical has been extracted from the plant. In the products that have been studied, the dosage varied between 2.4 and 2.6 g daily. Ask your pharmacist to recommend the optimum dose.

Drug Interactions

- If you are taking any medication that is broken down by or changed in the liver: Stop taking devil's claw because it can slow down the way the liver breaks down some medications. Check with your pharmacist to make sure that you are not taking any drugs that are changed by the liver. Some examples are Prilosec, Prevacid, Voltaren, Motrin, Elavil, Mevacor, and Halcion.

- If you are already taking medication or supplements that slow the way blood clots (e.g., Coumadin): Do not take devil's claw because it can make these medications even stronger, which might cause bleeding or bruising.

- If you are taking medications to decrease stomach acid: Devil's claw may work against these medications by increasing the amount of stomach acid that is produced. Some examples of these medications are Pepcid, Tagamet, Nexium, Prevacid, and Prilosec.

Side Effects

- May cause upset stomach, diarrhea and headache.

- If you have heart disease or blood pressure problems: Do not take devil's claw because it may lower blood pressure and heart rate. Discuss using this supplement with your doctor.

- If you are a child, pregnant, or breastfeeding: There is not enough information available to suggest that children or women who are pregnant or breastfeeding can safely take this medication.

- If you have diabetes: Discuss using devil's claw with your doctor or dietitian before you start to take it. Devil's claw can lower blood sugar levels. Its effect will be added to the effect of your other medications, and that could cause your blood sugar levels to get too low.

- If you have gallstones: Taking devil's claw might increase the amount of bile that is produced and aggravate your condition.

- If you tend to have stomach ulcers or produce too much stomach acid: Do not take devil's claw. This supplement increases the production of stomach acid and could aggravate your condition.

Ginger

Ginger has historically been used to treat rheumatism. Considerable research has been done in recent years to determine the exact dose to take for the best results. Studies seem to show that ginger can be used quite effectively to help manage the pain of osteoarthritis. Some studies have compared taking ginger to taking NSAIDs (non-steroidal anti-inflammatory drugs, such as ibuprofen). The results showed that both ginger and NSAIDs gave people with arthritis similar pain relief.

Ginger can also be used as an ingredient in topical ointments. Studies have compared various formulations of ointments containing ginger to similar products whose active ingredient is either diclofenac or salicylate. The studies found that all of the ointments were equally effective in reducing morning stiffness and pain.

Ginger oil has been used as a massage oil in the treatment of knee OA. A massage with a specific formulation of ginger oil was found to reduce pain but did not reduce morning stiffness.

Although there have been some studies on using ginger to help people with rheumatoid arthritis, there is not enough evidence to determine ginger's usefulness for managing the pain, stiffness, or inflammation caused by RA.

A number of studies show that ginger can be useful for preventing nausea and vomiting after surgery.

> **Ginger has historically been used to treat rheumatism.**

Therapeutic Dose

The specific dose depends on the formulation being used. Please check with your pharmacist to ensure that you take the correct dose of your ginger supplement.

Drug Interactions

- Ginger can react with many drugs. Be cautious.
- If you are taking any medications or herbs that slow blood clotting: Avoid ginger.
- If you are taking medications to treat low blood sugar: Monitor blood sugar carefully, because ginger supplements can also lower blood sugar levels. Consult with your doctor, who may adjust your medications.

Side Effects

- Ginger can cause nausea and vomiting if taken in very large doses (more than 5 g).
- If you have a blood disorder: Do not take ginger, as it can make it harder for the blood to clot.
- If you use ginger ointment or ginger massage oil: Be aware that ginger can cause a skin irritation.

Willow Bark

Hippocrates advised patients to chew on the bark of the willow tree to help relieve pain and fever. The active ingredient in willow bark is salicin, which is part of the same family of chemicals as Aspirin. Salicin is transformed into salicylic acid during digestion.

Therapeutic Dose

120 to 240 mg daily.

Drug Interactions

- If you are taking blood thinners or NSAIDs: Do not take willow bark. Like other medicines that contain salicylic acid, this supplement can slow down the way the blood clots. Do not take this supplement with any medicine that contains salicylic acid or that contains chemicals that break down to produce salicylic acid. Do not take with acetazolamide (Diamox), salsalate (such as Disalcid), or Trisilate.

Side Effects

- If you are allergic to salicylic acid: Do not take this supplement.

- This supplement has the same side effects as Aspirin. It can cause stomach upset and bleeding.

- If you are planning surgery: Stop taking willow bark 2 weeks before surgery to make sure that there is no risk of extra bleeding.

- If you have kidney disease: Do not take willow bark. Some studies show that this supplement will slow the flow of blood to the kidney, which could further damage the kidneys.

- If you are a child, pregnant, or breastfeeding: There is not enough information available to suggest that children or women who are pregnant or breastfeeding can safely take this medication.

Nutritional Supplements for RA

Gamma-Linolenic Acid (including Borage Oil)

Gamma-linolenic acid (GLA) is one of the active ingredients in borage oil and evening primrose oil. It is an omega-6 fatty acid. In fact, it seems to decrease inflammation by helping decrease in the cells the amount of fatty acids that promote inflammation. This will lead to less pain, inflammation, and swelling in patients with RA. In addition, it will decrease the risk of heart disease, which is often another problem for people with RA.

Therapeutic Dose
3.2 g daily.

Drug Interactions
- If you are taking pharmaceutical or herbal medicines to thin your blood: Avoid taking GLA. When the two medicines are combined, the effect can be increased. This means that the blood can become too thin, causing excess bleeding and bruising.

- If you are taking medications that prevent seizures: Do not take GLA because it interacts with medicines in the phenothiazine family. This group includes Thorazine, Prolixin, Stelazine, and Mellaril, to name just a few.

Side Effects
Some minor digestive side effects, such as soft stools, gas, or even diarrhea, can occur when taking this supplement.

Medicinal Herbs for RA

Thunder God Vine

This herb is used in traditional Chinese medicine as an anti-inflammatory. It also seems to have the ability to down-regulate the immune system. Early studies show that using thunder god vine can reduce stiffness and pain; however, more studies are needed to confirm this effect.

Caution

Some parts of the plant (leaves, flowers, and skin of the root) are very poisonous. If the active ingredients are contaminated with these poisons during the manufacturing process, the supplements could actually cause serious illness or death.

Therapeutic Dose

In RA, this herb can be taken as a pill or applied as an ointment:

Pill: 180 to 570 mg daily for up to 20 weeks.

Topical: Apply 5 to 6 times daily on the skin of affected joints.

Drug Interactions

- If you are taking drugs to alter the activity of your immune system: Avoid this herbal medicine because it also affects immune system activity.

Side Effects

- Stomach upset, diarrhea, headache, and hair loss.

- If taken for more than 5 years, this herb may also decrease bone mineral density.

- If your immune system has been compromised: Avoid this herb.

- If you have osteoporosis or are at risk for developing osteoporosis: Avoid this supplement.

Early studies show that using thunder god vine can reduce stiffness and pain; however, more studies are needed to confirm this effect.

Did You Know?

Risk vs. Reward
A review of the scientific studies found that the side effects of thunder god vine outweigh the benefits.

Nutritional Supplements for OA and RA

Calcium

Calcium does not play a direct role in the treatment of OA or RA; rather, it is needed to maintain good bone health. Stronger, healthier bones are an advantage in arthritis because they can better support the weaker joints. As well, some of the anti-inflammatory medications that are taken to treat RA can weaken the bone. Taking calcium and vitamin D can combat this effect.

If you have a deficiency of calcium in your diet, your bones can become more fragile and osteoporosis can develop. Osteoporosis can cause joint pain parallel to osteoarthritis and can also lead to painful fractures.

> If you have a deficiency of calcium in your diet, your bones can become more fragile and osteoporosis can develop. Osteoporosis can cause joint pain parallel to osteoarthritis and can also lead to painful fractures.

Therapeutic Dose

Dosing recommendations vary based on how much calcium is in your diet, so consult with your doctor for the dose that is appropriate for you. Choose either calcium carbonate or calcium citrate supplements. Ask your doctor or pharmacist for a recommendation.

Drug Interactions

- If you are taking antibiotics: Avoid taking them at the same time of day as calcium supplements because some antibiotics change when they are taken at the same time as calcium. If you are taking tetracycline antibiotics, for example, it is best to take calcium either 2 hours before or 4 hours after taking the antibiotic. With other antibiotics, such as Cipro, take calcium 1 hour after taking the antibiotic.

- If you are taking a bisphosphonate (such as Fosamax, Didronel or Actonel) for bone health; thyroid medications; iron supplements; heart medications such as digoxin (Lanoxin), diltiazem (Cardizem), verapamil (Covera), or water pills; calcipotriene; or some medications for HIV: Consult with your doctor or pharmacist to see whether calcium supplements will interfere with the absorption of any of your medications. Ask for specific instructions on how to space out your calcium and your other medications.

Side Effects

There are rarely any side effects reported by people taking calcium supplements. Occasionally, patients can have some gas or burping. Calcium can cause reactions in patients with too little or too much phosphate in the blood or in patients who already have too much calcium in the blood. Excess calcium supplements have recently been reported to possibly increase the risk of heart attack in susceptible people.

Dimethyl Sulfoxide (DMSO)

To treat arthritis, DMSO is delivered as a cream that is rubbed on the affected joints. Studies indicate that DMSO may have an anti-inflammatory effect that reduces pain and joint damage while possibly increasing the formation of cartilage.

> **Studies indicate that DMSO may have an anti-inflammatory effect that reduces pain and joint damage while possibly increasing the formation of cartilage.**

Therapeutic Dose

OA: 25% DMSO gel applied three times daily.
　　45.5% DMSO solution applied four times daily.
RA: 60% to 90% DMSO solution applied two to four
　　times daily.

Safety

In a less refined form, DMSO is used as an industrial solvent. Make sure that the supplement you purchase is pure, with no harmful contaminants. DMSO easily penetrates the skin and can be found in the blood 5 minutes after it has been applied. Because it is absorbed so quickly, it can be very dangerous if it contains any impurities.

Drug Interactions

Research studies show that DMSO can cause the body to absorb many medications more efficiently. This could increase the strength of the medicine or cause you to have more side effects. Be very careful if you use DMSO while taking other medication. Do not use DMSO if you are taking medicines for diabetes, high blood pressure, or any other condition.

Side Effects

- DMSO contains sulfur, which may leave a garlicky taste in the mouth.

- Because it has been linked to liver and kidney problems, have blood tests on a regular basis.

- If you are pregnant or breastfeeding: There is not enough information available to suggest it is safe for women who are pregnant or breastfeeding.

Lactobacillus

Lactobacillus are a specific type of "good" bacteria that usually live in our intestines and our urinary tract. They are also found in yogurt and some cheeses and can be taken as a probiotic supplement. A recent study found that taking a probiotic supplement of a particular strain of *Lactobacillus casei* resulted in a reduction in the number of tender and swollen joints in women with RA, along with a reduction of some of the markers of inflammation. More research is needed in this area.

Therapeutic Dose

100 million colony-forming units (CFU) was used in the study

Drug Interactions

- Antibiotics: Antibiotics are used to eradicate unhealthy bacteria in the body. Unfortunately, they can also reduce the number of healthy bacteria. Make sure to take antibiotics at least 2 hours before or after taking any probiotic, to ensure the effectiveness of the probiotic.

- Immunosuppressants: All probiotic supplements, including *Lactobacillus*, are made of live bacteria. If your immune system is not working properly, it is possible that the bacteria could grow too much or in the wrong place in your body and make you sick. If you are taking prednisone, cortisone, or any other immunosuppressant medication, ask your doctor if it is safe for you to take a probiotic.

Side Effects

- *Lactobacillus* supplements could cause gas, bloating, or a skin rash.

- Bacterial overgrowth: Recent studies showed that some people who took probiotics had an overgrowth of bacteria in their intestines. This could lead to digestive problems.

Omega-3 Fatty Acids

One of the main functions of omega-3 fatty acids is to help regulate an overactive immune system. In RA, the entire body is in a constant state of inflammation, and the immune system starts to attack the body. One of the ways that RA is diagnosed is by determining the levels of C-reactive protein (CRP) in the blood.

There is some research that supports increasing the amount of omega-3 fatty acids in the diet to relieve some of the symptoms of RA. Omega-3 fatty acids in foods will have the same effect as omega-3 fatty acids in supplements. They act by slowing down the production of one of the enzymes that is responsible for the development of inflammation, cyclooxygenase (COX), thereby reducing inflammation. In people with RA, this may result in a reduction in pain, stiffness, and swelling.

Recent studies on rats have shown that omega-3 fats help to both relieve the pain and slow the progression of OA. Some studies have shown benefits when people with OA take omega-3 supplements, so we can assume that omega-3 from food is also useful.

Fish and Krill Oil Supplements

Although you can derive enough omega-3 EFAs from food sources to relieve arthritis symptoms, many people find it more convenient to consume some omega-3 fats from food and some from supplements. Many studies have shown that taking fish and krill oil supplements can help lower triglyceride levels, promote heart health, and manage the symptoms of rheumatoid arthritis and possibly osteoarthritis. When buying either type of supplement, choose enteric-coated tablets to eliminate the possibility of suffering from fishy-tasting burps.

Krill oil is a special form of fish oil made from krill, tiny relatives of shrimp. Studies show that krill oil helps reduce the pain of osteoarthritis. In one study, a specific formulation of krill oil, when taken at 300 mg daily, lowered levels of C-reactive protein (which is a marker for inflammation), reduced pain and stiffness, and improved function. It can take up to 30 days to feel the maximum benefit from this supplement.

Therapeutic Dose

OA: Right now we do not have a suggested dose for fish oil supplements for the treatment of OA. However, one study shows that OA symptoms can improve when patients consume 300 mg of a specific type of krill oil.

RA: Fish oil containing 3.8 g of EPA and 2 g of DHA. Check with your doctor, dietitian, or pharmacist to get some product recommendations.

Safety

Fish oil supplements are made from the oils of fatty fish that may contain contaminants, such as PCBs and dioxin, which can increase the risk of developing cancer. Mercury is stored in the muscle of fish (not the fat), so it is not likely to be found in fish oil supplements. Make sure that any fish oil supplements you choose are purified, which means that any contaminants have been removed. Always check to make sure that your fish oil supplements are fresh, because they can become rancid. Rancid supplements are not as potent, they are more likely to cause burping, and they have an unpleasant odor.

Make sure that any fish oil supplements you choose are purified, which means that any contaminants have been removed.

Drug Interactions

- If you are taking blood thinners (e.g., Coumadin) or other medications that slow blood clotting: Do not take this supplement. Both fish and krill oils may slow down the way the blood clots. This can magnify the effect of medications that are prescribed to slow blood clotting.

- If you are taking orlistat (Alli or Xenical): Taking orlistat and an oil-based supplement together can reduce the amount of supplement that is absorbed, which would make the supplement less effective. Orlistat reduces the amount of fat the body can absorb. Take the supplement either 2 hours before or 2 hours after taking the orlistat.

- If you are taking medicines to lower blood pressure: Do not take fish or krill oil. Fish oils also lower blood pressure, and the combined effect could make your blood pressure too low. Some examples of blood pressure medications are Capoten, Vasotec, Cozaar, Cardizem, Norvasc, Diovan, Hydrodiuril, and Lasix.

Side Effects

> If you are allergic to fish or seafood, avoid both fish oil and krill oil supplements.

- The most common side effects from taking this medication are related to indigestion: bad breath, burping, and loose stools.

- Exercise caution and do not exceed a dose of 3 g of fish oil daily. Larger doses may increase the risk of bleeding and bruising, and reduce the function of the immune system. Fish oil and krill supplements can increase bleeding. They should be avoided by people who have blood disorders.

- If you have high blood pressure and blood sugar levels: Consult your doctor to learn how to adjust your medication.

- If you are allergic to fish or seafood: Avoid both fish oil and krill oil supplements.

- If you are pregnant or breastfeeding: Fish oil supplements seem to be safe for these women, but there is not yet enough information to recommend krill oil to those who are pregnant or breastfeeding.

- If you are planning surgery: Stop taking fish and krill oil 2 weeks before surgery to avoid bleeding complications.

Superoxide Dismutase

This enzyme occurs naturally in the body and acts to break down damaging free radicals. It is believed that by slowing down free radical damage, the aging process can also be slowed down. By decreasing the amount of free radicals in the joint, there is less damage to the synovial fluid. If the synovial fluid stays healthy, the joint will be healthier.

Therapeutic Dose

To be effective, this supplement must be injected. Enzymes are digested by the stomach acids. Studies have not been done to show that superoxide dismutase pills are effective.

Drug Interactions

There are no known drug or herb interactions.

Side Effects

The only side effect seems to be pain at the site of the injection.

Vitamin D

Vitamin D is made by the skin in the presence of UVB rays from the sun. In some populations, especially where exposure to the sun is limited in the winter, vitamin D levels are often deficient. Until recently, this problem was solved because the body was able to use the extra vitamin D that was provided and stored in the summer months. However, people are now spending less time outside in the summer and wearing sunscreen when they do.

Vitamin D appears in two forms, vitamin D_2 and D_3. Vitamin D helps the body absorb calcium, and that in turn helps to keep bones and muscles strong. When treating RA, it is common to prescribe medicines that will down-regulate the immune system. Some of these medicines can cause your bones to become more porous, leading to osteoporosis. Taking vitamin D can help maintain bone mass. In older women, there also seems to be a link between not having enough vitamin D in the blood and having a greater chance of developing RA.

Therapeutic Dose

400 to 1000 IU daily. When taken in amounts of less than 4000 IU, vitamin D is generally safe. However, it is ideal to have blood levels of 25-hydroxy-vitamin D measured before taking a supplement. There is some vitamin D in the food you consume, and there will be some produced by your skin. To determine your specific dose, have your blood tested for vitamin D levels and then take the dosage of supplement that will bring these levels

---

Did You Know?

Vitamin D Deficiency
Recent studies estimate that between 50% and 75% of women over the age of 50 have low blood levels of vitamin D. Among seniors over 65 and people who are obese, up to 90% or more can have low blood levels of vitamin D. Recent studies have demonstrated that having higher blood levels of vitamin D is linked to having stronger bones, muscles, and fewer falls in seniors. Food manufacturers have begun to fortify some products with vitamin D.

---

to normal. Some studies performed in Italy found that people with autoimmune disorders needed very high doses of vitamin D supplements to get near the desired blood levels. This type of supplementation can only be done with the help and advice of your doctor.

Drug Interactions

- If you are taking Calcipotriene (topical Dovonex): Supplements could cause too much vitamin D to accumulate in the body, which could cause kidney problems.
- If you are taking heart medications and/or water pills (diuretics): Check with your doctor regarding the best dose of vitamin D for you.

Side Effects

- If too much vitamin D is stored in the body, it can become toxic. Be sure to monitor levels of vitamin D.
- If you have kidney disease, high blood levels of calcium, sarcoidosis, histoplasmosis, an overactive parathyroid gland or lymphoma: Consult your doctor before taking vitamin D supplements.

Medicinal Herbs for OA and RA

Cat's Claw

Cat's claw is native to South America but has become one of the most popular supplements sold in North America. Chemicals found in the bark of the cat's claw vine may have an anti-inflammatory effect and an impact on immune system function.

In OA, cat's claw is used because it has anti-inflammatory properties. In one study, patients reported less pain when they were performing physical activity. In RA, cat's claw may be useful because it seems to modulate the immune system. In another study, a specific extract was used alongside traditional medications and people who participated in the study showed a decrease in the number of swollen and painful joints.

Dose

OA: 100 mg daily of a specific freeze-dried extract of cat's claw reduced pain in one study.

RA: 20 mg taken three times daily. The extract used to treat RA is different from the one used for OA. The tetracyclic indole alkaloids can be removed from the cat's claw because they interfere with the actions of the chemicals that can help reduce pain and swelling in RA.

Drug Interactions

- If you are taking medications (such as cortisone) to regulate your immune system: Avoid cat's claw because it may interfere with the action of these drugs.

- If you are taking medication for low blood pressure: Avoid cat's claw because it may lower blood pressure.

- If you are taking medications (such as Mevacor, Allegra, or Nizoral) that are broken down in the liver: Avoid cat's claw because it can make them more efficient and possibly cause more side effects. Check with your pharmacist to make sure that any other medicines or herbs you are taking are not broken down in the liver.

If you have an autoimmune disorder, such as systemic lupus, avoid cat's claw because it may up-regulate the immune system.

Side Effects

- Headache, dizziness, and vomiting.

- If you have an autoimmune disorder, such as systemic lupus: Avoid cat's claw because it may up-regulate the immune system.

- If you have leukemia: Avoid cat's claw because it seems to prolong the life of leukemia cells.

- If you have low blood pressure: Avoid cat's claw because it may further lower your blood pressure.

- If you are planning surgery: Stop taking this supplement 2 weeks before surgery so that blood pressure levels remain stable during surgery.

- If you are pregnant or breastfeeding: There have not been enough studies to know whether this supplement is safe for women who are pregnant or breastfeeding.

Turmeric

Best known for its bright yellow color and flavor in mustards and curries, turmeric has been used as a medicine for centuries. Studies show that curcumin, the active ingredient in turmeric, may help to reduce pain, morning stiffness, walking time, and joint stiffness in patients with RA.

In another study, patients with OA in the knee took 500 mg of a specific turmeric extract twice daily. After 8 weeks, they had decreased pain and improved function in the joint.

Best known for its bright yellow color and flavor in mustards and curries, turmeric has been used as a medicine for centuries.

Therapeutic Dose

- OA: 500 mg daily of a specific formulation.
- RA: Dose will vary depending on the specific product.

Drug Interactions

- Turmeric interacts with many medications, including sulfasalazine, a medication that may be used to treat RA. Before taking a turmeric supplement, check with your pharmacist.

- If you are taking blood thinners (such as warfarin) or other drugs or herbs that also slow blood clotting: Do not take turmeric, as it might slow down blood clotting and lead to bruising or bleeding.

Side Effects

Avoid turmeric if you are pregnant because it has been known to stimulate labor.

- When taken at the amounts needed to reduce inflammation, turmeric may cause nausea, diarrhea, constipation, or reflux.

- If you are pregnant or breastfeeding: Avoid turmeric, as it has been known to stimulate labor. There is not much information available on its safety for women who are breastfeeding, so it is best to avoid it then too.

- If you have gallbladder problems: Do not take turmeric, because it can make them worse.

- If you are having surgery: Stop taking turmeric at least 2 weeks before, to reduce the chances of extra bleeding during and after the surgery.

- If you have diabetes: Turmeric can lower blood sugar levels.

- If you have iron deficiency: Turmeric can reduce iron absorption.

Quick Reference Guide to the Effectiveness and Safety of Nutritional and Herbal Supplements*

Supplement	May Be Effective For	Not Proven Effective For	Safety Concerns
Nutritional Supplements			
Calcium	Preventing osteoporosis		Can interact with some medications; consult with your pharmacist, doctor, or dietitian before taking
Chondroitin Sulfate	OA		Avoid with blood thinners
Collagen	OA		Avoid if you have an allergy to chicken or eggs, or are pregnant or breastfeeding
Dimethyl Sulfoxide		OA and RA	Interactions with many medications; check with your doctor or pharmacist before using
Gamma-Linolenic Acid		OA	Avoid with blood thinners, seizure medications
Glucosamine Sulfate	OA		Avoid with blood thinners, chemotherapy, fish allergy
Krill Oil		OA and RA; studies are promising but not enough have been done to make a recommendation	Caution with blood thinners, orlistat, and medications that lower blood pressure
Lactobacillus		RA	Avoid with antibiotics, immune system suppressants
Omega-3 Fatty Acids	OA and RA		Avoid with blood thinners, blood pressure–lowering medication, orlistat
SAMe	OA		Avoid with antidepressants, MAOIs, dextromethorphan, Levodopa, meperidine, pentazocine, tramadol
Superoxide Dismutase	OA and RA		None known
Vitamin D	Preventing osteoporosis		Can interact with some medications; consult with your pharmacist, doctor, or dietitian before taking

continued...

* This is intended as a quick reference guide. For more complete information, consult with your health-care provider. Always tell your doctor or pharmacist about all the medications and supplements you are taking.

Supplement	May Be Effective For	Not Proven Effective For	Safety Concerns
Herbal Supplements			
Boswellia	OA	RA	Interacts with medications that are broken down in the liver; may stimulate the immune system
Cat's Claw	OA and RA		May interact with immuno-suppressant medications and other medications; consult with your pharmacist
Devil's Claw	OA	RA	Interacts with many medications; check with a pharmacist before using
Ginger	OA	RA; studies are promising but not enough have been done to make a recommendation	May interact with blood thinners, other medications, insulin levels; check with your pharmacist before using
Thunder God Vine	RA		May interact with immunosuppressant drugs; avoid if you have osteoporosis
Turmeric	OA and RA		Can interact with many medications; check with your pharmacist before using; take with food to increase absorption
Willow Bark		OA; studies are promising but not enough have been done to make a recommendation	May interact with blood thinners and Aspirin; avoid if you are allergic to salicylic acid, have kidney disease, or are pregnant or breastfeeding

CHAPTER 11

Dietary Therapy

....

CASE HISTORY
Food Journals

Rose decided that she wanted to start anti-inflammatory eating, but she also had a weight problem and felt that making wholesale changes would be too much like following a diet. She did not want to follow a cyclical pattern of being on and off her diet. She wanted to make permanent changes.

After looking at the anti-inflammatory diet guide and comparing it to her food journal, she realized that she was eating way too many animal products and not enough fish or legumes. She was also only eating 2 portions of vegetables daily. So her goals for the first month of her plan were to eat fish once weekly, eat legumes once weekly, and eat 3 portions of vegetables daily. She worked on these habits for a month and found it easy to comply.

Rose then added three new habits to practice for the next month. She decided to add a second meal based on legumes per week, add another portion of fish, and try a new type of grains each week.

Like Rose, Maria kept a food journal for a period of 2 weeks. She looked at the journal with her dietitian and neither of them could see any patterns that could lead them to conclude that a particular food was causing her arthritis symptoms to be increased. Her dietitian noticed that Maria did not include a lot of details about how the food was prepared, if spices or thickening agents were added, or what cooking method was used. Maria kept a more detailed journal for the next 2 weeks. She was able to find a pattern that showed that when she consumed too many foods that were cooked at a high temperature or grilled (especially foods with animal protein), her symptoms were worse.

Does what you eat affect the symptoms of your arthritis? Can you manage these symptoms by eating the right foods? For years, patients have been telling their doctors that when they ate or drank certain foods (such as soft drinks and cakes), their pain increased, and when they ate other foods (such as beans and fish), they felt less pain. Until recently, physicians dismissed any connection between what you eat and how you feel, but more and more doctors are now taking diet into account when managing arthritis. For many people, dietary therapy has become a mainstream addition to a comprehensive treatment plan.

Pro-Inflammatory and Anti-Inflammatory Diets

Pro-inflammatory foods cause inflammation that may worsen the symptoms of arthritis, while consuming foods that are anti-inflammatory may reduce the severity of the symptoms.

A growing body of evidence indicates that eating whole foods and following a balanced eating plan can cause changes in blood markers for inflammation. And if inflammation is reduced, someone suffering from either OA or RA could experience less pain, swelling, and stiffness. These studies have begun to identify pro-inflammatory and anti-inflammatory foods. Pro-inflammatory foods cause inflammation that may worsen the symptoms of arthritis, while consuming foods that are anti-inflammatory may reduce the severity of the symptoms.

Did You Know?

Arthritis Progression

It is not yet known whether an anti-inflammatory diet slows down the progression of RA. It is also not known if consuming a diet that is rich in the nutrients that make up cartilage and the other components of the synovial fluid will slow down the progression of OA. But consuming a diet that helps to reduce inflammation and happens to be rich in nutrients can help to promote healthy joints and better overall health.

Food Groups

Dietitians usually divide food items into several groups:

1. Vegetables and fruits
2. Grain and grain products
3. Meat products and alternatives
4. Dairy products and alternatives
5. Dietary fats
6. Beverages
7. Sweets and sweeteners

Pro-Inflammatory Diets
The Western Diet

Scientists have been able to link high levels of C-reactive protein (CRP), a marker for inflammation, to a particular pattern of eating, one that has been dubbed the "Western" diet. The Western diet is thought to be a perfect recipe for inflammation, and it may instigate or exacerbate arthritis. This pro-inflammatory diet needs to be replaced with anti-inflammatory foods to help manage arthritis. Many of the foods, herbs, and spices that are associated with reducing inflammation are not present in the Western diet. Phytochemical, antioxidant, and fiber levels are inadequate to prevent arthritis.

Vegetables and fruits: Very few phytochemical-rich vegetables and fruits are found in the Western diet. Nutrient deficiencies and a lack of phytochemicals and fiber may lead to inflammation.

Grains and grain products: Breads, rice, pasta, and cereals are made predominantly from processed or refined white flours, not whole grains. These foods are high in refined sugars, such as sucrose (table sugar) and corn syrup, used in cakes, cookies, and candies. Some studies link refined grains and sugars to higher levels of inflammation.

Meat products and alternatives: The Western diet includes high levels of saturated fats derived from meat products. Saturated fats not only seem to be a factor in causing heart disease, they can also raise C-reactive protein (CRP) inflammation levels.

Dairy products and alternatives: Dairy products add to the amount of saturated fats in the Western diet and may contribute to raising CRP levels.

Dietary fats: The Western diet is high in omega-6 and low in omega-3 fatty acids. The ideal ratio of omega-6 to omega-3 EFAs in the diet is thought to be between 1:1 and 4:1, whereas the Western diet ratio is between 10:1 and 30:1. Omega-6 EFAs are believed to be pro-inflammatory. The Western diet is also high in trans fatty acids and saturated fat, most of which are pro-inflammatory.

Did You Know?

Low-Fiber Diet
The Western diet includes very little fiber, which is needed to support digestion. A lack of fiber is associated with higher levels of CRP.

The Western diet is generally high in omega-6 and low in omega-3 fatty acids.

Beverages: Fruit drinks and soda pop are the staple beverages of the Western diet. They are high in inflammation-causing refined sugars and contribute to weight gain and obesity, factors that exacerbate joint damage in osteoarthritis.

Sweeteners: The latest statistics show that the average North American consumes between 22 and 26 teaspoons (110 to 130 mL) of added sugar daily, almost triple the recommended limit of 8 teaspoons (40 mL) daily. Many of the foods that are high in sugars are also high in saturated and trans fats, which promote inflammation.

Nightshades

Although the Western diet as a whole has been shown to be pro-inflammatory, specific foods may be especially problematic for people with arthritis. Among these foods is a family of vegetables known as nightshades. Some patients have reported that when they removed nightshade foods from their diets, their arthritis symptoms improved. Others suggest that nightshade vegetables trigger their symptoms.

Although some doctors have confirmed individual cases where arthritis symptoms improved after removing nightshade vegetables from the diet, no clinical studies supporting this theory have been done to date. You may want to try eliminating these foods from your diet, but remember that some of them also contain important nutrients that are believed to fight inflammation. It is possible that some people are more sensitive to these foods than others, just as some people are allergic to peanuts but the vast majority of the population is not.

Did You Know?

A Potential Treatment

New research has isolated a chemical in the nightshade family of foods that holds promise as a treatment for arthritis.

Did You Know?

Cooking Away Potential Inflammation

Cooking foods that are members of the nightshade family can remove up to 50% of the potentially inflammation-causing alkaloid chemicals.

Nightshade Family of Vegetables and Fruits

- Potatoes
- Eggplants
- Tomatoes
- Tomatillos
- Tamarillos
- Cherries
- Huckleberries
- Pimentos
- Peppers (sweet and hot)
- Hot pepper sauce
- Paprika (spice from pepper)

Gluten-Free Diets

Some people with RA or OA believe that removing gluten from the diet will greatly improve their arthritis symptoms. There is, in fact, some truth to this premise. Celiac disease, or gluten intolerance, is an autoimmune disease that occurs in roughly 1% of the general population. However, in people with an autoimmune disease like rheumatoid arthritis, the risk is higher: as much as 15% of the population with arthritis also has celiac disease.

Celiac disease can be diagnosed by a blood test to determine the level of IgA tissue transglutaminase (tTG) antibody, and is often confirmed by a biopsy of the lining of the intestine. For these tests to be valid, it is important to continue eating foods containing gluten for the 6 weeks leading up to the tests. Following a gluten-free diet and then being tested for celiac disease will give you a false negative result.

Another group of people have non-celiac gluten sensitivity. They may have some similar symptoms as people with celiac disease, but there will be no changes to the blood markers or the intestinal cells. This makes it very difficult to diagnose non-celiac gluten sensitivity. Two large studies, one in England and the other in Italy, found that between 1% and 13% of the population has symptoms of non-celiac gluten sensitivity.

To date, there are no studies to suggest that everyone with arthritis must eliminate gluten, but if you feel you might benefit from following a gluten-free diet, start by seeing your doctor, who can recommend appropriate blood tests. You should also discuss the diet with your dietitian. Many of the gluten-free foods available are high in fat, sugar, and calories and low in fiber and other important nutrients. A dietitian can guide you to choices that will ensure that you consume all the nutrients you need.

Vegan Diets

Another way to avoid pro-inflammatory foods is to eat a vegan diet that contains absolutely no animal products. Only foods of plant origin are consumed. In the case of arthritis patients, the assumption is that meat, dairy, and eggs can contribute to inflammation and other symptoms of arthritis.

Vegan Studies

Studies of patients changing to a vegan diet have shown that about 30% of these patients felt improvement in most arthritis symptoms, with the exception of morning stiffness. These studies evaluated blood levels of inflammatory markers, such as C-reactive protein (CRP), and natural antibodies against phosphorylcholine (anti-PC), RA factor, weight, and the level of cholesterol in the blood.

The vegan diet appeared to have an anti-inflammatory effect on the body. The best news for patients with arthritis is that inflammation markers decreased. Levels of fat in the blood, used to predict heart disease, also decreased, which is good news because many people with arthritis also have heart disease. In all these studies, the body mass index (BMI) of the participants on the vegan diets decreased, which could help alleviate the symptoms of osteoarthritis.

If you think you can stick to a vegan eating plan, give this diet a try. There may be some surprising benefits. A vegan diet is associated with many health benefits, such as a reduced risk of developing heart disease and some types of cancer, as well as losing weight or maintaining a healthy weight. Even if it does not cause a remission of the symptoms of arthritis, adopting a vegan eating plan can still be a healthy choice.

20 Most Common Pro-Inflammatory Foods

The following chart lists 20 foods that are pro-inflammatory and should be eliminated or substituted to manage your arthritis.

Food Group	Food Item	Why Inflammation Increases	Substitute
Vegetables and fruits	Watermelon	High glycemic index	Apples
	Potatoes	High glycemic index; possibility of sensitivity in some people	Sweet potatoes
Grains	White bread	High glycemic index; sensitivity to wheat proteins in some people	Whole-grain sourdough bread (no wheat)
	Bagels	High glycemic index; sensitivity to wheat proteins in some people	Whole-grain bagels (no wheat)
	Granola	High in sugar; sensitivity to wheat proteins in some people	Whole-grain cereal, oatmeal made with pure oats, or buckwheat porridge
Meats	Hot dogs	High in saturated fats	Tofu dogs
	Bacon	High in saturated fats	Canadian (back) bacon
	Barbecued ribs	High in saturated fats, sugar, and advanced glycation end products (AGEs)	Braised brisket or pulled pork
	Grilled steak	High in AGEs	Poached salmon
Dairy	Cheddar cheese	High in saturated fats; milk protein may cause sensitivity in some	Goat's milk cheese
	Creamy cheeses	High in saturated fats; milk protein may cause sensitivity in some	Creamy goat's milk cheese
	Milk	High in saturated fats; milk protein may cause sensitivity in some	Fortified almond beverage, fortified coconut milk
	Ice cream	High in saturated fats and sugar; milk protein may cause sensitivity in some	Sorbet with no sugar or sweetener added
Beverages	Soda	High in sugar; no nutritional value	Water
	Fruit juice	Concentrated source of sugars, calories	Water or unsweetened tea
Fats	Lard	High in saturated fats	Canola oil, olive oil

continued...

Food Group	Food Item	Why Inflammation Increases	Substitute
Sweets and sweeteners	Jam	High glycemic index; high in sugar	Stewed fruit purée
	Sugar	High in concentrated sugar	Honey
	Candy	High in sugar	Fruit
	Cake	High in sugar; high in saturated fats	Fruit-based desserts

Anti-Inflammatory Diets

Beyond changing your pro-inflammatory dietary habits and eliminating specific foods, you can build a complete diet program to help manage your arthritis. There is growing scientific evidence that an anti-inflammatory diet can lead to a reduction in the symptoms of arthritis and may lead to slowing the progress of the disease.

In cases of OA, this diet may help to alleviate symptoms by including foods that reduce inflammation. The anti-inflammatory diet can also help slow the progress of OA by affecting the aging process, keeping cartilage healthy, and reducing the effects of wear and tear on the joints. In this way, you may actually be able to modify the course of the disease.

In RA, the anti-inflammatory diet can also alleviate symptoms, though research has not yet proven that it can influence the progression of RA.

Food Guides

In recent years there has been a shift from more prescriptive food guides that suggest the number of portions to eat from each food group to an emphasis on basic principles of healthy eating. In the United States and Canada, nutrition experts suggest following a few basic principles. The USDA's MyPlate recommendations are available at www.choosemyplate.gov, and Canada's Food Guide is available at food-guide.canada.ca.

Looking closely at these recommendations, we see a trend toward choosing foods that are minimally processed and nutrient-rich. There is also now an emphasis not only on *what* we eat, but on *how* we prepare and eat food. We are encouraged to do our own cooking and to spend time eating with family and friends.

Scientists have realized that healthy eating is probably a lot simpler than they may have made it out to be up to now. By choosing whole foods — like vegetables, fruits, pulses, cheeses, yogurts and unprocessed whole grains — we consume more nutrients and less unhealthy fats and sugars.

We are also seeing more emphasis on taking steps to ensure that we *can* eat minimally processed foods. That means acquiring skills like grocery shopping and cooking. And it is also important to be mindful while eating the healthy meals you have prepared, focusing on the aromas, flavors and textures of the food and enjoying the company of the people eating with you. Taking the time to enjoy your meal reduces stress, which is linked to many health issues, including increased inflammation.

Many of the studies on managing arthritis through diet are based on the Mediterranean diet, which is essentially a slightly more structured version of the above recommendations. The basis of the Mediterranean diet is enjoying food, from meal planning through grocery shopping and cooking to connecting with friends and family at mealtime. The diet focuses on vegetables, fruits, and whole grains, as well as healthy fats, like nuts, seeds, olives and avocados. The main source of protein is pulses. Some animal foods are consumed, including fish and seafood, poultry, eggs, and dairy, particularly fermented dairy products such as cheese and yogurt. Consumption of red meat, processed meats and other processed foods, especially sugary desserts, is limited.

Following this type of eating pattern has been associated with a decreased risk of heart disease, type 2 diabetes, high blood pressure, and even obesity. So not only can it help you to manage the symptoms of arthritis, but it can help to prevent many of the diseases that are more likely when you have diabetes.

Did You Know?

Pulses

The term "pulses" is the group name used for the dried seeds of some members of the legume family, including dried peas, lentils, beans and chickpeas. These foods are great sources of protein and fiber, and excellent sources of folate, which is an important nutrient, especially if you take methotrexate. They also contain iron and potassium, nutrients that are sometimes lacking in our diets.

Weight Management

It is very important to manage your weight when you have either OA or RA. Studies have found that weight loss of as little as 10 pounds (5 kg) is associated with improvements in RA. The evidence also suggests that when patients with OA lose a similar amount of weight, the progression of damage to the joint slows down.

When you are trying to manage your weight, focus on realistic goals. There is no evidence that eliminating any one food group will lead to long-term weight loss or weight maintenance. Instead, it is more effective to work to gradually improve the overall quality and quantity of what you eat.

Success should be defined as achieving your "best weight" — your weight when you achieve the healthiest anti-inflammatory eating habits while having the best physical activity and lifestyle pattern you can maintain. Most specialists in weight management suggest that losing between 5% and 15% of your current body weight and maintaining that weight loss can contribute to reducing your risk for developing many medical issues, such as heart disease, and may reduce the risk of developing OA of the knee and hip. Newer studies suggest that losing that amount of

One of the best ways to alleviate joint pain is to maintain a healthy weight.

weight can also play a role in reducing arthritis pain. By working toward following the anti-inflammatory Mediterranean eating pattern and increasing your level of physical activity, you are well on your way to finding your best weight.

Before attempting weight loss, it is important to ensure that you do not have any health concerns that could be affecting your weight. A lack of sleep is associated with weight gain, as are medical conditions like sleep apnea and an underactive thyroid. Some medications are also associated with weight gain, so be sure to discuss any possible challenges with your doctor.

Once you decide to lose weight, there are many options. Take the time to discuss them with your doctor. People with a BMI over 35 who also have heart disease, type 2 diabetes, or other health problems, including arthritis, may be candidates for weight-loss surgery or weight-loss medications. If your BMI is over 40, you do not need to have any medical problems to be eligible for these options.

Weight-loss surgery and medication are tools that can help you to reach your goals, but they are only part of the solution. These tools work best when they are accompanied by consultations with a dietitian to help you learn new anti-inflammatory eating habits, a kinesiologist to help you to become more active, and a psychologist to help you stay motivated and learn new ways to manage stress.

A multidisciplinary approach provides the best chance for long-term success. Whether or not you have access to this ideal range of help, it's important that *you* realize that weight management involves a lifestyle that includes healthy eating, healthy activity and a positive mindset.

> **Weight management involves a lifestyle that includes healthy eating, healthy activity and a positive mindset.**

Fasting with OA or RA

Recent studies have focused on time-restricted eating, a fasting modified diet, and intermittent fasting. Time-restricted eating involves fasting for 12 to 16 hours per day, with food being consumed during an 8- to 12-hour period. The fasting modified diet protocol includes following a specific low-calorie diet for 5 days per month and an anti-inflammatory diet the rest of the time. With intermittent fasting, a calorie-restricted diet is consumed 2 days a week and a regular anti-inflammatory diet is eaten the other days.

Most of the studies have been done on animals, and the few that have been done with humans have been small. But the results are promising. Eating a reduced amount of calories seems to be linked to lower levels of pro-inflammatory cytokines and reduced CRP levels.

This type of protocol should not be attempted without consulting your doctor or a registered dietitian, as fasting can result in weight changes, a need to adjust medication doses, and malnutrition.

Anti-Inflammatory Foods

Let's focus on the food groups again, but this time isolate anti-inflammatory alternatives to pro-inflammatory foods.

Vegetables and Fruits

An anti-inflammatory diet features abundant fruits and vegetables that are high in inflammation-fighting phytochemicals and antioxidants. Vegetables and fruits are great sources of vitamin E and vitamin C, which are the antioxidant vitamins that work together synergistically to decrease inflammation. They also provide fiber, which helps to reduce inflammation.

Grains and Grain Products

Whole-grain wheat is a good source of betaine, which is transformed in the body into choline. Studies show that people with high levels of choline have lower levels of inflammation markers in their blood. Other whole grains, such as oats, rice, barley, and buckwheat, also contain various phytochemicals that may contribute to reducing inflammation and some much-needed fiber. Grain products with a low glycemic index will also help to reduce inflammation.

Meat and Alternatives

Red-meat consumption has frequently been linked to higher levels of inflammation. An anti-inflammatory diet limits or eliminates high-fat meats. This list includes ribs, sausages, cold cuts, bacon, and other processed meats. Many studies have linked the consumption of these foods to a higher incidence

Eating adequate fiber helps lower levels of inflammation. A recent study showed that eating between 25 and 29 grams of fiber daily was linked to lower levels of heart disease, stroke, type 2 diabetes, obesity and some types of cancer. Most North Americans are still not consuming nearly enough fiber. Adding a few servings of whole grains will go a long way toward helping you meet the goals for fiber.

Fish and chicken, along with other foods that are part of the meat and alternatives group, are great sources of mineral antioxidants.

of both cancer and heart disease. By increasing inflammation, they may also make arthritis symptoms worse.

Pulses (dried legumes) are great alternative sources of protein. Unlike the fiber found in wheat products, which is insoluble, the fiber in legumes is soluble, helping waste products pass through the intestine. Soluble fiber helps control both blood sugar and blood cholesterol levels. Foods that are high in soluble fiber also have a lower glycemic index. Consuming more foods with a low glycemic index has been linked to lower levels of C-reactive protein (CRP) and other markers of inflammation in the blood.

Dried beans and peas also contain some potent phytochemicals, mainly from the polyphenol family of chemicals. One of the functions of these phytochemicals may be to decrease the formation of AGEs (advanced glycation end products), which cause inflammation in the joints.

Fish and White Meat

In an anti-inflammatory eating plan, most of the protein comes from dried beans, dried peas, and lentils. However, consuming fish and seafood, especially fatty fish, will increase omega-3 fatty acids in the diet. Aside from adding healthy fats, these foods also contribute complete proteins and some valuable minerals, notably zinc.

Other fish, such as cod and sole, as well as most seafood, contain smaller amounts of omega-3 fatty acids; eating them still adds some omega-3 EFAs to the diet.

Anti-Inflammatory Fatty Fish

- Salmon
- Trout
- Mackerel
- Herring
- Sardines
- Arctic char
- Anchovies

Q. What are free radicals and antioxidants?

A. Let's start with a review of some basic molecular chemistry. Molecules are made up of particles called atoms. Atoms are made up of neutrons, protons, and electrons. The electrons are paired, with one holding a negative charge and the other a positive charge.

Most molecules are stable, but internal or external forces can break the bonds holding the electron pairs, releasing or freeing electrons. When one of these free electrons comes into contact with a stable atom, it will steal the electron it needs from the stable atom or deposit any extra electrons into the stable atom. This starts a domino effect of free radical reactions — unless the free radicals can be neutralized by restoring the electron pairs. This process happens about 10,000 times every day within the trillions of cells in your body.

These free radical electrons oxidize at a high rate as they seek more stable atoms. Oxidized free radicals are believed to cause tissue damage at the cellular level — harming our DNA, mitochondria, and cell membranes. This oxidative reaction is similar to the process of a banana rotting or metal rusting, from the inside out, and over time, this damage can accumulate, leading to diseases and premature aging. Smoking, drinking alcoholic beverages, undergoing X-rays, exposing our skin to excessive sunlight, and other external factors increase the number of free radicals in the body.

Antioxidants break this chain of free radical production by restoring the electron pairs before tissue can be damaged. Antioxidants have the ability to surrender electrons without adding to the chain reaction. Antioxidants spare oxygen, effectively reducing oxidative stress.

Antioxidants can be found in all cells. Some antioxidants are nutrients (vitamins and minerals) and some are enzymes. For example, vitamin E and coenzyme Q10 protect the cell membrane, and vitamin C and glutathione protect the nucleus from oxidative stress.

Antioxidants

Antioxidants are vitamins and minerals responsible for protecting the body from damage caused by free radicals. Free radicals are contributing factors in RA, OA, heart disease, and cancer.

Kinds of Antioxidants

Vitamins: vitamin C, vitamin E, and vitamin A (beta carotene)

Minerals: selenium, zinc, and manganese

Enzymes: coenzyme Q10

Vitamin Antioxidants

There are two categories of vitamins: those that need fat to be absorbed (fat-soluble vitamins) and those that need water to be absorbed (water-soluble vitamins).

Vitamin E

Vitamin E is a fat-soluble vitamin that protects the cell walls from being attacked by free radicals.

Best food sources of vitamin E: Dark green leafy vegetables, such as Swiss chard, mustard greens, spinach, collard greens, and kale; nuts and nut butters; and seeds, such as raw sunflower seeds. Olive oil and olives are also good sources of vitamin E. Other vegetables that have smaller but significant amounts of vitamin E include bell peppers, Brussels sprouts, ripe tomatoes, and steamed broccoli. Even fruits contain some vitamin E. Choose papaya, kiwi, and blueberries if you want to add some variety in the diet.

Remember that the vitamin E in food will react with oxygen in the air. Keep food in sealed containers to preserve the most vitamin E. This vitamin is fat-soluble, so it is better absorbed when it is eaten with a meal that contains some fat. Cooking does not reduce the amount of vitamin E in food.

Did You Know?

Reduced Inflammatory Markers

To date, no studies have indicated that consuming large amounts, or megadoses, of these vitamins will have a positive effect on our health. However, many studies suggest that consuming adequate amounts of antioxidant vitamins in our food is linked to better health in general and a reduction of inflammatory markers, including some of the markers for arthritis.

Vitamin A (Beta Carotene)

Vitamin A is a fat-soluble vitamin that "grabs" toxic forms of oxygen that can promote the formation of free radicals. It is also thought to have a stimulant effect on the immune system.

Beta carotene is transformed into vitamin A in the body. Beta carotene is found in brightly colored fruits and vegetables, especially bright yellow and orange foods, and in some dark leafy greens.

Best food sources of beta carotene: Cooked carrots, pumpkin, sweet potatoes, collard greens, spinach, kale, turnip greens, winter squash, and cantaloupe. Fresh parsley, basil, chives, and thyme contain beta carotene, as do chili powder, fresh and dried chiles, and hot pepper sauce.

Vitamin C

Vitamin C is a water-soluble vitamin that works inside the cell, keeping the free radicals under surveillance, ready to grab them as soon as they are freed. It also works in tandem with vitamin E, helping it to become reactivated.

This vitamin is easily destroyed during storage and cooking. To get the most vitamin C from the food you eat, choose raw vegetables and fruit. If you cut the raw fruits or vegetables, store them in an airtight container. If you choose to cook them, use the smallest amount of water possible because the vitamin C is lost in the water. Steam the produce or cook it for the shortest time possible in the microwave oven. If possible, cook the potatoes in their skin — this also makes potatoes a great source of fiber.

Best food sources of vitamin C: Vitamin C is found in fruits and vegetables, especially oranges, papaya, grapefruit, cantaloupe, strawberries, kiwi, and mango. Green peppers, broccoli, tomatoes, Brussels sprouts, cauliflower, cabbage, and potatoes are also great sources of vitamin C.

Did You Know?

Consume Grapefruit Cautiously

Grapefruit is a great source of vitamin C, but it also contains chemicals that could interfere with how some medications work. Always ask your pharmacist if you can continue to eat grapefruit with the medication you are taking. Medications that do not do not mix well with grapefruit and grapefruit juice include some cholesterol-lowering medications and some blood pressure medications.

Mineral Antioxidants

The three antioxidant minerals — zinc, manganese, and selenium — are called trace elements because they are needed in such small amounts. However, in a typical North American diet, you may find less than a trace amount.

Manganese, zinc, and selenium can be removed from food during processing by removing the hull of grains and, in the case of legumes, during the soaking and cooking process.

Zinc and Manganese

Zinc and manganese are trace elements that contribute to the formation of the antioxidant enzymes. The formation of the antioxidant enzymes that boost the immune system will be hindered by the lack of these minerals.

Best food sources of zinc: Zinc is found in animal products like beef, lamb, and chicken. It can also be found in legumes, nuts, and whole grains.

Best food sources of manganese: Manganese is found in pineapples, nuts (e.g., almonds and pecans), legumes, oatmeal, and green and black tea.

Selenium

The amount of selenium in our foods depends on the amount of selenium in the soil that the plants grew in and in the food that the animals eat. Selenium is a trace mineral that plays a role as an antioxidant in preventing cells from being damaged by free radicals. This may be particularly important in RA because the cells from the immune system can be damaged. Selenium may help prevent this damage. Other studies have shown that people with RA had low blood levels of selenium. People with OA appear to have low blood levels of selenium as well.

Best food sources of selenium: Selenium is found in most meats, poultry, fish and seafood. It is also found in most grains and cereals. As well, it can be found in plant sources like nuts, pinto beans, asparagus, spinach, and garlic.

> The amount of selenium in our foods depends on the amount of selenium in the soil that the plants grew in and in the food that the animals eat.

Enzymes

Coenzyme Q10

Coenzyme Q10, also known as ubiquinone and CoQ10, is made in the body and is found in every cell. It helps the cells to make energy. As an antioxidant, it helps protect the fats and proteins in the cell walls from becoming oxidized. It also stops LDL cholesterol from becoming oxidized. The oxidized form of these substances is damaging to the body. Coenzyme Q10 also works with vitamin C to help vitamin E become reactivated. Although coenzyme Q10 is made by the body, after the age of 20, the amount we can make starts to decrease, so obtaining CoQ10 from our food becomes more important as we age.

Coenzyme Q10, also known as ubiquinone and CoQ10, is made in the body and is found in every cell. It helps the cells to make energy.

Best food sources of coenzyme Q10: Coenzyme Q10 is found in meat, fish, poultry, canola oil, and nuts. It is found in lesser amounts in vegetables, fruits, eggs, and dairy products. Coenzyme Q10 is fat-soluble, so foods that are boiled will not lose their CoQ10. Frying seems to decrease the amount of CoQ10 in foods. At the current time, it is not known how much CoQ10 we need to get from the diet.

Q. **Will eating fatty fish increase the amount of mercury in my diet?**

A. Many studies have indicated that consuming some types of fish can add to the amount of mercury in the diet. Mercury is stored in the body, and when too much is accumulated, it can become toxic. Species higher on the food chain have more mercury in their bodies. Shark, swordfish, tilefish, and king mackerel are likely to contain the most mercury. To determine the safety of eating these fish, consult with your local board of health and department of natural resources and fisheries. Levels of mercury and other toxins in fish depend considerably on where they lived and were caught.

Dietary Fats

In North America, red meat, high in saturated fat, is a staple food. Free-range beef, pork, lamb, and poultry, however, may have lower levels of saturated fats than conventionally raised animals. Recently, it has been discovered that the fat content of the meat from these animals is a reflection of the food they eat. New studies from Australia show that some types of lamb are actually good sources of omega-3 fatty acids. Scientists are currently looking at both old and new ways of feeding animals to determine whether this would have a favorable effect on the amount of saturated fat in the human diet.

In many cultures, the amount of fat in the diet is quite high. The calories in the Mediterranean diet, for example, are concentrated in the fats, up to 50% of the total calorie intake. However, these fats tend to be healthy monounsaturated and polyunsaturated fats, found in olives and olive oil, avocado oil, avocados, pumpkin seeds, almonds and almond oil, pecans, and hazelnuts. Polyunsaturated fats include omega-3 and omega-6 EFAs. Add flax seeds and flax oil, chia seeds, walnuts and walnut oil, and canola oil to increase omega-3 levels in your diet — and help reduce inflammation in your body.

These foods provide not only beneficial oils but also key nutrients. Nuts, for example, provide magnesium and fiber that will also control inflammation. These foods also contain phytochemicals that may fight inflammation.

Bad Fats and Good Fats

There are three basic kinds of fat: saturated, unsaturated, and trans fats.

There are three basic kinds of fat: saturated, unsaturated, and trans fats. Fruits, vegetables, nuts, seeds, meat, eggs, and dairy typically contain a mix of the different kinds of saturated and unsaturated fats, while trans fats are mostly man-made and occur in processed foods, rarely found in nature. Olive oil, for example, contains about 75% monounsaturated fat, with about 25% polyunsaturated and saturated fat. Each type of fat has a different role in the body.

1. Saturated Fatty Acids

These fats can raise levels of low-density lipoprotein (LDL) cholesterol, which has been linked to an increased risk for heart disease and cancers of the breast, colon, prostate, and pancreas. High intake of saturated fat appears to increase symptoms of arthritis. Recent studies have linked saturated fats to increased levels of the inflammation markers in the blood.

> ## Kinds of Fats
>
> **1.** Saturated fatty acids
> **2.** Trans fatty acids
> **3.** Unsaturated fatty acids
>   Monounsaturated fatty acids
>   Polyunsaturated fatty acids
>   Omega-3 fatty acids
>   Omega-6 fatty acids

Sources: Butter, cream, full-fat cheese, whole milk, fatty meats, and chicken skin. These fats tend to be solid at room temperature and come from animals. A few plant foods, such as palm kernel oil and coconut oil, are also high in saturated fat.

2. Trans Fatty Acids

These fats occur in nature in small amounts, but the biggest source of these fats is added to our diets in manufactured "partially hydrogenated" vegetable oils, a process that makes them more stable and solid at room temperature. Trans fats are unhealthy and increase the risk of heart disease. They raise LDL ("bad") cholesterol and lower HDL ("good") cholesterol. They seem to promote inflammation.

Sources: Foods made with partially hydrogenated vegetable oil (some cookies, cakes, crackers, pie crusts, and other baked goods) and some margarine.

Did You Know?

Trans Fat Ban
As of 2018, the use of trans fats in processed foods has been banned in both the United States and Canada. New products cannot contain trans fats.

3. Unsaturated Fatty Acids

There are two kinds of unsaturated fats. Both have been credited with preventing disease.

Monounsaturated Fatty Acids

These fats do not raise LDL but they may raise HDL, the "good" cholesterol.

Sources: Olive oil and canola oil are good sources, as well as avocados, almonds, cashews, peanuts, and sesame seeds.

Polyunsaturated fatty acids

Polyunsaturated fats are commonly abbreviated as PUFAs. There are two kinds of PUFAs that should be consumed regularly in the diet: omega-3 essential fatty acids (EFAs) and omega-6 EFAs.

Omega-3 Fatty Acids

Omega-3 fatty acids are part of the membrane that surrounds the cells in the body and make up some of the chemicals that control inflammation. Omega-3 essential fatty acids (EFAs) include alpha-linolenic acid (ALA), eicosapentaenoic acid (EPA), and docosahexaenoic acid (DHA). These three EFAs are believed to be therapeutic in arthritis when consumed in the optimum proportion. Two of them, EPA and DHA, are found in animal sources, and ALA is found in plant sources. ALA cannot be used by the body directly, but the body can convert ALA to EPA and DHA. Omega-3 fatty acids slow down cell division, control blood clotting, and decrease inflammation.

ALA sources: Flax seeds or flaxseed oil, canola oil, walnuts, and chia. There are also many foods available that have been fortified with ALA. Adding flax seeds to the feed of chickens has resulted in eggs that contain more omega-3 fats and less of the harmful saturated fats. Adding ground flax seeds to breads, breakfast cereal, and pasta can increase the amount of omega-3 fats in the diet significantly. Other foods that have been fortified with omega-3 fats include margarine, milk, juice, yogurt and soy beverages.

EPA sources: Fatty fish and fish oils (herring, salmon, sardines, trout, and mackerel), plus their fish oils. Fish are high in EPA due to the algae they consume, and algae-based products are on the market as vegetarian sources of EPA. Infants thrive on EPA, and human breast milk also contains EPA.

DHA sources: Probably the best source of omega-3 fatty acids is fatty fish, including salmon, mackerel, sardines, herring, trout, anchovies, oysters, and Arctic char. Yogurt, orange juice, cheese, and milk may have fish oils added to them but do not have a fishy taste. For people who do not eat fish, these supplemented foods are important, but some are not appropriate for vegetarians or for people with a fish, seafood, or iodine allergy. Some of these products will contain DHA from algae. Although this may be appropriate for both vegetarians and those with a fish and seafood allergy, they will not be useful for people who are allergic to iodine.

> Omega-3 fatty acids slow down cell division, control blood clotting, and decrease inflammation.

Omega-6 Fatty Acids

The most common omega-6 fat in our diet is linoleic acid, which has been shown to help prevent heart disease. However, other omega-6 fatty acids have been found to be precursors to inflammatory compounds in the body. Omega-3 fatty acids are known to help balance the inflammatory effects of omega-6 fatty acids. When omega-3 fatty acids are deficient, the beneficial effects of omega-6 oils may be diminished. Because corn, soy, sunflower, and cottonseed oils are widely used in the production of commercial and processed foods, many people consume excessive amounts of omega-6 and insufficient amounts of omega-3 oils.

Omega-6 sources: Corn, sesame, sunflower, soy, and cottonseed oil. Omega-6 fatty acids are commercially available as evening primrose, borage, and currant oil. These oils can be used to prepare salad dressings, and in some cases of deficiency, omega-6 oils are prescribed as nutritional supplements. Omega-6 fatty acids are not heat stable and should not be used to fry foods.

Herbs and Spices

Though researchers have not identified the exact mechanism of action, there is a growing body of evidence showing that herbs and spices can add a significant amount of powerful anti-inflammatory phytochemicals to our diets. They should be used regularly. Herbs and spices contain different active ingredients, making it important to consume different varieties to get the most benefit. Most herbs retain their phytochemical content if they are dried, so use dried herbs if you do not have access to fresh plants.

Anti-Inflammatory Herbs and Spices

- Curry
- Ginger
- Turmeric
- Rosemary
- Savory
- Garlic
- Oregano
- Cinnamon
- Allspice

Phytochemicals

Phytochemicals are chemical compounds occurring naturally in plants. They are part of the system plants have devised to defend themselves against harm. In human nutrition, the word "phytochemical" means a plant chemical that can influence health. Scientists believe that phytochemicals may play a role in arthritis development and management as anti-inflammatory agents.

Phytochemical Families

- Polyphenols
- Terpenes
- Sulfides
- Saponins

- Betalains
- Organosulfides
- Indoles
- Anthocyanins

Phytochemical Actions

Initially, it was thought that all phytochemicals acted as antioxidants, but research is suggesting that some phytochemicals behave in ways that can directly interfere with the development of disease in the body. A number of phytochemicals have been investigated for their role in reducing inflammation and slowing the degenerative processes that result in the development of heart disease, diabetes, and cancer. New research shows that phytochemicals may also play a role in the development of the various forms of arthritis. Scientists have started to look to these nutrients for clues about how the cycle of inflammation gets turned on. At this time, most of the studies have been done in animals; more studies in humans are needed.

Scientists are now studying phytochemicals known to help protect the body from developing arthritis, cancer, heart disease, eye disease, and even aging, to help them develop a better understanding about their active ingredients and how these can then be best used to help reduce inflammation. One study looked at how the phytochemical resveratrol acted in rabbits that had arthritis. They were able to determine a specific pathway that would shut down inflammation and reduce the damage to the cartilage in the knee joint. Resveratrol is well known for its ability to reduce the oxidation of LDL ("bad") cholesterol and prevent heart disease. It is found in the pigment of red grapes, and it is believed to be one of the reasons that red wine is linked to better heart health.

The phytochemicals curcumin, ellagic acid, gallic acid, genistein, gingerol, and quercetin are being investigated to determine whether they play a role in the development or treatment of arthritis.

Sources of Phytochemicals

All plant foods contain phytochemicals that can help the body stay healthy. That is why it is so important to eat a variety of vegetables, fruits, nuts, and legumes every day. Below is a list of phytochemicals that seem to help reduce inflammation and joint symptoms in RA and OA.

Phytochemical	Food Source
Curcumin	Turmeric
Ellagic acid and gallic acid	Fruits, nuts
Genistein	Soybean and soy-based products, fava beans, chickpeas, other pulses and legumes
Gingerol	Ginger
Quercetin	Leafy vegetables, broccoli, red onions, peppers, tea, apples, grapes, berries

Beverages

Both tea and coffee contain some anti-inflammatory phytochemicals. They also contain caffeine, which can be difficult for some to tolerate, particularly for those who are taking NSAIDs. Try water-washed decaffeinated coffee and green and white tea. Limit your consumption of these beverages to three to four 8-oz (250 mL) cups daily.

Q. **Are alcoholic beverages okay to drink on an anti-inflammatory diet?**

A. Red wine and dark beers contain resveratrol, a phytochemical that is anti-inflammatory. Studies have linked the consumption of resveratrol to decreases in RA symptoms. Resveratrol is present in red grapes and red grape juice, as well as berries, peanuts, and turmeric. It has also been linked to lower LDL cholesterol levels. For women, one drink of red wine daily has been found to promote heart health, while men can consume up to two drinks daily. Consuming more alcoholic beverages than this has been linked to an increased risk of developing high blood pressure and an increased risk of developing certain types of cancers.

Sweeteners

Honey and maple syrup have been found to contain some phytochemicals. Using them to prepare desserts and to sweeten drinks may be preferable to using table sugar (sucrose). However, all sugars have a high glycemic index and raise blood sugar levels quickly, so use them with caution. Dark chocolate and cocoa powder are also sources of great taste and nutrients. Consuming small amounts of dark chocolate that contains at least 70% cocoa can have some health benefits. Adding plain cocoa to milk, soy beverage, or fruits can do much to fulfill our need for a treat and at the same time add some phytochemicals to the diet — and it tastes good!

20 Most Common Anti-Inflammatory Foods

This chart lists 20 foods that are anti-inflammatory and should be added to or adapted in your diet to help manage your arthritis.

Food Group	Food Item	Why Inflammation Decreases	Cooking or Eating
Meat and alternatives	Salmon	Omega-3 fatty acids	Poach, cook at low temperature
	Anchovies	Omega-3 fatty acids	Avoid cooking at high temperatures
	Walnuts	Omega-3 fatty acids, antioxidant minerals, vitamin E	Add to salads, use as nut butter spread, sprinkle on fruit
	Almonds	Antioxidant minerals, vitamin E	Choose natural, not blanched, to add fiber to the diet
	Beans and lentils	Fiber, phytochemicals	Soups, stews, salads; use the flour in baked goods
Milk and milk products	Yogurt and kefir	Probiotics	Add honey to yogurt for a great dessert
Vegetables	Garlic family	Phytochemicals: sulfides, thiols	Raw or cooked; let sit before cooking or adding acid to preserve phytochemicals
	Cabbage family (broccoli, cauliflower)	Phytochemical: isothiocyantantes	Raw or steamed
	Purple vegetables (cabbage and potatoes)	Phytochemicals: anthocyanins, polyphenols	Raw or steamed
Fruits	Apples	Phytochemical: quercitin	Raw or cooked
	Blueberries	Phytochemical: anthocyanins	Raw or cooked
	Purple/red grapes	Phytochemicals: proanthocyanidins, flavan-3-ols	Raw or cooked
Herbs and spices	Turmeric	Phytochemical: phenolic acid	Dry or fresh, raw or cooked
	Ginger	Phytochemical: flavonols	Dry or fresh, raw or cooked
	Cinnamon	Phytochemical: hydroxycinnamic acids	Dry or fresh, raw or cooked
Beverages	Green tea	Phytochemical: flavon-3-ols	Hot or iced
	Grape juice	Phytochemical: resveratrol	Small amounts
Fats and oils	Extra virgin olive oil	Phytochemical: tyrosol esters; omega-3 fatty acids	Do not overheat
	Olives	Phytochemical: tyrosol esters; omega-3 fatty acids, fiber	
	Avocado	Omega-3 fatty acids, fiber	Raw

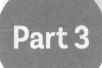

ARTHRITIS DIET PROGRAM

CHAPTER 12

Arthritis Diet Principles and Practices

··

CASE HISTORY
Surgery Postponed

When he was referred to our clinic, Ralph complained of pain due to OA in his knees. His OA was originally diagnosed using X-rays, and an MRI confirmed that there was no other cause for his knee pain. Ralph started out using a cream that contained NSAIDs to manage his pain. He also used some ice and heat, and used a brace when he went walking for long periods of time.

Ralph was now considering knee replacement surgery. At his visit with the surgeon, the nurse weighed him and measured his height. At five foot nine, he weighed 275 pounds, and his BMI was 40.6, which is classified as obese. After examining Ralph and looking at his X-rays, the surgeon suggested that losing about 10% to 15% (27.5 to 41.5 pounds) of his body weight would help him feel better.

He was referred to us as dietitians who specialize in weight management. Ralph decided to embark on a program to help manage his weight, integrate anti-inflammatory eating strategies into his diet, and strengthen his muscles to be ready for surgery.

Since he refused to eat fish, the doctor and dietitian both suggested that Ralph start taking fish oil supplements to ensure that he consumed enough omega-3 fatty acids. Our kinesiologist designed an exercise program for him that would strengthen his leg muscles and improve his cardiovascular fitness.

After he lost the first 15 pounds, Ralph noticed he was more mobile and in less pain. As he continued to gradually lose weight, he kept noticing improvements in his strength and mobility. When he reached his "best weight" of 235 pounds, even though he was still overweight he felt much better and was able to postpone his knee replacement surgery for a few years.

Anti-inflammatory diets adapt readily to the management of arthritis. Just such an eating plan is presented here for you to follow step by step. This plan assumes that most people with arthritis or people prone to arthritis are eating a Western diet to start. Here, you will find tips on changing your eating habits, shopping for anti-inflammatory foods, and creating monthly menu plans from more than 150 arthritis-friendly recipes.

But before you start cooking, you will need to prepare yourself for some significant changes in your eating habits.

Challenging Changes

It is empowering to understand that what you eat has an impact on your health. It can also be intimidating. For some people, following an anti-inflammatory diet will require wholesale changes to their lifestyle, and others may need only a few small adjustments to their current eating habits. Do I like making big changes or do I prefer to make small, gradual changes? Do I like structure or do I prefer to "do my own thing"? These are just a few of the questions you need to ask yourself.

> It is empowering to understand that what you eat has an impact on your health. It can also be intimidating.

Take Stock

Before making any changes to your diet, take a bit of time to reflect on what you would like to change, how quickly you would like to make the changes, and how changing your eating habits might affect other areas of your life. Always speak to your doctor and dietitian before making any wholesale changes in your diet. That way, any follow-up can be scheduled and medications can be adjusted if necessary.

Assess Your Situation

Are you ready for change? Assess your current eating habits so you can decide when and where to start your nutrition makeover. Ask yourself:

- Do I mind eating more vegetables and fruit?
- Can I give up eating white breads and desserts?
- Do I like lentils and beans?
- Can I give up eating red meat on a regular basis?
- Do I like to eat fish, especially fatty fish?
- Do I have the desire, energy, and stamina to shop for and cook with anti-inflammatory foods?

Keep a Food Journal

Keeping a food diary or journal of your current eating habits and arthritis symptoms will help you decide how you would like to proceed. Write down exactly what you eat, how much you eat, and how you feel both emotionally and physically before and after eating specific foods. Make sure you include as much detail as you can about what you are eating and feeling. Write down how many NSAIDs or other pain medications you are taking and how your food choices may be affecting them. Note how you prepared the food and how the way you prepared the food may have instigated arthritis symptoms.

Talk to Your Family

Food is a family affair. Any changes you might choose to make to your diet will ultimately have an effect on your family, your friends, and even your situation at work. You will need support from your family and friends if you would like to change the amount of cooking that you are doing. Changing what you are eating may involve taking more time to do grocery shopping, more time to prepare food, and more time to clean up. You may have to learn to pace yourself and ask your family and friends to help you complete some parts of the job.

Dietary Goals

Pick a maximum of three changes you would like to make and work on them for a month. It seems to take at least 30 tries for a behavior to become a habit. Avoid falling into the trap of choosing goals that are not specific enough, such as "I will eat a more balanced diet" or "I will do more exercise." These goals are difficult to evaluate, and it is easy to get discouraged.

Sample Monthly Dietary Goals

1. This month, I will consume oatmeal or whole-grain bread for breakfast on a daily basis.
2. This month, I will consume sweet potatoes or quinoa instead of white potatoes.
3. This month, I will start aquafit for arthritis two times weekly.

Did You Know?

Journaling

Psychologists tell us that keeping a journal is essential to making any changes that are to be long-lasting. Ideally, write in your journal on a daily basis, though some people find it useful to give themselves a day or two off every week. Once you have accumulated a week or two of journal entries, you will be ready to get started on changing your diet. Once you start making changes, keep track of the food you eat and the symptoms you feel so you can evaluate your progress.

HOW TO
Set Goals

Goals should be SMART:

S: Specific
M: Measurable
A: Attainable
R: Relevant
T: Trackable

10-Step Arthritis Diet Plan
Limit Red Meat

Step 1

Eating less animal food will help to reduce the amount of greenhouse gasses that are produced.

The World Cancer Research Fund recommends a maximum of 1 pound (500 g) of red meat per week. Be sure to choose lean meats and limit them to one-quarter of your plate. Lean meats contain not only protein but also iron, zinc, and B vitamins. Eating lean meat can give your diet a nutritional boost. However, limit or eliminate high-fat, smoked, or processed meats — cold cuts, sausages, and bacon, for example. Many studies have linked the consumption of these foods to a higher incidence of cancer and heart disease. By increasing inflammation, they may also make arthritis symptoms worse. Meat products are also among the foods that have the highest levels of AGEs, which lead to more inflammation.

Selection: Lean meats include round, chuck, sirloin, and tenderloin beef cuts, and the leanest cuts of lamb and pork are the tenderloin, the loin chop, and the leg. Extra-lean or lean ground meats are available. Wild game like bison and venison are also considered lean. Remove any extra fat before cooking.

Tips for Preparing and Serving Meat

- Do not cook meats at a high temperature without liquids (to prevent the formation of AGEs, which may increase inflammation). Cook meats at lower temperatures (medium-high and lower) to make stews, soups, braised dinners, or casseroles. Marinating meats in an acid (e.g., vinegar or lemon juice) also reduces AGEs.

- For an anti-inflammatory meal, fill only one-quarter of your plate with meat. Fill the rest with vegetables, fruits and whole grains.

- To keep portions small, prepare meat casseroles and stir-fries. Smaller portions of meat go further that way.

- Look for lean or extra-lean ground beef or ground sirloin to make spaghetti sauce, hamburgers, and casseroles.

Include Fish and Poultry

Step 2

Choose foods from this group 3 to 5 times a week. A recent study found that consuming fish at least twice a week reduced RA disease activity. Each additional portion of fish consumed during the week further reduced disease activity. Select fatty fish, such as salmon, trout, sardines, or mackerel, if available. Choose to eat poultry without the skin. To balance your plate, make sure that about one-quarter of it contains foods that are a good source of protein.

Preparation tips: Fish and poultry are great in soups and stews, baked or broiled. Prepare extra and freeze individual portions to make meal preparation easier when you do not feel like cooking.

Shopping tips: Choose fish that is fresh, frozen or canned.

Replace Red Meat with Beans and Other Legumes and Nuts

Step 3

Dried beans, peas, and lentils, also known as pulses, are good sources of fiber, protein, and phytochemicals. Although Canada is among the world leaders in the production of lentils and other pulses, these foods are rarely found in the typical Western diet, though they are typically consumed in the Mediterranean countries, in Europe, and in Asia. Nuts and nut butters are also an excellent source of protein and healthy fats and are packed with vitamins, minerals, and phytochemicals.

Eating a more plant-based diet has been associated with better health and longevity. Eating dried chickpeas, peas, beans and lentils more often is not only good for you, it is good for our planet. Eating less animal food will help to reduce the amount of greenhouse gasses that are produced.

Amino acid supplement: Meat, fish, chicken, and eggs contain all the amino acids that the body needs to build and repair muscles, cells, and other tissues. Unfortunately, with the exception of soy, legumes do not. For the body to be able to use the protein in legumes effectively, it has to be mixed with other foods that contain the missing amino acids. One way to do this is to consume grain products with the legumes. Another is to include a small amount of animal protein in the meal.

Q. Do pulses cause gas and flatulence?

A. Consuming pulses has been linked to increased flatulence and it is often cited as a reason why people do not like to eat dried beans and peas. But it is not necessary to have this problem. Try these tips to reduce gas and flatulence:

- Add small amounts of dried beans to your meals, then slowly increase the amount you are eating. Any big increase in fiber in your diet is likely to cause gas, bloating, and discomfort. Gradually increase your serving size until you can eat the desired amount without any difficulty.

- Soak dried beans and peas before cooking. Beans can cause gas because they contain some types of sugar that cannot be digested, but soaking them overnight can remove some of these sugars. Throw out the soaking water and cook the beans in fresh water. If soaking the beans intimidates you, start by using canned legumes but rinse them before using. This will remove some of the sodium (salt) and help reduce the amount of indigestible sugars in the pulses.

- If you still have a problem, you can try taking Beano, a natural enzyme supplement that will digest the sugars that your body can't.

Serving Tips

- Look for family favorite recipes for baked beans or chili.
- Join "Meatless Mondays" (www.meatlessmondays.com) or try the Half-Cup Habit (pulses.org/nap/half-cup-habit).
- Choose some great lentil or minestrone soup recipes for lunch.
- Purchase ready-made chilis or soups. These are great to add to a lunch box and are often low in fat and calories.
- Use recipes that contain meat as well as pulses.
- Add pulse flour to recipes for muffins and quick breads. This will add fiber and phytochemicals to a hearty snack or breakfast.
- Legumes are often quite bland. Pick recipes that add taste and spice.
- Certain legumes, like chickpeas and lentils, are easily mixed into a salad, but many meat-based dishes are tasty when legumes are substituted instead — try a bean burrito or vegetarian chili.

Increase Servings of Vegetables and Fruits

An anti-inflammatory diet is rich in vegetables and fruits. Although specific recommendations vary by country, most dietitians agree that to consume all the nutrients necessary for good health, longevity, and lower levels of inflammation, you should aim to fill half your plate with vegetables and fruits at each meal. Remember that all the vegetables and fruits do not have to be on the same plate. If you have a bowl of vegetable soup, some salad with your meal, and a fruit as part of your dessert, you have about the equivalent of half a plate of vegetables and fruits.

Preparation tips: To preserve the most nutrients, steam vegetables and fruits for a shorter time at moderate heat. If you do choose to boil them, use the leftover water to make gravy or add it to soups to make sure that you get the benefit of all the nutrients.

Serving tips: Make sure that your plate is very colorful. The more colors you include, the more nutrients you are likely to be consuming. Orange and dark green leafy vegetables are high in beta carotene, a potent phytochemical. These vegetables include broccoli, Swiss chard, beet greens, kale, collard greens, carrots, and squash. Dark blue and red fruits are rich in phytochemicals, so add in plums, red grapes and red grape juice, blueberries, and raspberries.

Storage tips: If fresh produce is not available, use frozen and, as a last resort, canned. Frozen produce is likely to have as many nutrients, including phytochemicals, as fresh. Ensure that vegetables and fruits are properly stored at the correct temperatures. Although some nutrients may be destroyed in the cooking process, others, such as lycopene, seem to be activated by heating.

Drink options: Juice can be a good option. Approximately 1/2 cup (125 mL) of juice contains the same number of nutrients as 1 serving of vegetables or fruits. It also comes packaged with about 1 tablespoon (15 mL) of natural sugar. The concentrated amount of sugar, combined with the fact that there is no fiber in juice, means that the GI of juice is high and your blood sugar levels will go up quickly. Keep juice portions small and add them to your diet only on an occasional basis.

> **Most dietitians agree that to consume all the nutrients necessary to manage inflammation, you need to eat at least half a plate of vegetables and fruits at each meal.**

Eat Whole Grains

The anti-inflammatory eating plan contains a significant amount of whole grains. There are an abundance of whole-grain products available at your supermarket. These products may be based on commonly used grains like wheat, rye, oats, and barley, but can also include Kamut, spelt, quinoa and even buckwheat. In an anti-inflammatory eating plan, pulses are included in this group to encourage you to eat them more often, either as a side dish or by using their flours as an ingredient in pastas or baked goods. Aim to balance your meal by making sure about one-quarter of your plate contains whole grains.

Aim to balance your meal by making sure about one-quarter of your plate contains whole grains.

Shopping tips: Look for whole grains or sprouted grains as the main ingredients. Read the labels on the grain packages and look for ground flax seeds, a great source of ALA, an omega-3 fatty acid. The omega-3 fatty acid in the flax seeds is not available to the body if the seeds are not ground. When purchasing breads and baked goods, look for the smallest amounts of added fats, oils, and sugars. Breakfast cereals should have as little added sugar as possible. Check the ingredient list, not just the Nutrition Facts tables. Some sugars are naturally occurring so will contribute to the amount of sugar that is shown on the Nutrition Facts panel. Fiber per portion of bread or breakfast cereal should be a minimum of 4 g.

Moderate Dairy Products and Eggs

This food group includes milk, cheese and yogurt (low-fat or regular) and eggs. These foods are important sources of protein and minerals like calcium and magnesium. Eggs are an inexpensive, nutrient-dense food that is heart-healthy. You can choose foods from this group on a daily basis.

Two large new studies suggest that the fat in dairy products is not associated with an increased risk of heart disease, especially in people over the age of 65. Fats found in fermented dairy products may actually decrease inflammation.

Shopping tips: If you are concerned about your weight, one way to reduce your caloric intake is to choose lower-fat milk, cheese and yogurt or kefir. Choose plain yogurt so that you can easily turn it into a savory dip or a sweet dessert.

Select Healthy Fats and Oils

Step 7

Omega-3 fatty acids and monounsaturated fats can help reduce inflammation. They are easy to use and bring great taste, not to mention a host of other nutrients, to your plate. For example, the skin of nuts contains magnesium and fiber. Try to eat these foods every day.

Serving tips: Always choose cold-pressed oils, and do not heat them to high temperatures because this will reduce their health benefits.

Tips for Adding Healthy Fats to Your Diet

- Use olive oil and canola oil in cooking. If you want a buttery taste, add a small amount of butter to the canola oil.
- Dip bread in olive oil instead of spreading butter on it.
- Use olive oil or another monounsaturated oil in salad dressings.
- Add ground flax seeds to recipes (cereals, muffins, and quick breads).
- Include slices of avocado in sandwiches or use it as a spread.

Add Herbs and Spices

Step 8

Herbs and spices can add a significant amount of powerful anti-inflammatory phytochemicals to your diet. Most herbs retain their phytochemicals if they are dried, so use dried herbs if you do not have access to fresh. You can keep a window box of fresh herbs in your home. They will add a wonderful fragrance to your living space. Store dried herbs and spices away from the heat. Garlic and other members of the garlic family (onions, leeks, shallots, and green onions) can impart benefits either raw or cooked, so enjoy them any way you like.

Herbs and spices can add a significant amount of powerful anti-inflammatory phytochemicals to your diet.

Serving tips: Look for recipes that call for herbs and spices. If you are not accustomed to using them, start by using smaller amounts in your recipes and gradually add more as you get acquainted with the taste. Dried herbs and spices need to be added at the beginning of the cooking process, and fresh or frozen herbs should be added at the end.

Storage: Buy small quantities of herbs and spices and replenish them on a regular basis. They need to be replaced when they no longer pass the sniff test. Open the jar and sniff. If the characteristic aroma is not there, it is likely that the nutrient value is also no longer present.

Step 9 — Drink Up

What we drink can also contribute to inflammation. The best drink is water, but an occasional glass of juice and some tea or coffee are also good. Both tea and coffee contain some anti-inflammatory phytochemicals. They also contain caffeine, which can be difficult for some people to tolerate, particularly if they are taking NSAIDs. Try water-washed decaffeinated coffee and black, green, or white tea. Limit your consumption of these beverages to three to four 8-ounce (250 mL) cups daily.

Both regular and diet soft drinks should be avoided. Neither contains any redeeming nutritional qualities, and the high sugar content of regular soft drinks is linked to increased inflammation. Diet soft drinks do not add any nutrition to the diet, and some studies have suggested that their consumption is linked to high blood pressure.

Although consuming some alcoholic beverages may promote heart health, you should consume them in moderation, which is 2 alcoholic beverages daily for men and 1 for women.

How much to drink: A total fluid intake of 6 cups (1.5 L) per day for women and 8 to 12 cups (2 to 3 L) per day for men. One alcoholic beverage is considered to be 12 ounces (341 mL) of regular beer, 18 ounces (511 mL) of light beer, 3 to 4 ounces (90 to 125 mL) of wine, or 1½ ounces (45 mL) of hard liquor.

Step 10 — Avoid Sweet Treats and Desserts

Sugar is now thought to be a cause of heart disease, obesity, and other noncommunicable diseases and may contribute to increased levels of inflammation. Most sweet treats and desserts add few if any nutrients to the diet. When we fill up on these treats, we do not have enough room for the foods we need to eat to ensure good health and lower levels of inflammation.

If you must serve sweets, take your inspiration from the Mediterranean diet, where prepared desserts are reserved for special occasions. For daily desserts, serve fruits and perhaps add a simple treat of yogurt sweetened with a bit of honey. Use small amounts of added sugar to make nutritious foods tastier; for example, add a bit of maple syrup to your breakfast oatmeal.

Beware of using artificial sweeteners. The evidence from scientific studies shows that foods made with artificial sweeteners are not associated with weight loss; in fact, participants either maintained their weight or gained weight when they ate these foods.

Q. **Does chocolate affect arthritis symptoms?**

A. Dark chocolate and cocoa powder are good sources of anti-inflammatory phytochemicals. Consuming small amounts of dark chocolate that contains at least 70% cocoa can have some health benefits. Adding plain cocoa to milk, soy beverage, or fruits can do much to fill our need for a treat while adding some phytochemicals to the diet.

Your Road Map to an Anti-Inflammatory Diet

Here is a quick guide to the changes you can make to your diet to help you to manage the pain and inflammation of arthritis. Before you make any changes, start by taking an objective look at your existing diet, your current lifestyle and how much you are willing to change. Remember, it is better to take small steps toward a big goal. If your goal is to eat more fish, you could start by having a tuna sandwich once a week and graduate to eating fish 4 times a week over a period of months or even years.

Here is a road map to the big goals you can keep in mind when you are setting smaller goals:

1. Limit consumption of red meat to about 1 pound (500 g) per week, spreading it across three meals. Red meat includes the meat from any animal that has four legs.

2. Include fish and poultry in your diet. Studies show eating fish and seafood at least twice a week reduces CRP levels. Try to eat fish, especially fatty fish, at least that often.

3. Replace red meat with pulses and nuts.

4. Fill half your plate with vegetables and fruits at each meal. Choose vegetables more often if you are concerned about how many calories you eat.

5. Eat more whole grains. Fill up one-quarter of your plate with whole grains at each meal.

6. Eat moderate amounts of eggs and dairy products, which add important nutrients to your diet.

Did You Know?

The Vital Role of Pulses

The legume family of plant foods includes soybeans, fresh peas, fresh beans, and peanuts, as well as pulses. Pulses include dried beans, peas, lentils and chickpeas. The Food and Agriculture Organization of the United Nations designated 2016 as "The Year of the Pulse" to highlight the vital role pulses play in our diet.

7. Select healthy fats and oils, including olive oil, flax seeds, avocados, and nuts.

8. Add herbs and spices to your meals for great flavor and extra phytochemicals.

9. Drink lots of water and avoid sugar-sweetened beverages.

10. Limit your consumption of sweet treats and desserts. This is one place where less is best. Consuming these foods often is linked to an increase in the development of obesity, heart disease, and type 2 diabetes, and may be linked to increased levels of inflammation.

Portion Size

The best way to make sure your portion is not super-sized is to use your fist as a guideline. Each member of your family can "right-size" their portion by using their own fist to evaluate their foods. Here is a handy guide to appropriate portion sizes:

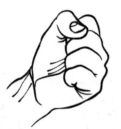

GRAINS/STARCHES/FRUITS
Choose an amount the size of your fist for grains, starches or fruit.

MILK/DAIRY ALTERNATIVES
Drink up to 1 cup (250 mL) of low-fat milk with a meal.

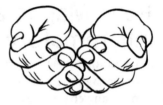

VEGETABLES
Portion as much as you can hold in both hands. Choose brightly colored vegetables.

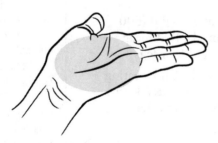

MEAT/PROTEINS
Choose an amount the size of the palm of your hand and the thickness of your little finger.

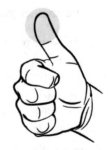

FATS
Limit fat to an amount the size of the tip of your thumb.

Based on "Handy Portion Guide" (www.guidelines.diabetes.ca/docs/patient-resources/handy-portion-guide.pdf), from *Beyond the Basics: Meal Planning for Healthy Eating, Diabetes Prevention and Management* © Canadian Diabetes Association, 2014.

CHAPTER 13

Arthritis Diet Cooking Tips

A**rthritis can make** it difficult to enjoy your time in the kitchen, causing physical challenges in the preparation of food. For people with arthritis, grocery shopping and simple kitchen tasks, such as mixing, chopping, and handling heavy pans, can be challenging. To help regain your independence in the kitchen, try following these helpful tips.

Grocery Shopping

1. Prepare a strategic grocery list.
Shop in a store where you are familiar with the layout. Prepare your grocery list so that items where you will begin your shopping are at the top of your list. This will decrease both the time and the energy you spend grocery shopping.

2. Wear comfortable shoes
Before going to the grocery store, make sure you are wearing cushioned, slip-proof shoes. This will make your trip less painful and more enjoyable.

3. Ask for help
If you find grocery shopping too tiring, ask someone to come with you. They can reach for items or save you some steps by walking ahead of you to find foods a couple of aisles away. Have your groceries delivered if they are too heavy to carry home. You can even order your groceries online for same-day or next-day delivery. This saves you time and conserves your energy for cooking or having fun.

> **Ordering your groceries online saves you time and conserves your energy for cooking or having fun.**

4. Use a reacher/grabber
Reachers/grabbers are helpful tools that extend your reach. They can be purchased from medical supply stores and some chain stores. They are useful when human help is not close by. Not only can they help in reaching for items at the grocery store, they can also be helpful at home for reaching items on higher shelves.

5. Buy trimmed and precut foods

Grocery stores now sell salads, fruits, and vegetables that have already been washed and cut for you. Raw meats can often be bought in thin slices. Although they are priced a bit higher, the convenience may be worth the cost.

6. Use a grocery cart

Make it easier on yourself. Even if you are planning to buy only a few items, a grocery cart can help provide stability while walking.

7. Use cloth bags

Plastic bags may be painful if your hands are sensitive, and paper bags may be too difficult to carry. Invest in good-quality, environmentally friendly grocery bags that have sturdy long handles and can be hung on a wheelchair or walker. If you have wrist issues, you can carry them in the middle of your arm where your bone is the strongest.

8. Take a break

After returning home, it might be a good idea to take a break. Put your perishables away first, then take a break before tackling the remaining items.

Kitchen Design

Try these tips to make your kitchen more user-friendly.

1. Make your doors easier to open

For appliances in the kitchen that have doors, such as the refrigerator, microwave, and oven, try attaching a ribbon or scarf to the handle in a loop. If you find it too difficult to open the door with your hands, hook your arm through the ribbon or scarf and use the weight of your entire body to open the door.

2. Organize shelving for convenience

Because we store most of our food products, dishware, and cooking utensils on shelves, it is a good idea to make your kitchen shelves easily accessible. If you are planning to remodel part of your kitchen, a helpful design is to use pullout shelves. This will allow you to easily access kitchen items stored at the back of shelves.

Ensure that your shelves are set up conveniently and strategically. The most commonly used items should be displayed at the front of shelves or near you, and infrequently used items should be stored at the back or higher on the shelves.

It is a good idea to keep pots, pans, plates, and glasses at a level where they are easy to reach.

3. Downsize
Too much clutter in your cupboards can be a safety risk if you are constantly sorting through them and moving heavy items. Move items you don't use often, such as dishware that only comes out on special occasions, to a separate area. This will provide you with much-needed room in preparing your meals.

4. Keep a kitchen stool or chair nearby
Depending on how complicated a recipe is, cooking can be a long process. Whenever possible, try sitting when preparing food, to help relieve the pain in your legs, especially when a lot of preparation work is required. If you need to be standing while cooking, take breaks and sit to rest your legs or back every so often. An adjustable-height office chair with wheels might be useful for moving from one part of the kitchen to the other. Raising and lowering the height can also be useful in different parts of the kitchen.

Whenever possible, try sitting when preparing food, to help relieve the pain in your legs or back, especially when a lot of preparation work is required.

5. Soak your hands
Fill the sink with warm soapy water while cooking. When your hands begin to hurt, soak your hands for a few minutes before finishing the task you are working on.

Wheelchair Access

1. Remove cabinets from under the counters
Standard counters can be difficult for you to use because the cabinets below are often in the way. Removing the base cabinets is a good idea to provide access to the sink and work area.

2. Countertops
Countertops should be as continuous as possible to make it easier to slide items between workstations.

3. Refrigerators and freezers
A side-by-side refrigerator/freezer, rather than a unit with a top or bottom freezer, can allow you easy access to all parts of the fridge.

4. Sinks
If you suffer back strain when you lean to reach items at the bottom of the sink, install a wooden, wire, or plastic rack. And leave the area below the sink empty. Many kitchens are designed with garbage disposal under the sink, but it may be useful to relocate your garbage to a separate area.

5. Ovens

A standard stove with an oven below the burners may create problems for you because you need to reach a long distance to pull out the contents. Switching to a countertop convection or microwave oven may be a good idea because these appliances have side-opening doors. A toaster oven is another alternative for heating smaller items.

6. Stove operating controls

These controls should be placed either at the front or on the side. It might be dangerous for you to reach for rear controls, which are located behind burners.

7. Storage

Kitchen storage can often be a problem, especially if your base cabinets have been removed. One recommendation is to use a rolling storage cart to transport utensils and equipment from one part of the kitchen to another. Using hooks for pots and pans, hangers for glassware, and lazy Susans in corner areas can help maximize your storage space.

8. Use a lapboard

A lapboard attached to your wheelchair or placed on your knees is an easy way to transfer items throughout the kitchen.

Cooking Tools

Acquire some arthritis-friendly tools to use around the kitchen.

1. Grabbers/reachers

For those with difficulties in reaching products in your cupboards or pantry, a grabber or reacher can help by allowing you to extend your reach.

2. Scissors

Rather than trying to rip packages open with your hands, keep scissors handy in an easily accessible drawer or on a hook in the kitchen.

3. Rubber mats

Rubber mats can be used to stand on when preparing foods or cooking. The padding can help relieve back and leg pain from standing on hard floors.

4. Food processors

If you are having trouble with manual cooking tasks such as chopping, cutting, and slicing, a food processor may be what you need in the kitchen. A food processor will automatically chop, shred, or slice the foods you load in. If you are considering purchasing one, make sure you choose one that has an easily removable blade, bowl, and lid. If you are on a budget, mini food processors are also available.

5. Appliances

Instead of tucking your pieces of equipment in the cupboard, display them on the counter with all the attachments. This will remind you to use the equipment instead of spending your energy chopping away.

> Instead of tucking your pieces of equipment in the cupboard, display them on the counter with all the attachments.

6. Slow cookers and pressure cookers

Slow cookers and pressure cookers can help people with arthritis cook nutritious meals, such as soups, stews, and roasts, with very little work. Most recipes for these machines are relatively simple and do not require many ingredients or much preparation, making your life that much easier. Save on cleanup time by choosing a cooker that can also brown the food before cooking.

7. Specialty knives

Cutting can put extra strain on the joints. Consider purchasing an ergonomically designed knife with a large handle. This will let you use your body weight to maneuver the knife while maintaining leverage and stability. Another alternative is a mezzaluna, or rocker knife, a two-handed tool that can add strength and control to your food preparation. You may also want to consider an electric knife, which is usually lightweight, powerful, and safe. Make sure you regularly sharpen your knives to make it easier to cut foods.

8. Pots and pans

Pots and pans are often heavy and can be difficult to manage for people with arthritis, especially if the pots have only one handle. Using a pot or pan with two handles can help distribute the weight more evenly between your hands and wrists and decrease your risk of injuring yourself in the kitchen. Store your pots and pans on hooks on the wall or use a pot hanger suspended from the ceiling so the pots are at chest level. You won't need to bend for your pots and pans anymore.

> Using a pot or pan with two handles can help distribute the weight more evenly between your hands and wrists and decrease your risk of injuring yourself in the kitchen.

9. Jar opener

For those who have difficulty opening jars, an electric jar opener is a godsend. No hand strength or strenuous twisting is required.

10. Specialty peelers

Instead of using a peeler to discard the flesh of certain fruits and vegetables, invest in a fruit and vegetable peeler that not only peels but also cores and slices with the turn of a knob.

11. Lightweight cooking tools

Use ergonomic, lightweight cooking tools, including spatulas, spoons, ladles, and whisks, that have easy grips and non-slip handles. Many types are available. Choose one that feels comfortable in your hand, improves manual dexterity, and reduces pain in the joints.

12. Specialty cooking appliances

From air fryers to spiralizers, there are now specialized kitchen appliances to do just about anything. Before you invest money in these tools, take the time to evaluate just how often you will use them. Ask yourself how each tool will help you. For example, some air fryers come with a paddle that stirs the food, making them a more versatile option as they can be used for stir-fries and risottos in addition to preparing low-fat versions of foods that would traditionally be deep-fried.

Table Tools

Try these helpful tools at the table.

1. A rubber mat

Setting up your plate on a rubber mat will decrease the chance of its slipping. Dycem, a non-slip plastic material, can also be used to stabilize your dishware.

2. A rubber drink holder

To reduce joint stress and prevent your glass from slipping, place a rubber drink holder around your glass. Not only will this make it easier to hold on to, but it will decrease the pressure along the thumb side of the hand, a pressure that may contribute to deformity.

To reduce joint stress and prevent your glass from slipping, place a rubber drink holder around your glass.

3. A straw

If it is too painful to lift a glass to your mouth, use a straw instead.

4. A scooper plate

If you have trouble scooping food from your plate, a plate with a contoured rim allows food to be trapped and pushed easily onto utensils. There are also versions that have a non-skid base to prevent the plate from sliding.

5. Utensils with grips

Arthritis can sometimes cause individuals to have a weak grasp. Spoons, forks, and knives with grips allow utensils to stay in your hands while you're eating. Look for utensils that also have safety caps, which can protect the fingers while cutting.

6. A spreadboard

A spreadboard can be useful if you have difficulties spreading condiments on your bread. It holds your bread in place.

Food Storage

Use these methods to store your foods properly.

1. Food storage containers

Make sure you have food storage containers that are easy for you to open and stack. This can be especially useful for products that come in heavy bags, such as flour, rice, and oats. There is a wide selection of plastic storage containers with easy-to-open lids, so choose one that is most convenient for you. Store foods you eat regularly in ready-to-eat condition. For example, if you like to nibble on carrots throughout the day, it is a good idea to clean, peel, and cut them in batches ahead of time so they are readily available through the week.

> **Make sure you have food storage containers that are easy for you to open and stack.**

2. Herbs and spices

Instead of storing herbs and spices on a shelf, try storing them in a spice rack on the counter or in a kitchen drawer that is at waist level. You may also want to consider placing your herbs and spices on a lazy Susan in a cupboard, which makes them easily accessible.

3. Bagged items

When small food bags have been opened, use clips instead of elastics or twist ties to reseal the bag.

Dish-Washing Strategies

1. Soak your dishes

For pots, pans, and dishware that have difficult-to-remove stains, soak them in warm soapy water. Then scrub them gradually so the food is easier to remove.

2. Keep your cleaning supplies for the kitchen in the kitchen

Store your cleaning detergents and soaps in a nearby cupboard. This will reduce unnecessary trips to and from other rooms to gather supplies.

3. Use the dishwasher

If you have a dishwasher, use it to wash and dry dishes. Check to see whether your pots, pans, storage containers, and serving dishes and utensils can be washed in the dishwasher.

4. Let your dishes air-dry

For those who do not have a dishwasher, try the following tip. Instead of drying your dishes with a cloth following a wash, try letting your dishes air-dry before putting them away. Not only will this save you energy, but it will reduce the pressure on your back and legs from standing and take the strain off your upper body joints from drying dishes and putting them away.

Q. I don't like grocery shopping, and I don't like cooking. What should I do?

A. Meeting your nutrition needs can be a challenge if you don't like meal planning, grocery shopping, and cooking. For the person who likes to cook and cannot, or who isn't proficient and doesn't want to start cooking, it is easy to give in to the temptation to order food from the nearest restaurant. But there are ways to get the nutrition you need while doing the least amount of cooking possible or, if you choose, no cooking at all. It just takes a bit of thinking outside the box. Here are some strategies.

1. **Purchase precut/trimmed foods**
   Grocery stores now offer many fresh foods that are already precut and ready to cook, including mixed greens and vegetables ready for dipping or cooking. Meat, fish, and poultry come ready to go into the pan. These can be marinated or already shaped into a meatloaf or hamburger patties. Take a look around your grocery store to see what is available.

2. **Use a meal delivery service**
   Most major cities have several companies that will deliver precooked meals. They may deliver freshly cooked meals on a daily basis or frozen meals on a weekly basis. If you are over 65, Meals on Wheels may be a good alternative for you.

   If you like to cook but do not want to spend time grocery shopping, you might want to try a service that delivers a meal kit containing everything you need to prepare a meal. Some of the food is chopped and sliced, making preparation even easier. Many people find that these kits simplify menu planning, grocery shopping and preparation while making it easy to try new foods. Some grocery stores also sell meal kits.

3. **Get to know a local restaurant**
   Going to the same restaurant all the time can actually be a good idea. Sometimes the owners get to know you, and if you ask, they might be willing to prepare meals to meet your special requirements.

4. **Batch cook**
   Some people prepare all their meals for the week on the weekend, then freeze all the portions for the week. The cooking is limited to a once-a-week occurrence. The rest of the time, just reheat and eat!

continued...

5. Hire a personal chef

Many of us have no qualms about hiring someone to clean our house for us, but the suggestion that someone be hired to do the cooking often causes quite a stir. A personal chef usually offers to either come into your home to do the cooking or prepare a week of meals for you and bring them to your home (in which case these meals might be frozen). Some personal chefs will work from their own menus, and others will be happy to choose recipes and menus tailored to your needs. Some people hire a housekeeper, who will prepare food to your specifications and do the grocery shopping, as well as some other tasks around the house.

6. Join a dinner club

This is a great option for couples and singles. Some groups meet three to four times weekly. Each day, one of the members is responsible for preparing a meal for the other members. It is often easier to prepare a meal for a crowd, and the company is always fun.

7. Consider community kitchens

The concept of a community kitchen is actually very old. And up until recently, the women of a community or family would routinely get together to cook.

A community kitchen involves getting a group of people together to prepare some meals together. The group makes a menu, and each person does some grocery shopping. Then everyone gets together and the fun starts. Sharing the tasks makes it easier and less physically demanding.

Nourishing yourself should be a priority because it will help you stay healthier, feel better, and manage your weight. Not feeling up to cooking or grocery shopping is not a reason to abandon healthy eating! It is an opportunity to get creative and find a way to accomplish your goal of healthy eating while taking into account your circumstances. Your health-care team, in particular your dietitian, will know what services are available in your area and will be able to steer you in the right direction. A community kitchen, for example, can be a formal group or as informal as getting together with friends and family to do a bit of cooking.

CHAPTER 14

Arthritis Diet Menu Plans

Menu planning can be fun. Save the menus you like in a binder or file box so you can reuse them. The best thing to do is to follow the menus that have been provided. Using the menus exactly as they are will provide structure and stability. It will give you an opportunity to concentrate on how you feel and how your body is reacting to the new eating plan without expending a lot of energy on making menus and figuring out what to eat.

Once you are familiar with the foods that are part of an anti-inflammatory way of eating, you can make up your own menus and adapt your own shopping list. That way, shopping is easier for you, or it can easily be done by a family member or caregiver. It could even be done online, if you like.

Cooking Prep
Stock Up

Keep at least three menus with simple and easy-to-prepare recipes posted on the pantry or refrigerator door. Make sure you have all the ingredients on hand, either in the pantry or in the freezer. That way, if you are ever too tired to cook a meal you had planned, you can just make up this easy-to-prepare meal.

Plan for Leftovers

On days when you feel good, it is a smart idea to make extra food. Try doubling your recipes to create leftovers, which can easily be frozen. Freeze in individual portions to make defrosting easier and faster. On days when you don't feel well enough to cook, reheat the nutritious meal waiting for you in the freezer.

Take Advantage of Good Days

Wash all your fruits and vegetables on days you are feeling well. That way, on the days where you feel weaker, this step is already done. You can purchase special containers that keep your produce fresh.

If time permits, you may also want to prepare for the following day's meal. On the next day, this can sometimes make a world of difference.

4-Week Menu Plan

Here is a 4-week menu plan you can follow, or use as a guide to making your own menus. The recipes included were chosen to showcase the wide variety of foods that can help reduce inflammation. Ease of preparation and low cooking temperatures to reduce AGEs were also part of the selection criteria. The first 2 weeks of the menu plan feature a Mediterranean-style diet that is high in vegetables, fruits, grains, and healthy oils, with limited animal protein but lots of fatty fish. The next 2 weeks are vegan, but in most of these meals, it would be very easy to add some animal protein.

Each menu is designed to meet the energy requirements for women (1800 calories) and men (2300 calories). These levels were chosen to help people maintain their current weight. Losing weight would require fewer calories for most individuals, so consult a dietitian for help in adapting the menus for weight loss. For those who choose to follow the vegan menu, make sure that you consult your dietitian and your doctor to discuss your options for supplementing your diet with iron and vitamin B_{12}, as it might be a challenge to meet your nutrition needs with your diet.

Remember that food and eating not only nourish our bodies but also our souls. We derive pleasure from shopping for and preparing our food, and from the sight and smells of food cooking in our kitchens. Keep that in mind as you plan and prepare your meals.

Make nourishing yourself a priority!

> Remember that food and eating not only nourish our bodies but also our souls. We derive pleasure from shopping for and preparing our food, and from the sight and smells of food cooking in our kitchens. Keep that in mind as you plan and prepare your meals.

Mediterranean-Style Menus (2 weeks)

Calories per day for women: 1800
Calories per day for men: 2300
For recipes from the book, the serving size is 1 serving unless otherwise noted.

Meal	Menu Plan for Women	Menu Plan for Men
Day 1: Monday		
Breakfast	Mushroom Egg Scramble (page 174) 2 slices whole-grain bread 1/2 cup (125 mL) reduced-fat yogurt 2 tbsp (30 mL) ground flax seeds (flaxseed meal)	Mushroom Egg Scramble (page 174) 2 slices whole-grain bread 1/2 cup (125 mL) reduced-fat yogurt 2 tbsp (30 mL) ground flax seeds (flaxseed meal)
Morning Snack	1 cup (250 mL) blueberries	1 cup (250 mL) blueberries 1 whole-grain cereal bar 2 oz (60 g) reduced-fat Cheddar cheese
Lunch	Moroccan Lentil Soup (page 211) 2 cups (500 mL) mixed salad greens 1/2 cup (125 mL) whole wheat croutons 1 tbsp (15 mL) olive oil–based salad dressing	Moroccan Lentil Soup (page 211) 2 cups (500 mL) mixed salad greens 1/2 cup (125 mL) whole wheat croutons 1 tbsp (15 mL) olive oil–based salad dressing
Afternoon Snack	1 mango	1 mango 2 clementines 1 cup (250 mL) 1% milk
Dinner	Maple Ginger Salmon (page 268) 1 cup (250 mL) cooked whole wheat couscous 1 cup (250 mL) chopped red and orange bell peppers 1 apple	Maple Ginger Salmon (page 268) 1 cup (250 mL) cooked whole wheat couscous 1 cup (250 mL) chopped red and orange bell peppers 1 apple
Evening Snack	Melon Balls with Warm Ginger Sauce (page 332) 1 cup (250 mL) 1% milk	Melon Balls with Warm Ginger Sauce (page 332) 1 cup (250 mL) 1% milk
Day 2: Tuesday		
Breakfast	1 Orange Cranberry Flax Muffin (page 177) 1 cup (250 mL) 1% milk	1 Orange Cranberry Flax Muffin (page 177) 1 cup (250 mL) 1% milk
Morning Snack	1/4 cup (60 mL) unsalted almonds	1/4 cup (60 mL) unsalted almonds
Lunch	Roasted Vegetable Lasagna (page 240) 3-inch (7.5 cm) whole wheat baguette 2 prunes 1/4 cup (60 mL) reduced-fat feta cheese	Roasted Vegetable Lasagna (page 240) 3-inch (7.5 cm) whole wheat baguette 2 prunes 1/4 cup (60 mL) reduced-fat feta cheese

Meal	Menu Plan for Women	Menu Plan for Men
Afternoon Snack	$\frac{1}{2}$ cup (125 mL) reduced-fat Greek yogurt	$\frac{1}{2}$ cup (125 mL) reduced-fat Greek yogurt 1 cup (250 mL) raspberries $\frac{1}{2}$ cup (125 mL) unsweetened granola
Dinner	Red Lentils with Garlic and Cilantro (page 244) Marinated Asparagus (page 221) 1 cup (250 mL) cooked brown rice	Red Lentils with Garlic and Cilantro (page 244) Marinated Asparagus (page 221) 1 cup (250 mL) cooked brown rice
Evening Snack		1 grapefruit
Day 3: Wednesday		
Breakfast	Cranberry Quinoa Porridge (page 179) 1 cup (250 mL) 1% milk	Cranberry Quinoa Porridge (page 179) 1 cup (250 mL) 1% milk
Morning Snack	1 banana 4 whole wheat crackers	1 banana 4 whole wheat crackers $\frac{1}{4}$ cup (60 mL) hummus
Lunch	1 Tuna Lettuce Pocket (page 235) 1 cup (250 mL) cooked wild rice 2 oz (60 g) reduced-fat Swiss cheese 1 cup (250 mL) baby carrots	1 Tuna Lettuce Pocket (page 235) 1 cup (250 mL) cooked wild rice 2 oz (60 g) reduced-fat Swiss cheese 1 cup (250 mL) baby carrots
Afternoon Snack	7-oz (200 mL) yogurt beverage	$\frac{1}{2}$ cup (125 mL) dried mangos 1 whole-grain cereal bar 7-oz (200 mL) yogurt beverage
Dinner	Baked Beans and Rice Casserole (page 253) 1 cup (250 mL) Brussels sprouts	Baked Beans and Rice Casserole (page 253) 1 cup (250 mL) Brussels sprouts 1 peach
Evening Snack	$\frac{1}{4}$ cup (60 mL) unsalted peanuts	$\frac{1}{4}$ cup (60 mL) unsalted peanuts 1 cup (250 mL) 1% milk
Day 4: Thursday		
Breakfast	1 whole-grain bagel $\frac{1}{2}$ cup (125 mL) cottage cheese 1 apple	1 whole-grain bagel $\frac{1}{2}$ cup (125 mL) cottage cheese 1 apple
Morning Snack	2 prunes	2 prunes
Lunch	Tofu Vegetable Pilaf (page 258) 1 cup (250 mL) broccoli	Tofu Vegetable Pilaf (page 258) 1 cup (250 mL) broccoli 1 cup (250 mL) chopped cantaloupe $\frac{1}{4}$ avocado
Afternoon Snack		
Dinner	Mediterranean-Style Mahi-Mahi (page 266) Spiced Spinach (page 315) 1 cup (250 mL) cooked quinoa	Mediterranean-Style Mahi-Mahi (page 266) Spiced Spinach (page 315) 1 cup (250 mL) cooked quinoa 1 cup (250 mL) grapes

Meal	Menu Plan for Women	Menu Plan for Men
Evening Snack		2 oz (60 g) reduced-fat Cheddar cheese 1 slice whole wheat bread
Day 5: Friday		
Breakfast	¼ cup (60 mL) dry Hot Cereal with Multigrains (page 180), cooked 1 cup (250 mL) 1% milk	¼ cup (60 mL) dry Hot Cereal with Multigrains (page 180), cooked 2 tbsp (30 mL) ground flax seeds (flaxseed meal) 1 banana 1 cup (250 mL) 1% milk
Morning Snack	½ cup (125 mL) cucumber sticks 2 tbsp (30 mL) Green Olive Tapenade (page 191) 4 whole-grain crackers	½ cup (125 mL) cucumber sticks 2 tbsp (30 mL) Green Olive Tapenade (page 191) 4 whole-grain crackers
Lunch	1 Chickpea Tofu Burger with Coriander Mayonnaise (page 262) 1 whole-grain bun Cauliflower with Capers (page 309) ½ cup (125 mL) reduced-fat Greek yogurt	1 Chickpea Tofu Burger with Coriander Mayonnaise (page 262) 1 whole-grain bun Cauliflower with Capers (page 309) ½ cup (125 mL) reduced-fat Greek yogurt
Afternoon Snack	1 cup (250 mL) 1% milk	1 cup (250 mL) chopped honeydew melon 1 cup (250 mL) 1% milk
Dinner	Cod Provençal (page 264) 1 cup (250 mL) cooked brown rice	Cod Provençal (page 264) 1 cup (250 mL) cooked brown rice
Evening Snack	1 whole-grain cereal bar	1 whole-grain cereal bar Wine-Poached Pears (page 331)
Day 6: Saturday		
Breakfast	Buttermilk Buckwheat Pancakes (page 175) 1 cup (250 mL) strawberries 1 cup (250 mL) 1% milk	Buttermilk Buckwheat Pancakes (page 175) 1 cup (250 mL) strawberries 1 cup (250 mL) 1% milk
Morning Snack	¼ cup (60 mL) dried fruit ¼ cup (60 mL) cashews	¼ cup (60 mL) dried fruit ¼ cup (60 mL) cashews
Lunch	Three-Bean Chili (page 252) 1 cup (250 mL) cooked whole wheat couscous	Three-Bean Chili (page 252) 1 cup (250 mL) cooked whole wheat couscous ½ avocado
Afternoon Snack		3-inch (7.5 cm) whole wheat baguette 2 oz (60 g) reduced-fat Swiss cheese
Dinner	Udon Noodles with Tofu and Gingered Peanut Sauce (page 261) 7-oz (200 mL) yogurt beverage	Udon Noodles with Tofu and Gingered Peanut Sauce (page 261) 7-oz (200 mL) yogurt beverage
Evening Snack		1 mango

Meal	Menu Plan for Women	Menu Plan for Men
Day 7: Sunday		
Breakfast	2 slices multigrain bread 2 tbsp (30 mL) peanut butter ½ cup (125 mL) reduced-fat Greek yogurt 1 cup (250 mL) blackberries	2 slices multigrain bread 2 tbsp (30 mL) peanut butter ½ cup (125 mL) reduced-fat Greek yogurt 1 cup (250 mL) blackberries
Morning Snack	¼ cup (60 mL) dried cranberries 1 cup (250 mL) 1% milk	¼ cup (60 mL) dried cranberries 1 cup (250 mL) 1% milk ½ cup (125 mL) unsweetened granola
Lunch	Hearty Black and White Bean Soup (page 212) Soba Noodle Salad with Edamame (page 228)	Hearty Black and White Bean Soup (page 212) Soba Noodle Salad with Edamame (page 228)
Afternoon Snack	1 cup (250 mL) 1% milk	1 grapefruit 1 cup (250 mL) 1% milk
Dinner	Buckwheat Pilaf with Paprika-Seasoned Chicken (page 295) 2 Veggie Kabobs (page 316)	Buckwheat Pilaf with Paprika-Seasoned Chicken (page 295) 2 Veggie Kabobs (page 316)
Evening Snack		1 cup (250 mL) cherries
Day 8: Monday		
Breakfast	1 whole wheat English muffin 1 poached egg ½ cup (125 mL) reduced-fat yogurt 1 cup (250 mL) mixed berries	1 whole wheat English muffin 1 poached egg ½ cup (125 mL) reduced-fat yogurt 1 cup (250 mL) mixed berries
Morning Snack	1 cup (250 mL) grapes	1 cup (250 mL) grapes 4 whole-grain crackers 2 oz (60 g) reduced-fat Cheddar cheese
Lunch	4 Rainbow Lettuce Wraps (page 238) 1 medium potato, boiled 2 oz (60 g) reduced-fat Swiss cheese 1 pear	4 Rainbow Lettuce Wraps (page 238) 1 medium potato, boiled 2 oz (60 g) reduced-fat Swiss cheese 1 pear
Afternoon Snack	½ cup (125 mL) sliced cucumbers 1 cup (250 mL) 1% milk	½ cup (125 mL) sliced cucumbers ¼ cup (60 mL) dried cranberries 1 cup (250 mL) 1% milk
Dinner	Peachy Glazed Trout (page 271) Quinoa and Corn Salad with Cumin Lime Dressing (page 231)	Peachy Glazed Trout (page 271) Quinoa and Corn Salad with Cumin Lime Dressing (page 231)
Evening Snack	½ cup (125 mL) reduced-fat yogurt	½ cup (125 mL) reduced-fat yogurt 1 cup (250 mL) chopped cantaloupe
Day 9: Tuesday		
Breakfast	1 cup (250 mL) cooked oatmeal 1 cup (250 mL) 1% milk 1 banana	1 cup (250 mL) cooked oatmeal 1 cup (250 mL) 1% milk 1 banana

Meal	Menu Plan for Women	Menu Plan for Men
Morning Snack	2 oz (60 g) goat cheese 4 whole-grain crackers	2 oz (60 g) goat cheese 4 whole-grain crackers 1 cup (250 mL) honeydew
Lunch	Zuppa di Pesce (page 216) 1 cup (250 mL) baby carrots	Zuppa di Pesce (page 216) 1 cup (250 mL) baby carrots
Afternoon Snack	7-oz (200 mL) yogurt beverage	2 clementines 7-oz (200 mL) yogurt beverage
Dinner	Mediterranean Kasha Casserole with Sun-Dried Tomatoes (page 255) Autumn Harvest Salad (page 224)	Mediterranean Kasha Casserole with Sun-Dried Tomatoes (page 255) Autumn Harvest Salad (page 224)
Evening Snack		4 reduced-fat graham crackers 1 cup (250 mL) 1% milk

Day 10: Wednesday

Meal	Menu Plan for Women	Menu Plan for Men
Breakfast	½ cup (125 mL) unsweetened granola ¼ cup (60 mL) unsalted pecans 1 cup (250 mL) 1% milk 2 kiwifruits	½ cup (125 mL) unsweetened granola ¼ cup (60 mL) unsalted pecans 1 cup (250 mL) 1% milk 2 kiwifruits
Morning Snack	½ mango ½ cup (125 mL) reduced-fat yogurt	½ mango ½ cup (125 mL) reduced-fat yogurt 4 Melba toasts
Lunch	Hot Sweet Potato Salad (page 222) ½ cup (125 mL) wax beans	Hot Sweet Potato Salad (page 222) ½ cup (125 mL) wax beans ¼ cup (60 mL) unsalted sunflower seeds
Afternoon Snack	½ cup (125 mL) reduced-fat cottage cheese	½ cup (125 mL) reduced-fat cottage cheese 6-inch (15 cm) whole wheat pita
Dinner	Buttery Mung Dal (page 248) 1 piece naan ½ cup (125 mL) dried apricots	Buttery Mung Dal (page 248) 1 piece naan ½ cup (125 mL) dried apricots
Evening Snack	1 cup (250 mL) 1% milk	1 pear 1 cup (250 mL) 1% milk

Day 11: Thursday

Meal	Menu Plan for Women	Menu Plan for Men
Breakfast	2 slices whole-grain bread 2 eggs, boiled ½ cup (125 mL) reduced-fat yogurt 1 cup (250 mL) cherries	2 slices whole-grain bread 2 eggs, boiled ½ cup (125 mL) reduced-fat yogurt 1 cup (250 mL) cherries
Morning Snack	¼ cup (60 mL) reduced-fat feta cheese 4 whole-grain crackers	¼ cup (60 mL) reduced-fat feta cheese 4 whole-grain crackers 2 apricots
Lunch	Quinoa with Almonds (page 322) 2 cups (500 mL) mixed salad greens 1 tbsp (15 mL) olive oil–based salad dressing	Quinoa with Almonds (page 322) 2 cups (500 mL) mixed salad greens 1 tbsp (15 mL) olive oil–based salad dressing

Meal	Menu Plan for Women	Menu Plan for Men
Afternoon Snack	1 orange 1 cup (250 mL) 1% milk	1 orange 4 whole-grain crackers 1 cup (250 mL) 1% milk
Dinner	1/2 serving Lamb and White Bean Ragoût (page 286) 1 cup (250 mL) steamed green beans 1 cup (250 mL) 1% milk	1/2 serving Lamb and White Bean Ragoût (page 286) 1 cup (250 mL) steamed green beans 1 cup (250 mL) 1% milk
Evening Snack	1 cup (250 mL) fruit nectar	1 cup (250 mL) chopped papaya 1 cup (250 mL) fruit nectar
Day 12: Friday		
Breakfast	2 servings Banana Cake with Lemon Cream Frosting (page 324) 1 cup (250 mL) 1% milk	2 servings Banana Cake with Lemon Cream Frosting (page 324) 1 banana 1 cup (250 mL) 1% milk
Morning Snack	1 cup (250 mL) chopped watermelon 1/4 cup (60 mL) unsalted watermelon seeds	1 cup (250 mL) chopped watermelon 1/4 cup (60 mL) unsalted watermelon seeds
Lunch	Vegetable Fried Rice (page 318) 1 cup (250 mL) tofu, sautéed 1 cup (250 mL) fruit nectar	Vegetable Fried Rice (page 318) 1 cup (250 mL) tofu, sautéed 1 cup (250 mL) fruit nectar
Afternoon Snack	7-oz (200 mL) yogurt beverage	6-inch (15 cm) whole wheat pita 7-oz (200 mL) yogurt beverage
Dinner	Spinach Pasta (page 259) 3 oz (90 g) grilled skinless chicken breast 1/2 cup (125 mL) sliced bell peppers	Spinach Pasta (page 259) 3 oz (90 g) grilled skinless chicken breast 1/2 cup (125 mL) sliced bell peppers
Evening Snack	1 cup (250 mL) 1% milk	1 peach 1/2 cup (125 mL) dates 1 cup (250 mL) 1% milk
Day 13: Saturday		
Breakfast	Banana Raspberry Tapioca Pudding (page 334) 2 slices whole-grain bread 2 tbsp (30 mL) peanut butter	Banana Raspberry Tapioca Pudding (page 334) 2 slices whole-grain bread 2 tbsp (30 mL) peanut butter 3/4 cup (175 mL) 100% fruit juice
Morning Snack	2 prunes 1/2 cup (125 mL) reduced-fat yogurt	2 prunes 1/2 cup (125 mL) reduced-fat yogurt 4 reduced-fat graham crackers
Lunch	Slow Cooker Squash Couscous (page 256) 1 cup (250 mL) 1% milk	Slow Cooker Squash Couscous (page 256) 1 cup (250 mL) 1% milk
Afternoon Snack	1 cup (250 mL) 1% milk	1 tangerine 1 cup (250 mL) 1% milk

Meal	Menu Plan for Women	Menu Plan for Men
Dinner	Rice with Shrimp and Lemon (page 277) 1 cup (250 mL) baked kale	Rice with Shrimp and Lemon (page 277) 1 cup (250 mL) baked kale
Evening Snack		1 cup (250 mL) 1% milk
Day 14: Sunday		
Breakfast	1 cup (250 mL) cooked oatmeal 1 cup (250 mL) 1% milk 1 cup (250 mL) blueberries	1 cup (250 mL) cooked oatmeal 1 cup (250 mL) 1% milk 1 cup (250 mL) blueberries
Morning Snack	$\frac{1}{2}$ cup (125 mL) cottage cheese	$\frac{1}{2}$ cup (125 mL) cottage cheese 2 slices whole-grain bread
Lunch	2 servings Hot-and-Sour Vegetable Curry (page 314) $\frac{1}{2}$ cup (125 mL) chickpeas, cooked	2 servings Hot-and-Sour Vegetable Curry (page 314) $\frac{1}{2}$ cup (125 mL) chickpeas, cooked
Afternoon Snack	$\frac{1}{2}$ cup (125 mL) reduced-fat yogurt $\frac{1}{4}$ cup (60 mL) almonds	$\frac{1}{2}$ cup (125 mL) reduced-fat yogurt $\frac{1}{4}$ cup (60 mL) almonds 1 cup (250 mL) cranberries
Dinner	1 Terrific Chicken Burger (page 298) 1 whole-grain bun 1 cup (250 mL) steamed broccoli 1 medium potato, boiled	1 Terrific Chicken Burger (page 298) 1 whole-grain bun 1 cup (250 mL) steamed broccoli 1 medium potato, boiled 1 cup (250 mL) strawberries
Evening snack	Baked Peaches with Almond Crust (page 329) 1 cup (250 mL) 1% milk	Baked Peaches with Almond Crust (page 329) 1 cup (250 mL) 1% milk

Vegan Menus (2 weeks)

Calories per day for women: 1800
Calories per day for men: 2300
For recipes from the book, the serving size is 1 serving unless otherwise noted.

Note: A B₁₂ supplement is recommended if a vegan diet is followed.

Meal	Menu Plan for Women	Menu Plan for Men
Day 15: Monday		
Breakfast	Apple Berry Muesli, vegan variation (page 182) ¼ cup (60 mL) sliced almonds	Apple Berry Muesli, vegan variation (page 182) ¼ cup (60 mL) sliced almonds
Morning Snack	1 cup (250 mL) blueberries 2 oz (60 g) fortified soy cheese	1 cup (250 mL) blueberries 2 oz (60 g) fortified soy cheese 1 whole-grain cereal bar
Lunch	Moroccan Lentil Soup (page 211) 2 cups (500 mL) mixed salad greens ½ cup (125 mL) whole wheat croutons 1 tbsp (15 mL) olive oil–based salad dressing	Moroccan Lentil Soup (page 211) 2 cups (500 mL) mixed salad greens ½ cup (125 mL) whole wheat croutons 1 tbsp (15 mL) olive oil–based salad dressing
Afternoon Snack		2 clementines 1 cup (250 L) fortified rice, almond, or soy milk
Dinner	Curried Vegetables with Tofu (page 257) 1 cup (250 mL) cooked whole wheat couscous	Curried Vegetables with Tofu (page 257) 1 cup (250 mL) cooked whole wheat couscous
Evening Snack	Melon Balls with Warm Ginger Sauce (page 331) 1 cup (250 mL) fortified rice, almond, or soy milk	Melon Balls with Warm Ginger Sauce (page 331) 1 cup (250 mL) fortified rice, almond, or soy milk
Day 16: Tuesday		
Breakfast	2 slices whole-grain bread 2 tbsp (30 mL) peanut butter 1 peach ½ cup (125 mL) fortified soy or rice yogurt	2 slices whole-grain bread 2 tbsp (30 mL) peanut butter 1 peach ½ cup (125 mL) fortified soy or rice yogurt
Morning Snack	2 tbsp (30 mL) Tofu Mayonnaise (page 196) 4 multigrain crackers	2 tbsp (30 mL) Tofu Mayonnaise (page 196) 4 multigrain crackers
Lunch	Roasted Vegetable Lasagna (page 240) 3-inch (7.5 cm) whole wheat baguette 2 prunes 1 cup (250 mL) fortified rice, almond, or soy milk	Roasted Vegetable Lasagna (page 240) 3-inch (7.5 cm) whole wheat baguette 2 prunes 1 cup (250 mL) fortified rice, almond, or soy milk
Afternoon Snack	½ cup (125 mL) fortified soy or rice yogurt	½ cup (125 mL) fortified soy or rice yogurt 1 cup (250 mL) raspberries ½ cup (125 mL) unsweetened granola

Meal	Menu Plan for Women	Menu Plan for Men
Dinner	Red Lentils with Garlic and Cilantro (page 244) Marinated Asparagus (page 221) 1 cup (250 mL) cooked brown rice	Red Lentils with Garlic and Cilantro (page 244) Marinated Asparagus (page 221) 1 cup (250 mL) cooked brown rice 1 cup (250 mL) fruit nectar
Evening Snack		1 grapefruit

Day 17: Wednesday

Meal	Menu Plan for Women	Menu Plan for Men
Breakfast	2 servings Cranberry Quinoa Porridge (page 179) 1 cup (250 mL) fortified rice, almond, or soy milk	2 servings Cranberry Quinoa Porridge (page 179) 1 cup (250 mL) fortified rice, almond, or soy milk
Morning Snack	1 banana 4 whole wheat crackers	1 banana 4 whole wheat crackers 2 tbsp (30 mL) hummus
Lunch	Tofu Vegetable Pilaf (page 258) 1 cup (250 mL) kale, cooked	Tofu Vegetable Pilaf (page 258) 1 cup (250 mL) kale, cooked 1 cup (250 mL) chopped cantaloupe ½ avocado
Afternoon Snack	½ cup (125 mL) fortified soy or rice yogurt	½ cup (125 mL) fortified soy or rice yogurt ½ cup (125 mL) unsweetened granola ¼ cup (60 mL) dried cranberries
Dinner	Baked Beans and Rice Casserole (page 253) 1 cup (250 mL) collard greens, cooked	Baked Beans and Rice Casserole (page 253) 1 cup (250 mL) collard greens, cooked 1 peach
Evening Snack	¼ cup (60 mL) unsalted peanuts	¼ cup (60 mL) unsalted peanuts

Day 18: Thursday

Meal	Menu Plan for Women	Menu Plan for Men
Breakfast	1 multigrain bagel 2 oz (60 g) fortified soy cheese 1 apple 1 cup (250 mL) fortified rice, almond, or soy milk	1 multigrain bagel 2 oz (60 g) fortified soy cheese 1 apple 1 cup (250 mL) fortified rice, almond, or soy milk
Morning Snack	2 prunes ¼ cup (60 mL) unsalted sunflower seeds	2 prunes ¼ cup (60 mL) unsalted sunflower seeds
Lunch	Quinoa à la Med (page 254) ½ cup (125 mL) tempeh 1 cup (250 mL) fortified rice, almond, or soy milk	Quinoa à la Med (page 254) ½ cup (125 mL) tempeh 1 cup (250 mL) fortified rice, almond, or soy milk
Afternoon Snack	Rice Pudding (page 333)	Rice Pudding (page 333)
Dinner	Split Yellow Peas with Zucchini (page 242) 1 cup (250 mL) cooked quinoa	Split Yellow Peas with Zucchini (page 242) 1 cup (250 mL) cooked quinoa 1 cup (250 mL) grapes
Evening Snack	2 oz (60 g) fortified soy cheese	2 oz (60 g) fortified soy cheese 1 slice whole wheat bread

Meal	Menu Plan for Women	Menu Plan for Men
Day 19: Friday		
Breakfast	½ cup (125 mL) dry Hot Cereal with Multigrains (page 180), cooked 1 cup (250 mL) fortified rice, almond, or soy milk 1 banana	½ cup (125 mL) dry Hot Cereal with Multigrains (page 180), cooked 1 cup (250 mL) fortified rice, almond, or soy milk 1 banana
Morning Snack	1 cup (250 mL) cucumber sticks 2 tbsp (30 mL) Green Olive Tapenade (page 191) 4 multigrain crackers	1 cup (250 mL) cucumber sticks 2 tbsp (30 mL) Green Olive Tapenade (page 191) 4 multigrain crackers
Lunch	1 Herbed Nut and Bean Patty (page 249) 1 multigrain bun ½ cup (125 mL) fortified soy or rice yogurt 1 cup (250 mL) mixed salad greens 1 tbsp (15 mL) olive oil–based salad dressing	1 Herbed Nut and Bean Patty (page 249) 1 multigrain bun ½ cup (125 mL) fortified soy or rice yogurt 1 cup (250 mL) mixed salad greens 1 tbsp (15 mL) olive oil–based salad dressing
Afternoon Snack	1 cup (250 mL) fortified rice, almond, or soy milk	1 cup (250 mL) chopped honeydew melon 1 cup (250 mL) fortified rice, almond, or soy milk
Dinner	Zucchini with Yellow Mung Beans (page 250) 1 roti or chapati	Zucchini with Yellow Mung Beans (page 250) 1 roti or chapati 1 cup (250 mL) fortified rice, almond, or soy milk
Evening Snack		¼ cup (60 mL) walnuts 1 cup (250 mL) fruit nectar
Day 20: Saturday		
Breakfast	1 cup (250 mL) cooked oatmeal 1 cup (250 mL) strawberries 1 cup (250 mL) fortified rice, almond, or soy milk	1 cup (250 mL) cooked oatmeal 1 cup (250 mL) strawberries 1 cup (250 mL) fortified rice, almond, or soy milk
Morning Snack	¼ cup (60 mL) unsalted cashews	¼ cup (60 mL) unsalted cashews ¼ cup (60 mL) dried fruit
Lunch	Easy Borscht (page 203) Three-Bean Chili (page 252) 1 cup (250 mL) cooked whole wheat couscous	Easy Borscht (page 203) Three-Bean Chili (page 252) 1 cup (250 mL) cooked whole wheat couscous ½ avocado
Afternoon Snack	1 cup (250 mL) fortified rice, almond, or soy milk	1 cup (250 mL) fortified rice, almond, or soy milk
Dinner	Udon Noodles with Tofu and Gingered Peanut Sauce (page 261) 1 cup (250 mL) fortified rice, almond, or soy milk	Udon Noodles with Tofu and Gingered Peanut Sauce (page 261) 1 cup (250 mL) fortified rice, almond, or soy milk
Evening Snack		1 mango

Meal	Menu Plan for Women	Menu Plan for Men
Day 21: Sunday		
Breakfast	2 slices multigrain bread 2 tbsp (30 mL) peanut butter 1/2 cup (125 mL) fortified soy or rice yogurt 1 cup (250 mL) blackberries	2 slices multigrain bread 2 tbsp (30 mL) peanut butter 1/2 cup (125 mL) fortified soy or rice yogurt 1 cup (250 mL) blackberries
Morning Snack	1/4 cup (60 mL) dried cranberries 1 cup (250 mL) fortified rice, almond, or soy milk	1/2 cup (125 mL) unsweetened granola 1/4 cup (60 mL) dried cranberries 1 cup (250 mL) fortified rice, almond, or soy milk
Lunch	Hearty Black and White Bean Soup (page 212) Soba Noodle Salad with Edamame (page 228)	Hearty Black and White Bean Soup (page 212) Soba Noodle Salad with Edamame (page 228)
Afternoon Snack	1 cup (250 mL) fortified rice, almond, or soy milk	1 grapefruit 1 cup (250 mL) fortified rice, almond, or soy milk
Dinner	Lemon-Dill White Bean Salad (page 227) 1 whole wheat pita 2 Veggie Kabobs (page 316) 1 apple	Lemon-Dill White Bean Salad (page 227) 1 whole wheat pita 2 Veggie Kabobs (page 316) 1 apple
Evening Snack		1 cup (250 mL) cherries
Day 22: Monday		
Breakfast	Poached Peaches with Lavender Custard (page 330) 1 whole-grain English muffin 2 oz (60 g) fortified soy cheese	Poached Peaches with Lavender Custard (page 330) 1 whole-grain English muffin 2 oz (60 g) fortified soy cheese
Morning Snack	1 banana 1 whole-grain cereal bar	1 banana 1 whole-grain cereal bar 1/2 cup (125 mL) almonds
Lunch	Slow Cooker Squash Couscous (page 256), made with olive oil instead of margarine 2 cups (500 mL) arugula 1 tbsp (15 mL) olive oil–based salad dressing	Slow Cooker Squash Couscous (page 256), made with olive oil instead of margarine 2 cups (500 mL) arugula 1 tbsp (15 mL) olive oil–based salad dressing 2 tbsp (30 mL) ground flax seeds (flaxseed meal)
Afternoon Snack	1 cup (250 mL) fortified rice, almond, or soy milk	1/4 cup (60 mL) dried figs 1 cup (250 mL) fortified rice, almond, or soy milk
Dinner	Golden Curried Pineapple Rice (page 321) 1 cup (250 mL) cooked lentils 1 cup (250 mL) Swiss chard, cooked	Golden Curried Pineapple Rice (page 321) 1 cup (250 mL) cooked lentils 1 cup (250 mL) Swiss chard, cooked
Evening Snack	1 cup (250 mL) fortified rice, almond, or soy milk	1 blood orange 1 cup (250 mL) fortified rice, almond, or soy milk

Meal	Menu Plan for Women	Menu Plan for Men
Day 23: Tuesday		
Breakfast	2 Date and Nut Pinwheels (page 327) ½ cup (125 mL) fortified soy or rice yogurt ½ cup (125 mL) unsweetened granola	2 Date and Nut Pinwheels (page 327) ½ cup (125 mL) fortified soy or rice yogurt ½ cup (125 mL) unsweetened granola
Morning Snack	¼ cup (60 mL) Seasoned Chickpeas and Almonds (page 190)	¼ cup (60 mL) Seasoned Chickpeas and Almonds (page 190) 2 plums 1 cup (250 mL) fortified rice, almond, or soy milk
Lunch	½ cup (125 mL) Italian White Bean Spread (page 193) 1 whole wheat pita 2 cups (500 mL) mixed salad greens 1 tbsp (15 mL) olive oil–based salad dressing	½ cup (125 mL) Italian White Bean Spread (page 193) 1 whole wheat pita 2 cups (500 mL) mixed salad greens 1 tbsp (15 mL) olive oil–based salad dressing
Afternoon Snack	½ cup (125 mL) fortified soy or rice yogurt	½ cup (125 mL) fortified soy or rice yogurt 1 cup (250 mL) chopped honeydew melon
Dinner	Mushroom and Barley Soup (page 207) 1 cup (250 mL) cooked brown rice ½ cup (125 mL) tempeh	Mushroom and Barley Soup (page 207) 1 cup (250 mL) cooked brown rice ½ cup (125 mL) tempeh
Evening Snack		1 grapefruit ¼ cup (60 mL) unsalted pistachios
Day 24: Wednesday		
Breakfast	1 cup (250 mL) cooked oatmeal ½ cup (125 mL) fortified soy or rice yogurt 1 Citrus Cocktail (page 182), made with soy yogurt instead of yogurt	1 cup (250 mL) cooked oatmeal ½ cup (125 mL) fortified soy or rice yogurt 2 tbsp (30 mL) ground flax seeds (flaxseed meal) 1 Citrus Cocktail (page 182), made with soy yogurt instead of yogurt
Morning Snack	Black Olive Pâté (page 192) 6 Melba toasts	Black Olive Pâté (page 192) 6 Melba toasts
Lunch	Pasta Fagioli Capra (page 214) 1 cup (250 mL) fortified rice, almond, or soy milk	Pasta Fagioli Capra (page 214) 1 cup (250 mL) red grapes 1 cup (250 mL) fortified rice, almond, or soy milk
Afternoon Snack	½ cup (125 mL) fortified soy or rice yogurt ¼ cup (60 mL) almonds	½ cup (125 mL) fortified soy or rice yogurt ¼ cup (60 mL) almonds 2 clementines
Dinner	Quinoa Beet Potato Salad (page 226) 2 tofu sausages 1 cup (250 mL) Brussels sprouts, steamed	Quinoa Beet Potato Salad (page 226) 2 tofu sausages 1 cup (250 mL) Brussels sprouts, steamed

Meal	Menu Plan for Women	Menu Plan for Men
Evening Snack	1 cup (250 mL) fortified rice, almond, or soy milk	¼ cup (60 mL) hazelnuts 1 apple 1 cup (250 mL) fortified rice, almond, or soy milk

Day 25: Thursday

Meal	Menu Plan for Women	Menu Plan for Men
Breakfast	1 multigrain bagel 2 oz (60 g) fortified soy cheese 1 cup (250 mL) cherries	1 multigrain bagel 2 oz (60 g) fortified soy cheese 1 cup (250 mL) cherries
Morning Snack	1 cup (250 mL) chopped pineapple ½ cup (125 mL) fortified soy or rice yogurt	1 cup (250 mL) chopped pineapple ½ cup (125 mL) fortified soy or rice yogurt 1 whole-grain cereal bar
Lunch	Tabbouleh (page 230) 1 cup (250 mL) tofu 1 cup (250 mL) cooked whole wheat couscous	Tabbouleh (page 230) 1 cup (250 mL) tofu 1 cup (250 mL) cooked whole wheat couscous
Afternoon Snack	1 cup (250 mL) fortified rice, almond, or soy milk	1 pear 1 cup (250 mL) fortified rice, almond, or soy milk
Dinner	2 servings Zucchini with Yellow Mung Beans (page 250) 1 cup (250 mL) cooked brown rice	2 servings Zucchini with Yellow Mung Beans (page 250) 1 cup (250 mL) cooked brown rice
Evening Snack		2 plums 1 cup (250 mL) fortified rice, almond, or soy milk

Day 26: Friday

Meal	Menu Plan for Women	Menu Plan for Men
Breakfast	2 slices whole-grain bread 2 tbsp (30 mL) peanut butter 1 cup (250 mL) fortified rice, almond, or soy milk	2 slices whole-grain bread 2 tbsp (30 mL) peanut butter 1 cup (250 mL) chopped honeydew melon 1 cup (250 mL) fortified rice, almond, or soy milk
Morning Snack	1 nectarine 2 oz (60 g) fortified soy cheese	1 nectarine 2 oz (60 g) fortified soy cheese 4 whole-grain crackers
Lunch	2 cups (500 mL) mixed salad greens 1 tbsp (15 mL) Asian Dressing (page 196) ¼ cup (60 mL) sliced almonds ½ cup (125 mL) whole wheat croutons ¼ cup (60 mL) dried cranberries	2 cups (500 mL) mixed salad greens 1 tbsp (15 mL) Asian Dressing (page 196) ¼ cup (60 mL) sliced almonds ½ cup (125 mL) whole wheat croutons ¼ cup (60 mL) dried cranberries
Afternoon Snack	1 apple 1 cup (250 mL) fortified rice, almond, or soy milk	1 apple 1 cup (250 mL) fortified rice, almond, or soy milk
Dinner	Curry-Roasted Squash and Apple Soup (page 208) 1 cup (250 mL) cooked quinoa 1 cup (250 mL) cooked lentils	Curry-Roasted Squash and Apple Soup (page 208) 1 cup (250 mL) cooked quinoa 1 cup (250 mL) cooked lentils

Meal	Menu Plan for Women	Menu Plan for Men
Evening Snack		1 cup (250 mL) raspberries ¼ cup (60 mL) sliced almonds

Day 27: Saturday

Meal	Menu Plan for Women	Menu Plan for Men
Breakfast	1 whole-grain English muffin 2 oz (60 g) fortified soy cheese ½ cup (125 mL) fortified soy or rice yogurt 1 cup (250 mL) blackberries	1 whole-grain English muffin 2 oz (60 g) fortified soy cheese ½ cup (125 mL) fortified soy or rice yogurt 1 cup (250 mL) blackberries
Morning Snack	1 mango ½ cup (125 mL) fortified soy or rice yogurt	1 mango ½ cup (125 mL) fortified soy or rice yogurt 1 whole-grain cereal bar
Lunch	1 tofu burger 1 whole-grain bun 1 cup (250 mL) mixed salad greens 1 tbsp (15 mL) olive oil–based salad dressing	1 tofu burger 1 whole-grain bun 1 cup (250 mL) mixed salad greens 1 tbsp (15 mL) olive oil–based salad dressing
Afternoon Snack	1 cup (250 mL) chopped cantaloupe	1 cup (250 mL) chopped cantaloupe ¼ cup (60 mL) unsalted peanuts
Dinner	Rajasthani Mixed Dal (page 246), made with olive oil instead of ghee 1 cup (250 mL) cooked basmati rice 1 cup (250 mL) green peas, cooked	Rajasthani Mixed Dal (page 246), made with olive oil instead of ghee 1 cup (250 mL) cooked basmati rice 1 cup (250 mL) green peas, cooked
Evening Snack		1 orange

Day 28: Sunday

Meal	Menu Plan for Women	Menu Plan for Men
Breakfast	1 cup (250 mL) cooked oatmeal 1 cup (250 mL) strawberries 1 cup (250 mL) fortified rice, almond, or soy milk	1 cup (250 mL) cooked oatmeal 1 cup (250 mL) strawberries 2 tbsp (30 mL) ground flax seeds (flaxseed meal) 1 cup (250 mL) fortified rice, almond, or soy milk
Morning Snack	½ cup (125 mL) fortified soy or rice yogurt 2 tbsp (30 mL) ground flax seeds (flaxseed meal)	½ cup (125 mL) fortified soy or rice yogurt 2 tbsp (30 mL) ground flax seeds (flaxseed meal) 4 whole-grain crackers
Lunch	1 cup (250 mL) cooked mixed beans 1 cup (250 mL) cooked wild rice 1 cup (250 mL) broccoli	1 cup (250 mL) cooked mixed beans 1 cup (250 mL) cooked wild rice 1 cup (250 mL) broccoli
Afternoon Snack	1 cup (250 mL) fortified rice, almond, or soy milk	1 peach 1 cup (250 mL) fortified rice, almond, or soy milk
Dinner	Ginger-Laced Beet Soup with Orange (page 206) 1 whole wheat pita 2 tbsp (30 mL) hummus	Ginger-Laced Beet Soup with Orange (page 206) 1 whole wheat pita 2 tbsp (30 mL) hummus
Evening Snack		1 cup (250 mL) chopped watermelon 1 whole-grain cereal bar

RECIPES

Breakfasts and Beverages

Gluten-Free Flour Mix

If wheat products or eggs make your arthritis flare up, you might want to eliminate them from your diet. Using this easy recipe to make all your baked goods will allow you to enjoy your favorite treats!

TIP

Use this flour mix in place of wheat-based flours in cakes and other baked goods. One cup (250 mL) flour mix is the equivalent of 1 cup (250 mL) regular flour.

2 cups	finely ground brown rice flour	500 mL
¾ cup	potato starch (not potato flour)	175 mL
½ cup	tapioca flour	125 mL
1 tsp	xanthan gum	5 mL

1. In a large bowl, whisk together brown rice flour, potato starch, tapioca flour and xanthan gum until combined.
2. Transfer to an airtight container and store in a cool, dry, dark place (such as a cupboard) for up to 2 weeks.

Egg Replacements

Eggs thicken and bind ingredients in recipes. When whole eggs or egg whites are beaten or whipped, they hold air and cause the other ingredients to rise. Dishes such as puffy soufflés and angel food cakes rely on eggs for leavening.

Vegan egg replacement powders, available at natural food stores, are the best bet when egg whites for meringues or whipped egg whites are required. Vegan lecithin (from soybeans, peanuts and corn) can be used as an emulsifier to replace eggs in cooking. The following substitutes may be used in place of 1 egg as a thickener or binder:

- ½ mashed banana in baked goods that contain baking powder or soda
- 1 tbsp (15 mL) flax seeds or chia seeds dissolved in 2 tbsp (30 mL) water in baked goods and where ingredients need an emulsifier
- 2 tbsp (30 mL) cornstarch + ¼ cup (60 mL) water for soups and stews
- 2 tbsp (30 mL) arrowroot flour + ¼ cup (60 mL) water or other liquid, such as vegetable stock, broth or juice, for anything that needs to be dissolved before adding to the recipe
- 1 tbsp (15 mL) chickpea flour + 2 tbsp (30 mL) water as a binder in pancakes and baked products
- 1 tbsp (15 mL) soy powder + 2 tbsp (30 mL) water for batters and doughs

Nutrients per ¼ cup (60 mL)	
Calories	176
Fat	1 g
Carbohydrates	40 g
Protein	3 g

Mushroom Egg Scramble

This recipe makes a wonderfully nourishing breakfast or even a quick lunch. Using eggs that contain omega-3 fatty acids will help you get more of this inflammation-fighting nutrient in your diet.

TIP

Serve over whole wheat toast or toasted English muffin halves.

1 tbsp	butter or margarine	15 mL
2	large mushrooms, sliced	2
2	large eggs	2
2 tbsp	milk	30 mL
	Salt and freshly ground black pepper	

1. In a nonstick skillet over high heat, melt butter. Add mushrooms and cook, stirring often, for 5 minutes or until golden brown.

2. Whisk together eggs, milk, salt and pepper. Reduce heat to low. Pour egg mixture into skillet with mushrooms, stirring occasionally until eggs are set.

Nutrients per serving	
Calories	135
Fat	10 g
Carbohydrates	3 g
Protein	7 g

Buttermilk Buckwheat Pancakes

Makes 6 servings

Buckwheat is a great source of some amazing phytochemicals that help our bodies stay healthy. Spread each pancake with a bit of fruit butter and top with some ground nuts for a tasty, well-balanced breakfast.

TIPS

Buckwheat flour is available in natural food stores. If you don't have any, you can make your own by processing kasha or toasted buckwheat groats in a food processor until finely ground.

You can make this batter ahead and store it, covered, in the refrigerator for up to 2 days. The batter will thicken a bit, so you may need to add a little buttermilk to thin it out. Your pancakes will not be as airy as those made immediately after mixing, but they will still be delicious.

- **Food processor**

2½ cups	buttermilk	625 mL
2 tsp	baking powder	10 mL
1 tsp	baking soda	5 mL
½ tsp	salt	2 mL
1 tbsp	light (fancy) molasses	15 mL
1	large egg	1
2 cups	buckwheat flour (see tip, at left)	500 mL

1. In food processor, combine buttermilk, baking powder, baking soda and salt. Pulse to blend. Add molasses and egg and pulse to blend. Add buckwheat flour and pulse just until combined. Set aside for 5 minutes. Mixture should be of a pourable consistency. If necessary, add more flour or buttermilk and pulse until blended.

2. Heat a lightly greased nonstick skillet over medium heat until water dropped on the surface bounces before evaporating. Add about ¼ cup (60 mL) batter at a time and cook until bubbles appear all over the top surface, then flip and cook until bottom side is browned, about 1 minute per side. Keep warm. Continue with remaining batter.

Nutrients per serving	
Calories	92
Fat	2 g
Carbohydrates	16 g
Protein	4 g

Rhubarb Orange Muffins

Makes 12 muffins

Delicious and healthy —
who could ask for more?
Gluten-free sorghum
flour has a mild taste,
so it easily replaces
wheat in baked goods.

TIPS

When using frozen rhubarb,
it is easier to chop while still
partially frozen. The rhubarb
must be finely chopped;
otherwise, the finished
muffin will be crumbly.

Xanthan gum, which is made
from corn syrup, is used as
a thickener. It is available in
natural foods stores.

If you're making these
muffins for someone who
can't tolerate gluten, check
your baking powder, as some
brands contain wheat starch.
You may need to purchase a
gluten-free variety.

Nutrients per muffin	
Calories	172
Fat	8 g
Carbohydrates	24 g
Protein	3 g

- **12-cup muffin pan, lightly greased**

1¾ cups	finely chopped rhubarb	425 mL
⅓ cup	granulated sugar	75 mL
1⅓ cups	sorghum flour	325 mL
⅓ cup	quinoa flour	75 mL
⅓ cup	potato starch	75 mL
1½ tsp	xanthan gum	7 mL
1 tbsp	baking powder	15 mL
1 tsp	baking soda	5 mL
½ tsp	salt	2 mL
1	large egg	1
2 tbsp	finely grated orange zest	30 mL
⅔ cup	freshly squeezed orange juice	150 mL
3 tbsp	vegetable oil	45 mL
1 tsp	vanilla extract	5 mL
½ cup	chopped walnuts	125 mL

1. In a bowl, combine rhubarb and sugar. Mix well and set aside for 10 minutes.

2. In a large bowl, combine sorghum and quinoa flours, potato starch, xanthan gum, baking powder, baking soda and salt.

3. In a separate bowl, using an electric mixer, beat egg, orange zest, orange juice, oil and vanilla until combined. Stir in rhubarb, then dry ingredients just until combined. Stir in walnuts.

4. Divide batter evenly among prepared muffin cups. Let stand for 30 minutes. Meanwhile, preheat oven to 350°F (180°C).

5. Bake for 18 to 20 minutes or until firm to the touch. Remove from pan immediately and let cool completely on a wire rack.

VARIATIONS

Rhubarb Orange Bread: Spoon batter into a lightly greased 9- by 5-inch (23 by 12.5 cm) loaf pan and bake in preheated oven until a tester inserted in the center comes out clean, 55 to 65 minutes.

Substitute pecans or ¼ cup (60 mL) green pumpkin seeds for the walnuts.

Orange Cranberry Flax Muffins

Makes 18 muffins

Dried cranberries are packed with phytochemicals and anti-inflammatory nutrients. Whole cranberries (including dried) provide more nutrition than cranberry juices or drinks.

TIPS

Assemble the wet and dry ingredients in separate bowls on Friday night so that it takes less than a minute to finish the prep work in the morning. Be sure to refrigerate the wet ingredients.

These muffins freeze well. Wrap cooled muffins individually in plastic wrap, then seal in an airtight container or freezer bag and freeze for up to 1 month.

- Preheat oven to 375°F (190°C)
- Two 12-cup muffin pans, 18 cups lightly greased or lined with paper cups

¾ cup	dried cranberries, coarsely chopped	175 mL
1½ cups	orange juice, divided	375 mL
2 cups	all-purpose flour	500 mL
¾ cup	whole wheat flour	175 mL
½ cup	ground flax seeds (flaxseed meal)	125 mL
½ cup	granulated sugar	125 mL
2 tsp	grated orange zest	10 mL
2 tsp	baking powder	10 mL
1 tsp	baking soda	5 mL
1	large egg, beaten	1
¼ cup	canola oil	60 mL

1. In a small bowl, combine cranberries and ¼ cup (60 mL) of the orange juice. Set aside.

2. In a large bowl, combine all-purpose flour, whole wheat flour, flax seeds, sugar, orange zest, baking powder and baking soda.

3. In a medium bowl, whisk together egg, oil and the remaining orange juice until blended. Pour over flour mixture and stir until just combined. Fold in cranberry mixture.

4. Divide batter evenly among prepared muffin cups. Bake in preheated oven for 16 to 18 minutes or until tops are firm to the touch and a tester inserted in the center of a muffin comes out clean. Let cool in pans on a wire rack for 10 minutes, then transfer to rack to cool completely.

VARIATION

Substitute dried cherries or dried blueberries for the cranberries.

This recipe courtesy of dietitian Joan Rew.

Nutrients per muffin

Calories	162
Fat	5 g
Carbohydrates	27 g
Protein	3 g

Kasha Pudding
with Apple and Raisins

To get the same amount of vitamin D and calcium as cow's milk, make sure to use fortified rice or soy milk. Lower-fat cottage cheese contains 2% fat or less.

TIP

For breakfast, serve with fresh fruit (bananas, blueberries, peaches) and milk. As a satisfying afternoon snack or dessert, garnish with 1 cup (250 mL) drained natural yogurt.

MAKE AHEAD

Let cool completely, cover and refrigerate overnight. Reheat in a 350°F (180°C) oven for 15 to 20 minutes.

- Preheat oven to 375°F (190°C)
- 8-inch (20 cm) baking dish with lid or foil, lightly oiled

1 cup	rice or soy milk	250 mL
½ cup	kasha	125 mL
2	large eggs	2
1 cup	lower-fat cottage cheese	250 mL
½ cup	lower-fat plain yogurt	125 mL
1	small apple, finely chopped	1
¼ cup	raisins	60 mL
1 tsp	vanilla extract	5 mL
1 tsp	ground cinnamon	5 mL

1. In a small saucepan, bring milk to a boil over medium-high heat. Stir in kasha. Reduce heat and simmer, stirring occasionally, for 10 to 12 minutes or until all liquid has been absorbed. Transfer to a wire rack and let cool.

2. Meanwhile, in a large bowl, beat eggs. Stir in cheese and yogurt, mashing cheese with a fork to break up the curds.

3. Stir apple and raisins into kasha. Add vanilla and cinnamon. Using a spatula, scrape kasha mixture into cheese mixture and mix well. Spread into prepared baking dish.

4. Bake in preheated oven for 30 to 40 minutes or until lightly browned. Serve warm or at room temperature.

VARIATION

For a sweeter pudding, substitute ¼ cup (60 mL) chopped dates for the raisins.

Nutrients per serving	
Calories	169
Fat	3 g
Carbohydrates	26 g
Protein	10 g

Cranberry Quinoa Porridge

Makes 6 servings

This is a tasty, nutritious alternative to oatmeal porridge. There is about 3 grams of fiber in ¼ cup (60 mL) uncooked quinoa. If you'd like to add a fiber boost, sprinkle some flax seeds over the porridge.

TIP

Unless you have a stove with a true simmer, after reducing the heat to low, I recommend placing a heat diffuser under the pot to prevent the mixture from boiling. This device also helps to ensure the grains will cook evenly and prevents hot spots, which might cause scorching. Heat diffusers are available at kitchen supply and hardware stores and are made to work on gas or electric stoves.

3 cups	water	750 mL
1 cup	quinoa, rinsed	250 mL
½ cup	dried cranberries	125 mL
	Pure maple syrup or liquid honey	
	Milk or non-dairy alternative (optional)	

1. In a saucepan over medium heat, bring water to a boil. Stir in quinoa and cranberries and return to a boil. Reduce heat to low. Cover and simmer until quinoa is cooked (look for a white line around the seeds), about 15 minutes. Remove from heat and let stand, covered, about 5 minutes. Serve with maple syrup and milk or non-dairy alternative (if using).

VARIATIONS

Substitute dried cherries, dried blueberries or raisins for the cranberries.

Use red quinoa for a change.

Nutrients per serving	
Calories	137
Fat	2 g
Carbohydrates	28 g
Protein	4 g

Hot Cereal with Multigrains

Makes about 3 cups (750 mL)

Turn this great hot cereal into a cold muesli by adding ¾ cup (175 mL) milk, soy milk or almond milk to ¼ cup (60 mL) cereal. Let it stand to absorb some of the liquid while you are preparing for your busy day.

TIPS

Ingredients such as wheat flakes can be found in bulk or health food stores. Rye flakes or cracked wheat are good replacements for wheat flakes.

To release the health benefits of flax seeds, the hard outer coating must be broken down. You can buy ground flax seeds (flaxseed meal) or easily prepare your own. This is best done using a blender, a mini food processor or a coffee grinder.

Dried fruit such as apricots, raisins, cherries and cranberries are all excellent additions.

Nutrients per ¼ cup (60 mL) dry cereal mix	
Calories	86
Fat	3 g
Carbohydrates	15 g
Protein	4 g

- **Small blender or coffee grinder**

Dry Cereal Mix

2 cups	large flake (old-fashioned) rolled oats	500 mL
½ cup	wheat flakes	125 mL
½ cup	oat bran	125 mL
¼ cup	flax seeds, divided	60 mL

1. In a medium bowl, combine rolled oats, wheat flakes and oat bran.

2. Place half the flax seeds in blender. Process to fine meal. Combine flaxseed meal and remaining seeds with rolled oat mixture. Store in a tightly sealed container for several weeks or for longer storage in the refrigerator.

For a Single Serving

Microwave

1. In a microwave-safe serving bowl, combine ¼ cup (60 mL) Dry Cereal Mix, ¾ cup (175 mL) water and dash vanilla or maple extract. Microwave, uncovered, on High for 2 minutes. Stir. Microwave on Low for 3 minutes. Let stand for 2 minutes. Stir and serve.

Stovetop

1. In a small saucepan over medium heat, bring ¼ cup (60 mL) Dry Cereal Mix, ¾ cup (175 mL) water and dash vanilla or maple extract to a boil. Reduce heat to low. Cook, stirring occasionally, for 3 minutes or until desired consistency. Cover and remove from heat. Let stand for a few minutes. Stir and serve.

Orange-Spiked Power Cereal

> **Makes about 12 cups (3 L)**

Large-flake oats add texture and contribute to a lower glycemic index in this delicious cereal. The raisins, prunes and dates add lots of natural sweetness. Feel free to adjust the amount of agave nectar to suit your taste.

- **Preheat oven to 300°F (150°C)**
- **2 rimmed baking sheets**

4 cups	large-flake (old-fashioned) rolled oats	1 L
1 cup	chopped unsulfured prunes or dried apples	250 mL
1 cup	coarsely chopped almonds	250 mL
1 cup	unsweetened shredded coconut (optional)	250 mL
¾ cup	unsalted raw sunflower seeds	175 mL
½ cup	whole-grain teff	125 mL
½ cup	chopped unsulfured dried apricots	125 mL
½ cup	chopped raisins	125 mL
¼ cup	raw pumpkin seeds	60 mL
1 cup	agave nectar or brown rice syrup	250 mL
¼ cup	coconut oil	60 mL
½ cup	chopped dates	125 mL
2 tsp	ground cinnamon	10 mL
	Grated zest of 1 orange	

1. In a large bowl, combine oats, prunes, almonds, coconut (if using), sunflower seeds, teff, apricots, raisins and pumpkin seeds.

2. In a small saucepan, heat agave nectar and coconut oil over medium heat. Add dates, cinnamon and orange zest. Cook, stirring constantly, until dates are softened and mixture is thick, about 5 minutes. Pour over grains and mix well.

3. Divide mixture evenly between baking sheets and spread in a thin layer. Bake in preheated oven, stirring every 10 minutes, for 40 minutes or until grains and nuts are toasted and golden brown. Let cool on baking sheets, running a metal spatula under the grains to loosen them periodically as they cool.

4. Store cereal in an airtight container at room temperature for 2 to 3 weeks or in the refrigerator for up to 2 months.

VARIATIONS

Tailor this great-tasting snack to your own tastes by using any nuts, seeds and dried fruit.

Use lemon zest in place of the orange zest.

Nutrients per 1 cup (250 mL)	
Calories	495
Fat	23 g
Carbohydrates	68 g
Protein	11 g

Apple Berry Muesli

Makes 8 servings

Here's a filling and delicious way to start the day.

TIP

If you're using frozen berries, thaw them in the fridge overnight and drain liquid before adding to the yogurt mixture.

VARIATION

Turn this into a vegan meal by using soy yogurt in place of the yogurt, and a fortified vegan option, such as soy milk or coconut milk, in place of the milk.

2 cups	quick-cooking rolled oats	500 mL
2 cups	low-fat plain yogurt	500 mL
1 cup	milk	250 mL
3 tbsp	granulated sugar or liquid honey	45 mL
2	large apples, cored	2
	Juice of ½ lemon	
1 cup	chopped berries	250 mL
	Raisins and nuts (optional)	

1. In a medium bowl, combine oats, yogurt, milk and sugar. Set aside.

2. Grate apples, leaving the skin on. Sprinkle with lemon juice to prevent browning. Add apples and berries to yogurt mixture. Gently mix together. Refrigerate overnight. Serve topped with raisins and/or nuts, if desired.

This recipe courtesy of dietitian Sandra Gabriele.

Nutrients per serving			
Calories	201	Carbohydrates	36 g
Fat	3 g	Protein	8 g

Citrus Cocktail

Makes 2 servings

Make this cocktail with plain yogurt so the fruit flavors shine through. The yogurt helps slow the absorption of the sugars from the juices.

Nutrients per serving	
Calories	97
Fat	2 g
Carbohydrates	20 g
Protein	3 g

- **Blender**

½ cup	orange juice	125 mL
¼ cup	grapefruit juice	60 mL
12	strawberries, hulled and halved	12
1	½-inch (1 cm) piece gingerroot, sliced (optional)	1
¼ cup	natural or frozen yogurt	60 mL

1. In blender, combine orange juice, grapefruit juice, strawberries, ginger (if using) and yogurt. Cover and blend on Low for 30 seconds. Gradually increase speed to High and blend for 30 seconds or until smooth.

Cumin Mint Refresher

This refreshing drink is abundant in phytochemicals, which seem to promote good health and decrease inflammation.

TIP

This beverage can be refrigerated for up to 3 days. Always stir well before serving.

- **Blender**

1 cup	fresh mint leaves	250 mL
¼ cup	fresh cilantro leaves and soft stems	60 mL
1 tsp	chopped green chile pepper (preferably serrano)	5 mL
1 tsp	minced gingerroot	5 mL
⅓ cup	unsalted Thai tamarind purée	75 mL
2½ tsp	black salt (kala namak)	12 mL
2 tsp	toasted cumin seeds, powdered	10 mL
4	fresh mint leaves	4

1. In blender, combine 1 cup (250 mL) mint, cilantro, chiles and ginger. Spoon tamarind over top. Blend to a paste, scraping down sides of blender a couple of times. Transfer to a pitcher.

2. Add 4 cups (1 L) water, black salt and cumin and stir vigorously to mix well. Refrigerate until chilled, at least 3 hours, preferably 10 to 12 hours. Stir well a couple of times while in the refrigerator as herbs and spices tend to settle.

3. Stir just before serving. Pour into juice glasses. Garnish with mint and serve chilled.

Nutrients per serving	
Calories	33
Fat	0 g
Carbohydrates	8 g
Protein	1 g

Masala Chai

Store-bought chai tea can be filled with sugar. When making this recipe, feel free to use the alternative sweetener of your choice. You'll control the amount of sweetener while getting all the benefits of chai's great taste and good nutrition.

TIP

If making 4 cups (1 L) or more at a time, reduce tea to ¾ tsp (3 mL) per cup.

1½ cups	water	375 mL
½ cup	milk	125 mL
2	whole cloves	2
1	green cardamom pod, one side peeled open	1
1	thin slice gingerroot (about ½ inch/1 cm round)	1
4 to 5	2-inch (5 cm) pieces lemongrass (optional)	4 to 5
2 tsp	Indian black tea leaves	10 mL
2 tsp	granulated sugar, or to taste	10 mL

1. In a saucepan over medium-high heat, combine water, milk, cloves, cardamom, ginger and lemongrass (if using). Bring to a boil.

2. Add tea and sugar. Reduce heat to medium and simmer for 2 minutes. Remove from heat, cover and let tea steep for 3 to 4 minutes longer. (If using an electric stove, turn off heat, cover and leave on burner.) Strain into warmed teapot or cups.

Nutrients per ½ cup (125 mL)	
Calories	22
Fat	1 g
Carbohydrates	3 g
Protein	1 g

Appetizers and Snacks, Spreads and Sauces

Steamed Mussels with Vinaigrette

Mussels are a great source of omega-3 fatty acids and contain more iron than a similar-size portion of chicken or turkey. And brightly colored peppers are a great source of nutrients. Together, they add up to a fabulous appetizer, packed with nutrition.

TIP

Scrub mussels using a toothbrush. Using a dry towel, sharply pull out the fibrous beard (also known as byssal threads) toward the hinge end of the mussel. This will ensure that the mussel remains alive. Only begin cooking with mussels that are completely closed. Mussels should open during cooking.

24	mussels, scrubbed and debearded (see tip, at left)	24
1	roasted red bell pepper, peeled, seeded and finely chopped	1
1	roasted orange bell pepper, peeled, seeded and finely chopped	1
1	roasted yellow bell pepper, peeled, seeded and finely chopped	1
1	hard-cooked egg, chopped	1
¼ cup	olive oil	60 mL
¼ cup	red wine vinegar	60 mL
2 tbsp	chopped fresh parsley	30 mL
½ tsp	salt	2 mL
	Freshly ground black pepper	

1. In a large pot, bring 1 inch (2.5 cm) of water to a boil over high heat. Add mussels, cover and steam for 3 to 5 minutes or until mussels have opened. Drain mussels and discard any unopened mussels.

2. Remove one side of each shell and arrange the open-shelled mussels on a serving platter.

3. In a medium bowl, combine red, orange and yellow peppers, egg, oil, vinegar, parsley, salt and pepper to taste. Spoon over mussels. Cover and refrigerate until ready to serve. Refrigerated mussels should be eaten within 2 days.

Nutrients per serving

Calories	168
Fat	12 g
Carbohydrates	6 g
Protein	9 g

Crab and Smoked Salmon Tea Sandwiches

Makes 4 servings

Omega-3 fatty acids abound in these dainty sandwiches. If you're trying to avoid wheat, choose gluten-free bread or spread the fillings on gluten-free crackers.

TIP

Leaving the crusts on the bread or choosing whole-grain buns turns these sandwiches into a hearty casual meal.

6 oz	backfin (lump) crabmeat, shells picked out	175 g
3	green onions, finely chopped	3
3 tbsp	mayonnaise	45 mL
8	thin slices sandwich bread, one side buttered, divided	8
4	thin slices sandwich bread, toasted and both sides buttered	4
2 oz	cream cheese, softened	60 g
1 oz	smoked salmon, chopped	30 g
1 tbsp	chopped fresh dill	15 mL

1. Combine crabmeat, green onions and mayonnaise; spoon on the buttered sides of 4 of the untoasted bread slices. Top with toasted slices.

2. Combine cream cheese, smoked salmon and dill; spread on the exposed side of the toasted bread. Top with the remaining bread, buttered sides down.

3. Cut off crusts and slice each sandwich into 3 fingers.

Nutrients per serving	
Calories	395
Fat	17 g
Carbohydrates	43 g
Protein	18 g

Braised Endive and Tomato Gratinée

Makes 2 servings

Endive is extremely low in calories, which is a boon to people who are trying to manage their weight. Choose your favorite cheese and use it sparingly — in this recipe, the cheese is meant to be a great supporting component, not the star.

2	endives	2
2 tbsp	water	30 mL
1 tbsp	olive oil	15 mL
4	black olives, pitted and cut into thirds	4
2	cloves garlic, thinly sliced	2
2	sun-dried tomatoes, cut into thirds	2
1	ripe tomato, cut into $\frac{1}{2}$-inch (1 cm) wedges	1
Pinch	dried oregano	Pinch
Pinch	dried basil	Pinch
$\frac{1}{4}$ tsp	salt	1 mL
$\frac{1}{8}$ tsp	freshly ground black pepper	0.5 mL
2 oz	sharp cheese (such as pecorino, Parmesan or sharp/old Cheddar), shredded	60 g
	Few sprigs fresh basil or parsley, chopped	

1. Place endives into a small shallow pot with a lid. Add water, olive oil, olives, garlic, sun-dried tomatoes, tomato, oregano, basil, salt and pepper; cook over high heat for 1 to 2 minutes or until bubbling. Push the tomato wedges to the bottom of the pot around the endives, pushing the other ingredients into the ensuing liquid. Reduce heat to minimum, cover and cook undisturbed for 35 minutes or until soft and pierceable. (The recipe can prepared to this point up to 2 hours in advance.)

2. Carefully transfer endives to a small ovenproof dish. (They should fit snugly.) Cover endives with sauce. With a sharp knife, slice the endives halfway down and open up the cuts so that they are somewhat butterflied. Sprinkle shredded cheese evenly on the butterflied surfaces. Place under a hot broiler for 3 to 4 minutes, until the cheese is bubbling and beginning to char. Lift the endives carefully with a spatula onto 2 plates and pour sauce around them. Garnish with chopped basil or parsley. Serve immediately.

Nutrients per serving	
Calories	313
Fat	20 g
Carbohydrates	24 g
Protein	15 g

Lemon Rosemary Olives

Olives make a healthy and delicious snack. To reduce the sodium even more than you will by rinsing the olives, let them soak in cold water, changing the water two or three times. Olives prepared this way can be refrigerated for up to 1 week.

½ cup	kalamata olives	125 mL
½ cup	large green olives	125 mL
1 tbsp	chopped fresh thyme	15 mL
1 tbsp	chopped fresh rosemary	15 mL
½ tsp	grated lemon zest	2 mL
1 tbsp	freshly squeezed lemon juice	15 mL
1	clove garlic, thinly sliced	1
½ tsp	freshly ground black pepper	2 mL
1 tbsp	extra virgin olive oil	15 mL

1. Rinse kalamata and green olives to remove brine. Drain and pat dry.

2. In a bowl, combine olives, thyme, rosemary, lemon zest and juice, garlic and pepper. Add oil and mix well. Set aside for flavors to meld.

Nutrients per 2 tbsp (30 mL)	
Calories	39
Fat	4 g
Carbohydrates	1 g
Protein	0 g

Seasoned Chickpeas and Almonds

Makes about 4 cups (1 L)

Plain almonds can be boring, but this spicy combo of chickpeas and almonds is anything but! The garlic and garam masala add phytochemicals as well as a ton of flavor.

TIPS

You can use 2 cups (500 mL) cooked chickpeas, drained and rinsed, instead of canned.

Add another teaspoon (5 mL) of hot pepper flakes if you like heat.

- **Preheat oven to 400°F (200°C)**
- **Rimmed baking sheet, lightly oiled**

2 cups	whole almonds (unblanched)	500 mL
1	can (14 to 19 oz/398 to 540 mL) chickpeas, drained and rinsed	1
3	cloves garlic, coarsely chopped	3
2 tbsp	olive oil	30 mL
1 tbsp	freshly squeezed lime juice	15 mL
1 tbsp	garam masala	15 mL
1 tsp	hot pepper flakes	5 mL
	Sea salt and freshly ground black pepper	

1. In a bowl, combine almonds, chickpeas, garlic, oil, lime juice, garam masala, hot pepper flakes and salt and pepper to taste. Spread evenly on prepared baking sheet. Bake in preheated oven, stirring once, for 30 minutes. Test for crunchiness and return to the oven, testing every 5 minutes until the desired dryness is achieved. Let cool.

2. Store mixture in an airtight container in the refrigerator for up to 2 weeks.

VARIATION

Use your favorite spice blend in place of the garam masala.

Nutrients per ¼ cup (60 mL)	
Calories	151
Fat	12 g
Carbohydrates	8 g
Protein	5 g

Healthy Snack Mix

When you make your own snack mix, you can include only the types of nuts, dried fruits and seeds you prefer, and make sure that you achieve the perfect balance of all the elements. Plus, there's no added sodium or sugar.

1 cup	whole almonds	250 mL
½ cup	roasted peanuts	125 mL
½ cup	golden raisins	125 mL
½ cup	dark raisins	125 mL
½ cup	toasted wheat germ	125 mL
¼ cup	toasted sesame seeds	60 mL
¼ cup	roasted sunflower seeds	60 mL

1. In a large bowl, combine almonds, peanuts, golden raisins, dark raisins, wheat germ, sesame seeds and sunflower seeds.
2. Store at room temperature in an airtight container for up to 2 days.

Nutrients per 1 tbsp (15 mL)			
Calories	207	Carbohydrates	17 g
Fat	13 g	Protein	7 g

Green Olive Tapenade

Green olives are as nutritious as black olives. This spread is a great substitute for mayonnaise on a sandwich, or can be added to tuna or salmon to make a wonderful salad.

- **Food processor**

1 cup	pitted drained green olives	250 mL
¼ cup	fresh basil leaves	60 mL
2	cloves garlic, coarsely chopped	2
1 tbsp	drained capers	15 mL
¼ cup	extra virgin olive oil	60 mL
1 tbsp	freshly squeezed lemon juice	15 mL

1. In food processor, pulse olives, basil, garlic and capers until finely chopped. With the motor running, slowly add olive oil and lemon juice through the feed tube and process just until blended.
2. Transfer to a small serving bowl. Cover and refrigerate for at least 2 hours or for up to 3 days.

Nutrients per 1 tbsp (15 mL)			
Calories	44	Carbohydrates	1 g
Fat	5 g	Protein	0 g

Black Olive Pâté

Makes 6 servings

Black olives are a wonderful source of omega-3 fatty acids and contain a bevy of phytochemicals. Make sure to choose whole-grain bread.

TIPS

This versatile mixture is wonderful tossed with fresh, hot pasta. You can also try it as a topping for grilled fish or chicken, or as an omelet filling.

Don't choose kalamata olives for this preparation, as they are just a little too bitter.

Allow the pâté to come to room temperature before serving as a spread.

You can vary the recipe by adding a few sun-dried tomatoes, roasted red peppers, grilled eggplant or 1 or 2 dried chile peppers. A jar of this makes a wonderful gift for olive lovers.

- **Food processor (optional)**

1 cup	pitted black olives (preferably oil-cured)	250 mL
4	sprigs fresh flat-leaf (Italian) parsley	4
2 tbsp	fresh bread crumbs	30 mL
1 tbsp	butter	15 mL
1½ tsp	grated lemon zest	7 mL
2 tbsp	freshly squeezed lemon juice	30 mL
2 tbsp	extra virgin olive oil	30 mL
	Salt and freshly ground black pepper	
6	slices rustic country-style bread	6
	Olive oil	

1. In food processor, combine olives, parsley, bread crumbs, butter, lemon zest, lemon juice and olive oil; blend until a smooth paste forms. (Alternatively, with a sharp chef's knife, finely chop olives, parsley, bread crumbs and lemon zest; transfer to a bowl and blend in butter, lemon juice and olive oil.) Season to taste with salt and pepper.

2. Brush bread slices with a little olive oil. Grill or toast until golden. Spread each slice with about 2 tbsp (30 mL) of the olivada. Serve immediately.

Nutrients per serving	
Calories	186
Fat	10 g
Carbohydrates	22 g
Protein	4 g

Italian White Bean Spread

**Makes about
2 cups (500 mL)**

Enjoy this spread as a snack with whole-grain or gluten-free bread or crackers. Make sure to rinse the beans well, as rinsing canned beans can remove up to 50% of the sodium.

TIPS

Dip can be made up to 3 days ahead.

Instead of finely chopped fresh herbs, you can use frozen chopped herbs.

- **Food processor**

2 tbsp	olive oil	30 mL
1	small onion, finely chopped	1
2	large cloves garlic, finely chopped	2
1 tbsp	red wine vinegar	15 mL
1	can (19 oz/540 mL) white kidney beans, drained and rinsed	1
2 tbsp	finely chopped, drained, oil-packed sun-dried tomatoes	30 mL
1 tbsp	chopped fresh parsley	15 mL
1 tbsp	chopped fresh basil	15 mL
	Freshly ground black pepper	

1. In a small skillet, heat oil over medium heat. Cook onion and garlic, stirring occasionally, for 3 minutes or until softened (do not brown). Add vinegar and remove from heat.

2. In food processor, purée kidney beans and onion mixture until smooth.

3. Transfer to a bowl. Stir in sun-dried tomatoes, parsley and basil; season with pepper to taste. Cover and refrigerate.

VARIATION

Greek White Bean Spread: Instead of fresh basil, increase chopped parsley to 2 tbsp (30 mL) and add $\frac{1}{2}$ tsp (2 mL) dried oregano to the onions when cooking.

Nutrients per 1 tbsp (15 mL)	
Calories	26
Fat	1 g
Carbohydrates	3 g
Protein	1 g

Tunnato Spread

Makes about 1½ cups (375 mL)

The parsley in this spread contributes many nutrients that may help reduce inflammation. If you can't find tuna packed in olive oil, choose tuna packed in broth or water.

TIP

Don't confuse real mayonnaise with "mayonnaise-type" salad dressings, which are similar in appearance. Mayonnaise is a combination of egg yolks, vinegar or lemon juice, olive oil and seasonings. Imitators will contain additional ingredients, such as sugar, flour or milk. Make sure the label says mayonnaise and check the ingredients.

- **Food processor**

¾ cup	mayonnaise	175 mL
1	can (6 oz/170 g) tuna (preferably Italian), packed in olive oil, drained	1
20	fresh parsley leaves	20
	Crudités	

1. In food processor, combine mayonnaise, tuna and parsley. Process until smooth.

2. Transfer to a small bowl and serve surrounded by crudités for dipping. If not using immediately, cover spread and refrigerate for up to 3 days.

VARIATIONS

Tunnato-Stuffed Eggs: Hard-cook 4 eggs. Let cool and peel. Cut in half lengthwise. Pop out the yolks and mash with ¼ cup (60 mL) Tunnato Spread. Mound the mixture back into the whites. Dust with 1 tsp (5 mL) paprika, if desired. If you prefer a plated appetizer, simply cut the peeled cooked eggs in half, arrange them on a platter and spoon the sauce over top. Makes 6 to 8 servings.

Asparagus with Tunnato: Arrange 1 can or jar (16 oz/330 g approx.) white asparagus, drained, on a small platter or serving plate. Top with ¼ cup (60 mL) Tunnato Spread. Use fresh green asparagus in season, if desired. You can also turn this into a salad by spreading a layer of salad greens over a large platter. Arrange the asparagus over the greens and top with Tunnato Spread. Makes 4 servings.

Nutrients per 1 tbsp (15 mL)	
Calories	43
Fat	3 g
Carbohydrates	2 g
Protein	2 g

Fruit Purée (Butter Replacement)

**Makes about
1¾ cups (425 mL)**

This terrific vegan substitute for butter can even be used in baking, although it is quite sweet, so you may want to reduce the amount of sugar that the recipe calls for. To replace 1 cup (250 mL) butter, use ¾ cup (175 mL) fruit purée. If you prefer a milder flavor, replace the olive oil with canola oil.

TIPS

Lecithin, available in dried granules at natural food stores, is a fatty substance that occurs in both plant and animal tissues.

For a lighter-tasting butter substitute, omit the prunes and dates and use 4 apples.

- **Blender or food processor**

1 cup	water	250 mL
3	apples, peeled and cut into chunks	3
½ cup	pitted prunes	125 mL
¼ cup	chopped dates	60 mL
2 tbsp	organic cane sugar	30 mL
1 tbsp	lecithin granules (optional)	15 mL
1 tbsp	freshly squeezed lemon juice	15 mL
Pinch	sea salt	Pinch
3 tbsp	olive oil	45 mL

1. In a saucepan over high heat, bring water to a boil. Add apples, prunes, dates, sugar, lecithin (if using), lemon juice and salt. Reduce heat and simmer, stirring occasionally, for 1 hour or until very soft. Let cool.

2. Spoon fruit mixture into blender and, with the motor running, slowly pour oil through the feed tube. Blend until oil is completely incorporated into the mixture.

3. Store purée tightly covered in the refrigerator for up to 4 days.

Nutrients per 1 tbsp (15 mL)	
Calories	39
Fat	2 g
Carbohydrates	7 g
Protein	0 g

Asian Dressing and Dip

Makes about ½ cup (125 mL)

Drizzle this versatile dressing over salad or serve it as a dip with crudités. The best choice for the vegetable oil is canola oil, which contains omega-3 fatty acids and has a mild taste.

TIP

Bird's eye chiles are tiny, thin-skinned red Thai chiles that pack quite a heat. Add amounts that suit your taste.

3 tbsp	natural rice vinegar	45 mL
2 tbsp	freshly squeezed lime juice	30 mL
2 tbsp	granulated sugar	30 mL
1 tbsp	finely chopped gingerroot	15 mL
1 tbsp	finely chopped lemongrass	15 mL
2 tsp	fish sauce (nam pla)	10 mL
½ to 1	bird's eye (Thai) chile, seeded and finely chopped	½ to 1
¼ cup	vegetable oil	60 mL
1 tbsp	sesame oil	15 mL
	Kosher or sea salt	

1. In a small bowl, combine vinegar, lime juice, sugar, ginger, lemongrass, fish sauce and chile. Whisk in vegetable and sesame oils. Season with salt to taste.

Nutrients per 1 tbsp (15 mL)

Calories	90	Carbohydrates	4 g
Fat	9 g	Protein	0 g

Tofu Mayonnaise

Makes about 1 cup (250 mL)

Tofu mayonnaise can replace regular mayonnaise in any recipe. Check the package of tofu carefully, as this recipe will not be as smooth if made with firm or extra-firm tofu.

- **Blender or food processor**

1	clove garlic	1
8 oz	medium-soft or regular tofu, drained	250 g
2 tbsp	freshly squeezed lemon juice	30 mL
1 tbsp	olive oil	15 mL
1 tsp	Dijon mustard	5 mL
	Sea salt	

1. In blender, chop garlic. Add tofu, lemon juice, oil and mustard and process for 20 seconds or until smooth. Add salt to taste and process for 5 seconds to blend.

2. Transfer mixture to a clean container with lid. Store mayonnaise tightly covered in the refrigerator for up to 3 days.

Nutrients per 1 tbsp (15 mL)

Calories	17	Carbohydrates	1 g
Fat	1 g	Protein	1 g

Peanut Sauce

Peanut sauce tastes great on dumplings and makes a wonderful sauce for chicken or dressing for salad. It's also a good source of many phytochemicals. Choose natural peanut butter, as regular peanut butter may contain trans fats, sugar and salt.

MAKE AHEAD

Sauce can be made ahead, covered and refrigerated for up to 4 days or frozen for up to 4 weeks. Stir well after defrosting.

- **Food processor**

2 tbsp	vegetable oil	30 mL
2 tbsp	chopped gingerroot	30 mL
3	cloves garlic, chopped	3
4	green onions, chopped	4
½ cup	peanut butter	125 mL
½ cup	coconut milk	125 mL
¼ cup	coarsely chopped fresh cilantro	60 mL
2 tbsp	freshly squeezed lime or lemon juice	30 mL
1 tbsp	fish sauce (nam pla)	15 mL
1 tbsp	soy sauce	15 mL
1 tbsp	packed brown sugar	15 mL
½ tsp	hot pepper sauce	2 mL

1. In a small skillet, heat oil over medium heat. Add ginger, garlic and green onions. Cook for 2 minutes, stirring occasionally, until softened. Cool for 20 minutes.

2. In food processor, combine cooled ginger mixture, peanut butter, coconut milk, cilantro, lime juice, fish sauce, soy sauce, sugar and hot pepper sauce. Purée until smooth. (Sauce will be thick. For a slightly thinner sauce, add a small amount of water.)

Nutrients per 1 tbsp (15 mL)	
Calories	27
Fat	2 g
Carbohydrates	1 g
Protein	0 g

Barbecue Sauce

Commercial barbecue sauces contain a significant amount of sugar. Making your own allows you to control the amount and type of sweetener you use.

TIP

Store sauce in clean quart (1 L) or pint (500 mL) jars with lids in the refrigerator for up to 1 week or in freezer bags in the freezer for up to 2 months.

- Preheat oven to 400°F (200°C)
- 13- by 9-inch (33 by 23 cm) baking pan, lightly oiled
- Blender or food processor

6	large ripe tomatoes (about 4 lbs/2 kg)	6
1	onion, quartered	1
1	whole head garlic	1
3 tbsp	olive oil, divided	45 mL
1	can (5½ oz/156 mL) tomato paste	1
⅓ cup	blackstrap molasses	75 mL
1 tbsp	apple cider vinegar	15 mL
2 tbsp	freshly squeezed lemon juice	30 mL
1 tbsp	tamari or soy sauce	15 mL
1 tsp	mustard powder	5 mL
2 tbsp	fresh thyme leaves	30 mL
	Salt and freshly ground pepper	

1. Core tomatoes, cut in half, gently squeeze out and discard seeds and liquid. Arrange tomatoes, cut side down, in prepared baking dish. Add onion wedges to the pan.

2. Remove the loose, papery skin from the garlic head and slice and discard ¼ inch (0.5 cm) off the tips of the cloves in the entire head, leaving the whole head intact. Place the garlic head, cut side up, in the baking pan with tomatoes and onion. Drizzle about 1 tbsp (15 mL) of the oil over garlic head and remaining 2 tbsp (30 mL) oil over tomatoes and onion. Roast in preheated oven for 1 hour. Let cool slightly.

3. Slip skins off tomatoes and using a slotted spoon, transfer to blender. Add onion to blender. Reserve pan juices for another use or freeze for vegetable stock. Squeeze roasted garlic cloves into the blender. Process for 30 seconds or until smooth.

4. Pour tomato purée into a saucepan. Add tomato paste, molasses, vinegar, lemon juice, tamari, mustard and thyme. Bring to a boil over high heat. Reduce heat and simmer, stirring occasionally, for 45 minutes. Let cool. Add salt and pepper, to taste.

Nutrients per 1 tbsp (15 mL)	
Calories	11
Fat	1 g
Carbohydrates	2 g
Protein	0 g

Soups

Vegetable Stock

Makes about 5 cups (1.25 L)

It's great to have vegetable stock on hand in the freezer. In addition to its use as a base for soups and stews, it makes a tasty drink instead of plain water and can be used to add flavor to cooked vegetables.

- **8-quart (8 L) stockpot**
- **Fine sieve, lined with cheesecloth**

2	carrots, roughly chopped	2
2	stalks celery, roughly chopped	2
1	onion, roughly chopped	1
1	leek, top green leaves only, roughly chopped	1
1 cup	mushroom stems	250 mL
2	cloves garlic, smashed	2
6 cups	cold water	1.5 L
1	bay leaf	1
4	sprigs thyme	4
4	sprigs parsley	4
1 tsp	whole black peppercorns	5 mL
½ tsp	kosher or sea salt	2 mL

1. In stockpot, combine carrots, celery, onion, leek, mushrooms, garlic and water. Tie bay leaf, thyme and parsley in a bundle with kitchen string and add to pot with peppercorns and salt.

2. Bring to a boil over medium heat. Reduce heat to low and simmer until liquid is flavorful, about 30 minutes.

3. Remove pot from heat. Pour stock into a large bowl through prepared sieve. Discard solids. Simmer stock to reduce and intensify flavor, if needed. Let cool. Keep in refrigerator in a covered container for up to 4 days or freeze for up to 3 months.

Nutrients per 1 cup (250 mL)	
Calories	29
Fat	0 g
Carbohydrates	7 g
Protein	1 g

Chicken Stock

Chicken stock is a fabulous base for great soups and sauces. Chilling the broth in the refrigerator before use makes it easier to remove the fat that congeals on the top. Freeze stock in small containers so you can thaw it quickly and easily.

3 lbs	chicken bones (such as neck, backbones and wing tips)	1.5 kg
2	carrots, coarsely chopped	2
2	stalks celery, including leaves, chopped	1
1	large onion, chopped	1
½ tsp	dried thyme	2 mL
1	bay leaf	1
	Salt and freshly ground black pepper	

1. Place chicken bones in a large stockpot. Add water to cover (about 10 cups/2.5 L). Add carrots, celery, onion, thyme and bay leaf. Bring to a boil and skim. Simmer, covered, for 2 hours; strain through a fine sieve. Season with salt and pepper to taste.

Nutrients per 1 cup (250 mL)	
Calories	86
Fat	3 g
Carbohydrates	9 g
Protein	6 g

Chunky Southwest Vegetable Soup

Everyone's always looking for an easy way to add vegetables to their diet, and this soup fits the bill! Make a double batch and then freeze the extras in small containers.

TIPS

If you prefer your vegetables sautéed in oil, add 1 tbsp (15 mL) vegetable oil to the saucepan and heat over medium heat, then sauté the celery, onion, mushrooms, green pepper and jalapeño with the chili powder. But keep in mind that doing this will affect the nutrient analysis, since you are adding fat to the recipe.

Don't want to chop vegetables? Buy fresh or frozen vegetables that are already chopped.

1 cup	chopped celery	250 mL
1 cup	chopped onion	250 mL
1 cup	chopped mushrooms	250 mL
1/2 cup	chopped green bell pepper	125 mL
1 tbsp	minced seeded jalapeño pepper	15 mL
1 tsp	chili powder	5 mL
1	can (19 oz/540 mL) diced tomatoes (about 2 1/3 cups/575 mL)	540 mL

1. In a large saucepan, over medium heat, combine celery, onion, mushrooms, green pepper, jalapeño and chili powder. Add tomatoes, then fill can twice with water and add to saucepan; bring to a boil. Reduce heat, cover and simmer for 25 minutes.

VARIATION

If your family does not like heat, substitute 1 tbsp (15 mL) chopped fresh parsley for the jalapeño.

This recipe courtesy of Eileen Campbell.

Nutrients per serving	
Calories	49
Fat	0 g
Carbohydrates	11 g
Protein	2 g

Easy Borscht

Beets contain a bit more sugar than most vegetables, so many people avoid them. But they are a great source of betalains, which may help reduce inflammation.

TIP

You can also use prepared or homemade beef, chicken or vegetable stock or broth in this recipe. If it is not concentrated, use 2 cups (500 mL) broth and omit the water.

- **Food processor**

1 tbsp	vegetable oil	15 mL
1	onion, coarsely chopped	1
1 tbsp	minced garlic	15 mL
1	can (14 oz/398 mL) beets, with juice	1
1	can (10 oz/284 mL) condensed beef, chicken or vegetable broth (see tip, at left)	1
½ cup	water	125 mL
½	bag (10 oz/300 g) baby spinach (or 2 cups/500 mL tightly packed baby spinach)	½
2 tbsp	freshly squeezed lemon juice	30 mL
	Salt and freshly ground black pepper	
	Sour cream or vegan alternative	
	Finely chopped fresh dill	

1. In a large saucepan, heat oil over medium heat. Add onion and cook, stirring, until softened, about 3 minutes. Add garlic and cook, stirring, for 1 minute.

2. Add beets with juice, broth and water. Bring to a boil. Reduce heat to low and simmer for 10 minutes to combine flavors. Add spinach and cook, stirring, just until wilted. Stir in lemon juice. Season with salt and pepper to taste.

3. Place a strainer over a large bowl and strain soup. Transfer solids to food processor and add 1 cup (250 mL) of the liquid. Purée until smooth. Return puréed solids to saucepan and stir in remaining liquid. Reheat and serve hot or cover and chill thoroughly for at least 3 hours or for up to 3 days. Top individual servings with a dollop of sour cream and/or finely chopped dill.

Nutrients per serving

Calories	87
Fat	4 g
Carbohydrates	11 g
Protein	1 g

Tuscan Vegetable Soup

Make this tasty soup alone as a starter or to accompany a main-course salad, or add the toasts to create a full meal. Choose reduced-fat ricotta cheese to reduce the saturated fat in the recipe, as saturated fat can cause inflammation.

TIP

Reserve the white part of leeks for making stock.

- **Baking sheet**

Soup

1½ cups	dried cannellini beans (white kidney beans) or navy beans, soaked overnight in enough water to cover	375 mL
¼ cup	olive oil	60 mL
3	cloves garlic, finely chopped	3
2	stalks celery, finely chopped	2
2	sprigs fresh rosemary, leaves only, finely chopped	2
1	small onion, finely chopped	1
1	carrot, finely chopped	1
6 cups	Chicken Stock (page 201) or ready-to-use chicken broth	1.5 L
2 tbsp	tomato paste	30 mL
½	small head savoy cabbage, cored and shredded (about 6 cups/1.5 L)	½
2	leeks, green part only, washed and chopped	2
2	small zucchini, trimmed and finely chopped	2
	Salt and freshly ground black pepper	
12	fresh basil leaves, roughly chopped	12

Toasts

½ cup	extra virgin olive oil	125 mL
1	long Italian loaf of rustic country-style bread (or baguette) cut diagonally into 1-inch (2.5 cm) slices	1
1½ cups	ricotta cheese	375 mL
3 cups	grated Parmigiano-Reggiano cheese, divided	750 mL
¼ cup	chopped fresh flat-leaf (Italian) parsley	60 mL

Nutrients per serving	
Calories	691
Fat	39 g
Carbohydrates	55 g
Protein	35 g

TIP

Leeks can be gritty and need to be thoroughly cleaned before cooking. Peel off the tough outer layer(s) and cut off the root. Slice leeks according to recipe instructions and submerge in a basin of lukewarm water, swishing them around to remove all traces of dirt. Transfer to a colander and rinse under cold water.

1. *Soup:* In a large saucepan, combine drained beans with 6 cups (1.5 L) cold water. Bring to a boil; reduce heat to simmer and cook for 1 hour or until beans are tender. Meanwhile, in a large skillet, heat olive oil over medium heat. Add garlic, celery, rosemary, onion and carrot; cook for 10 minutes or until vegetables are softened.

2. When beans are tender, stir vegetable mixture into beans (do not drain), along with chicken stock, tomato paste and cabbage. Bring to a boil; reduce heat to simmer and cook for 10 minutes. Stir in leeks and zucchini; cook for 15 minutes longer or until vegetables are tender. Meanwhile, make the toasts.

3. *Toasts:* Preheat oven to 400°F (200°C). In a heavy skillet, heat olive oil over medium-high heat. In batches, cook bread slices for 1 minute per side, or until golden brown. Drain on paper towel.

4. Divide ricotta among toasts; spread over surface. Place on baking sheet. Sprinkle with some of the Parmigiano-Reggiano. Bake for 5 minutes or until cheese is golden. Sprinkle toasts with parsley.

5. Season soup to taste with salt and pepper. Stir in basil. Serve soup with cheese toasts, with remaining Parmigiano-Reggiano on the side.

Ginger-Laced Beet Soup with Orange

Makes 8 servings

This yummy soup is overflowing with nutrients, all with different health-promoting actions. Add some beneficial omega-3 fatty acids by choosing canola or olive oil.

- **Food processor**

2	onions, quartered	2
2	stalks celery, cut into 3-inch (7.5 cm) lengths	2
¼ cup	chopped gingerroot	60 mL
4	cloves garlic, chopped	4
1 tbsp	vegetable oil	15 mL
1 tbsp	finely grated orange zest	15 mL
	Salt and freshly ground black pepper	
4	large beets, peeled and quartered	4
4 cups	Chicken Stock (page 201), Vegetable Stock (page 200) or ready-to-use chicken or vegetable broth	1 L
1 cup	freshly squeezed orange juice	250 mL
½ cup	dried cranberries	125 mL
	Plain yogurt (optional)	

1. In food processor, pulse onions, celery, ginger and garlic until finely chopped, about 15 times, stopping and scraping down sides of the bowl once or twice.

2. In a large saucepan, heat oil over medium heat. Add onion mixture and cook, stirring, until softened, about 5 minutes. Add orange zest, and salt and pepper to taste. Cook, stirring, for 1 minute. Add beets and chicken stock and bring to a boil. Reduce heat and simmer until beets are tender, about 30 minutes. Remove from heat. Stir in orange juice and cranberries. Taste and adjust seasoning.

3. Place a strainer over a large bowl and strain soup. Transfer solids to food processor and add 1 cup (250 mL) of the liquid. Purée until smooth. If serving hot, return puréed solids to saucepan and stir in remaining liquid. If serving cold, add puréed solids to bowl, cover and refrigerate for at least 3 hours or for up to 3 days. To serve, ladle into bowls and top with a dollop of yogurt (if using).

Nutrients per serving	
Calories	91
Fat	2 g
Carbohydrates	17 g
Protein	2 g

Mushroom and Barley Soup

Barley is a wonderful grain. It contains soluble fiber, which helps keep us full longer and helps control blood sugar and cholesterol levels. If you decide to use pot barley because of its extra fiber content, you may need to add more broth to the soup, and it will take longer to cook.

TIPS

You can often find mushroom stock in your supermarket or health food store. If you can't find it, use vegetable stock instead and add an additional 4 oz (125 g) sliced mushrooms along with the 8 oz (250 g) called for in the recipe.

Choose canned diced tomatoes with or without seasonings for this soup.

2 tbsp	vegetable or olive oil	30 mL
1	large onion, finely chopped	1
4	cloves garlic, minced (about 1½ tbsp/22 mL)	4
2	carrots, peeled and thinly sliced	2
1	stalk celery, finely chopped	1
8 oz	mushrooms, thinly sliced	250 g
4 cups	mushroom stock (see tip, at left)	1 L
4 cups	Vegetable Stock (page 200) or ready-to-use vegetable broth	1 L
1	can (14 oz/398 mL) diced tomatoes, with juice	1
1 cup	pearl barley, rinsed and drained	250 mL
2 tsp	dried thyme	10 mL
1 tsp	white wine vinegar	5 mL
¼ tsp	freshly ground black pepper, or to taste	1 mL
1	bay leaf	1
	Salt	

1. In a large pot, heat oil over medium heat for 30 seconds. Add onion and cook, stirring, for 3 minutes or until softened. Add garlic, carrots, celery and mushrooms and cook, stirring frequently, for 7 minutes or until mushrooms start to brown.

2. Add mushroom and vegetable stocks, tomatoes, barley, thyme, vinegar, pepper, bay leaf and salt to taste. Stir well and bring to a boil. Reduce heat to medium-low and simmer, uncovered, for 30 minutes or until barley is tender. Remove bay leaf before serving.

VARIATIONS

Replace thyme with half the amount of dried rosemary.

If you like spice, add hot pepper sauce to taste before serving.

Nutrients per serving

Calories	166
Fat	4 g
Carbohydrates	30 g
Protein	4 g

Curry-Roasted Squash and Apple Soup

Makes 8 servings

This pretty, fragrant soup is wonderful any time of year, but especially in the fall, when squash and apples are plentiful. But what really makes this soup a winner is the flavorful spices, in particular the turmeric and coriander, which are known for their phytochemical content.

MAKE AHEAD

The soup can be made ahead, cooled, covered and refrigerated for up to 2 days or frozen for up to 2 months (thaw overnight in the refrigerator). Freeze in individual portions for easy defrosting. Reheat over medium heat until steaming and season to taste before serving.

VARIATION

Replace squash with 2 large sweet potatoes, peeled and cut into ½-inch (1 cm) pieces.

Nutrients per serving	
Calories	155
Fat	7 g
Carbohydrates	24 g
Protein	2 g

- **Preheat oven to 450°F (230°C)**
- **Rimmed baking sheet, ungreased**
- **Immersion blender or upright blender**

2 tsp	salt	10 mL
1 tsp	ground coriander	5 mL
1 tsp	ground cumin	5 mL
½ tsp	ground turmeric	2 mL
¼ tsp	ground cinnamon	1 mL
¼ tsp	freshly ground black pepper	1 mL
¼ cup	vegetable oil	60 mL
2 tbsp	cider vinegar or white wine vinegar	30 mL
4	cloves garlic	4
2	tart apples, peeled and chopped	2
1	butternut squash, peeled and cut into ½-inch (1 cm) pieces (about 8 cups/2 L)	1
1	large onion, chopped	1
6 cups	water (approx.)	1.5 L
½ tsp	garam masala, divided	2 mL
	Salt and freshly ground black pepper	

1. In a small bowl, combine salt, coriander, cumin, turmeric, cinnamon, pepper, oil and vinegar.

2. On baking sheet, combine garlic, apples, squash and onion. Drizzle with spice mixture and toss to coat evenly. Roast in preheated oven, stirring twice, for about 45 minutes or until softened and golden brown.

3. Transfer roasted vegetables to a large pot. Add water and bring to a boil over medium-high heat. Reduce heat and simmer, stirring occasionally, until vegetables are very soft and liquid is reduced by about one-third, about 30 minutes. Remove from heat.

4. Using an immersion blender in pot or transferring soup in batches to an upright blender, purée until very smooth. Return to pot, if necessary.

5. Reheat over medium heat until steaming, stirring often. Thin with a little water, if necessary, to desired consistency. Stir in half the garam masala and season to taste with salt and pepper. Ladle into warmed bowls and serve sprinkled with remaining garam masala.

Pumpkin and Coconut Soup

Makes 6 servings

The combination of pumpkin, coconut and shrimp makes a luscious soup. Serve a salad alongside, add some fruit for dessert, and you have a complete meal. Choose fortified coconut milk for the added calcium and vitamin D.

TIP

If fresh pumpkin is not in season, use butternut squash. You can find fresh or frozen squash all year round.

- **Food processor or mortar and pestle**

1 lb	pumpkin, peeled and cut into 1-inch (2.5 cm) pieces	500 g
2 tbsp	freshly squeezed lime juice	30 mL
2	shallots, peeled	2
2	cloves garlic, peeled	2
½ tsp	chopped fresh red or green chile pepper	2 mL
½ tsp	shrimp or anchovy paste	2 mL
2 tsp	fish sauce (nam pla)	10 mL
1 tsp	granulated or brown sugar	5 mL
12 oz	small shrimp, peeled and deveined, divided	375 g
3 cups	coconut milk	750 mL
2 cups	Chicken Stock (page 201), fish stock or water	500 mL
½ cup	fresh sweet Thai basil leaves	125 mL

1. In a bowl, combine pumpkin and lime juice. Let stand while preparing paste.

2. In a food processor or using a mortar and pestle, combine shallots, garlic, chiles, shrimp paste, fish sauce, sugar and half the shrimp. Purée or pound to a paste.

3. In a saucepan, combine coconut milk and chicken stock. Stir in paste. Heat to just below boiling, stirring often.

4. Add pumpkin and simmer for 15 minutes, or until pumpkin is just tender. Do not overcook or pumpkin will fall apart.

5. Add remaining shrimp and cook for 3 to 4 minutes, or until just cooked.

6. Stir in basil just before serving.

Nutrients per serving	
Calories	326
Fat	26 g
Carbohydrates	14 g
Protein	14 g

Mulligatawny Soup

Makes 6 servings

This creamy soup is a real treat. Using real cream adds taste and texture, but also adds saturated fat. To compensate, make sure to eat this soup with a vegetarian- or fish-based entrée.

TIP

Use frozen cauliflower florets and/or chopped onion in this recipe for convenience. If you run out, 1 medium onion produces about 1 cup (250 mL) finely chopped onion.

- **Food processor, blender or immersion blender**

2 tbsp	butter	30 mL
1 cup	finely chopped onion	250 mL
	Freshly ground black pepper	
1 tbsp	curry powder	15 mL
1 tsp	salt	5 mL
1	can (19 oz/540 mL) sliced potatoes, drained (or 2 cups/500 mL cooked chopped potatoes)	1
4 cups	cauliflower florets	1 L
6 cups	Vegetable Stock (page 200) or Chicken Stock (page 201) or ready-to-use vegetable or chicken broth	1.5 L
2 cups	chopped cooked chicken	500 mL
½ cup	heavy or whipping (35%) cream	125 mL
¼ cup	mango chutney	60 mL

1. In a large saucepan, melt butter over medium heat. Add onion and cook, stirring, until softened, about 3 minutes. Add pepper to taste, curry powder and salt, and cook, stirring, for 1 minute.

2. Add potatoes, cauliflower and vegetable stock. Bring to a boil. Reduce heat to low. Cover and cook until cauliflower is tender and flavors are combined, about 15 minutes.

3. Using a slotted spoon, transfer solids to food processor. Add ½ cup (125 mL) of the cooking liquid and process until smooth. (You can also do this in the saucepan, using an immersion blender.)

4. Return mixture to saucepan over low heat. Add chicken, cream and chutney and heat gently until mixture almost reaches a simmer. Ladle into bowls and serve immediately.

Nutrients per serving	
Calories	279
Fat	17 g
Carbohydrates	21 g
Protein	12 g

Moroccan Lentil Soup

Makes 5 servings

Here's a fabulous way to introduce lentils and chickpeas — great sources of protein and soluble fiber — into your diet. Add the optional spices for flavor and phytochemicals.

TIPS

You can replace the vegetable stock with beef or chicken stock for non-vegetarians.

Turmeric, paprika, cumin and cayenne pepper are frequently added to this soup to provide a more authentic North African flavor. Add the spices to the onions while they soften. At serving time, garnish with chopped cilantro for color.

1	large onion, chopped	1
	Seasonings (optional; see tip, at left)	
1 cup	dried red lentils	250 mL
4 cups	Vegetable Stock (page 200) or ready-to-use vegetable broth	1 L
1	can (19 oz/540 mL) chickpeas, drained and rinsed	1
	Salt and freshly ground black pepper	

1. In a large saucepan over medium heat, sauté onion with a little water or oil until softened. Stir in seasonings (if using). Add lentils and vegetable stock.

2. Bring to a boil over high heat. Reduce heat, cover and cook slowly, stirring occasionally, for 30 minutes or until lentils are soft.

3. Stir in chickpeas. Season with salt and pepper to taste.

Nutrients per serving	
Calories	249
Fat	2 g
Carbohydrates	43 g
Protein	15 g

Hearty Black and White Bean Soup

Here's a thick, chunky and tasty soup the whole family can enjoy. Remember to rinse the beans well to remove as much sodium as possible, or look for frozen beans: they are just as convenient and nutritious, but they contain less sodium.

TIPS

Beans are a nutritious alternative to meat and are high in iron and folate.

If you're using 19-oz (540 mL) cans of beans, add an additional 2 cups (500 mL) vegetable stock, 2 tsp (10 mL) red wine vinegar and a pinch more dried basil and chili powder.

If you prefer a smoother soup, purée the tomatoes in a food processor or blender before adding to soup in step 2.

Nutrients per serving	
Calories	202
Fat	3 g
Carbohydrates	33 g
Protein	10 g

- **Food processor or blender**

1½ tbsp	olive oil	22 mL
1	large onion, finely chopped	1
3	cloves garlic, minced	3
2	carrots, peeled and thinly sliced	2
2	stalks celery, coarsely chopped	2
4 cups	Vegetable Stock (page 200) or ready-to-use vegetable broth	1 L
1	can (28 oz/796 mL) diced tomatoes, with juices	1
2	cans (each 14 to 19 oz/398 to 540 mL) black beans, drained and rinsed	2
1	can (14 to 19 oz/398 to 540 mL) white beans, drained and rinsed	1
2 tbsp	red wine vinegar	30 mL
1½ tbsp	chili powder	22 mL
1 tbsp	dried basil	15 mL
	Salt and freshly ground black pepper	

1. In a large pot, heat oil over medium heat for 30 seconds. Add onion and garlic and cook, stirring, for 3 minutes or until softened. Add carrots and celery and cook, stirring, for 3 minutes.

2. Stir in vegetable stock and tomatoes and bring to a boil. Reduce heat to medium-low and cook, uncovered, for 10 minutes or until vegetables are tender.

3. Meanwhile, in food processor, process half of the black beans to achieve a thick paste-like consistency. Stir into soup. Add the remaining black beans and white beans.

4. Add red wine vinegar, chili powder, basil, salt and pepper to taste. Stir well. Reduce heat to low, cover and simmer for 15 minutes or until the flavors meld.

VARIATIONS

Purée the entire soup to completely blend flavors. This will give you a thick, rich result.

Add two sliced smoked soy sausages, thawed if frozen, after the soup has finished cooking. Cook for 5 minutes longer or until sausages are heated through. Garnish with chopped fresh basil or cilantro, to taste.

Mediterranean Seafood Soup

Makes 6 servings

Here's an inviting soup that's fragrant with garlic and brimming with fresh seafood in a rich wine and tomato broth. Even better: seafood is typically low in fat and cholesterol and provides a bounty of important nutrients.

TIP

For a less expensive version of this recipe, replace shrimp and scallops with an equal quantity of mild fish.

VARIATION

For a change, add steamed mussels. Place 1 lb (500 g) mussels in a saucepan with ¼ cup (60 mL) white wine or water. Place over high heat; cover and steam for 3 to 5 minutes or until shells open. Strain liquid and use as part of the fish stock called for in recipe. Discard any mussels that do not open. Add mussels to soup just before serving (leave in the shells, if desired).

2 tbsp	olive oil	30 mL
1	Spanish onion (about 1 lb/500 g), chopped	1
3	cloves garlic, finely chopped	3
1	red bell pepper, finely chopped	1
1	green bell pepper, finely chopped	1
1	large stalk celery, including leaves, chopped	1
1	bay leaf	1
1 tsp	salt	5 mL
1 tsp	paprika	5 mL
¼ tsp	hot pepper flakes	1 mL
¼ tsp	saffron threads, crushed	1 mL
1	can (19 oz/540 mL) tomatoes, with juice, chopped	1
4 cups	fish stock or ready-to-use chicken broth (approx.)	1 L
1 cup	dry white wine or vermouth or stock	250 mL
1 lb	halibut or other mild white fish, cubed	500 g
8 oz	medium shrimp, peeled and deveined, with tails left on	250 g
8 oz	scallops, halved if large	250 g
⅓ cup	finely chopped fresh parsley	75 mL

1. In a Dutch oven or large saucepan, heat oil over medium-high heat. Add onion, garlic, red and green peppers, celery, bay leaf, salt, paprika, hot pepper flakes and saffron; cook, stirring often, for 5 minutes or until vegetables are softened.

2. Add tomatoes with juice, stock and wine. Bring to a boil; reduce heat to medium-low and simmer, covered, for 30 minutes. (Recipe can be prepared to this point up to a day ahead, or frozen for up to 3 months; when reheating, bring back to a full boil.)

3. Stir in halibut, shrimp, scallops and parsley; cover and simmer for 3 to 5 minutes or until fish is opaque. Serve immediately in warm soup bowls.

Nutrients per serving	
Calories	308
Fat	8 g
Carbohydrates	18 g
Protein	33 g

Pasta Fagioli Capra

This long-time favorite is truly a meal in a bowl. If you're avoiding wheat products, try substituting your favorite gluten-free pasta.

TIP

A traditional favorite soup, pasta fagioli combines beans, pasta and vegetables to make a delicious meal-in-a-bowl. Italian-born Toronto chef Massimo Capra, of Mistura Restaurant, uses different types of beans. The actual combination of beans can be varied to suit your taste and may either be canned, dried, fresh or frozen. If using canned beans, rinse and drain well.

3 tbsp	extra virgin olive oil	45 mL
1	stalk celery, finely chopped	1
1	small onion, finely chopped	1
1	small carrot, finely chopped	1
6	cloves garlic, finely chopped	6
1	sprig fresh thyme, leaves only, finely chopped	1
2	bay leaves	2
1 cup	chopped plum (Roma) tomatoes (canned or fresh)	250 mL
¼ cup	cooked romano beans	60 mL
¼ cup	cooked black-eyed peas	60 mL
¼ cup	cooked cannellini (white kidney) beans or navy beans	60 mL
¼ cup	cooked large lima beans	60 mL
¼ cup	cooked chickpeas	60 mL
6 cups	Vegetable Stock (page 200) or ready-to-use vegetable broth	1.5 L
	Salt and freshly ground black pepper	
	Freshly grated nutmeg	
1 cup	maccheroni (the straight, short variety) or ditalini or tubetti	250 mL
½ cup	cooked, peeled fava beans	125 mL
¼ cup	roughly chopped fresh flat-leaf (Italian) parsley	60 mL
	Olive oil	
6	slices of rustic country-style bread brushed with olive oil and grilled or oven-toasted	6

1. In a large saucepan, heat olive oil over medium heat. Add celery, onion, carrot, garlic, thyme and bay leaves; cook for 5 minutes or until vegetables are softened. Stir in tomatoes; cook, stirring, for 3 minutes.

Nutrients per serving	
Calories	285
Fat	8 g
Carbohydrate	44 g
Protein	10 g

TIP

When purchasing ready-to-use broths, be sure to read the Nutrition Facts table and nutritional claims. As elevated levels of sodium can contribute to hypertension and cardiovascular disease, select broths that have no added salt or are at least low in sodium.

2. Stir in romano beans, black-eyed peas, kidney beans, lima beans and chickpeas. Add vegetable stock and bring to a boil. Reduce heat to simmer and cook for 15 minutes, skimming any foam that rises to the top. Season to taste with salt, pepper and nutmeg.

3. Stir in pasta and fava beans; return to a simmer and cook, stirring occasionally, for 10 minutes or just until pasta is tender.

4. Stir in parsley. Drizzle with olive oil and serve immediately with toasts.

Zuppa di Pesce

Makes 6 servings

This meal-worthy Italian-style fish stew is a wonderful source of lean protein. Using the slow cooker makes it easy to prepare: you can start the soup when your energy levels are highest, then serve it later in the day when you are tired.

TIPS

If you don't have mild chile powder, substitute 1 tsp (5 mL) sweet paprika mixed with a pinch of cayenne pepper.

Use firm white fish such as halibut, snapper, monkfish or sea bass.

If you prefer, substitute an extra cup (250 mL) of water plus 1 tbsp (15 mL) lemon juice for the white wine.

For best results, when asking for trimmings, be sure to use non-oily fish, which means no salmon.

- **Minimum 5-quart slow cooker**
- **Cheesecloth**

3 tbsp	extra virgin olive oil, divided	45 mL
1 tbsp	freshly squeezed lemon juice	15 mL
1 tsp	fennel seeds, toasted and ground	5 mL
1 tsp	coarse salt (preferably sea salt)	5 mL
1 tsp	mild chile powder (such as Aleppo)	5 mL
2 lbs	assorted skinless fish fillets, cut into chunks (see tip, at left)	1 kg
2	onions, finely chopped	2
4	stalks celery, diced	4
4	cloves garlic, minced	4
2	bay leaves	2
1 tsp	dried oregano	5 mL
½ tsp	cracked black peppercorns	2 mL
1 cup	dry white wine	250 mL
1	can (28 oz/796 mL) tomatoes, with juice, chopped	1
2 lbs	fish trimmings (see tip, at left)	1 kg
6 cups	water	1.5 L
16	Garlic Crostini (see tip, at right)	16
½ cup	finely chopped parsley	125 mL

1. In a bowl, combine 2 tbsp (30 mL) of the olive oil, lemon juice, fennel seeds, salt and chile powder. Mix well. Add fish chunks and toss until coated. Cover and refrigerate for 2 hours or overnight, stirring occasionally.

2. In a skillet, heat remaining 1 tbsp (15 mL) of olive oil over medium heat. Add onions and celery and cook, stirring, until softened, about 5 minutes. Add garlic, bay leaves, oregano and peppercorns and cook, stirring, for 1 minute. Add white wine and bring to a boil. Boil for 2 minutes. Stir in tomatoes with juice. Transfer to slow cooker stoneware.

Nutrients per serving	
Calories	475
Fat	10 g
Carbohydrates	50 g
Protein	38 g

TIP

To make Garlic Crostini:
Preheat broiler. In a small bowl, combine ¼ cup (60 mL) extra virgin olive oil with 2 cloves garlic, peeled and put through a press. Stir well. Brush 12 baguette slices on both sides with infused oil and toast under broiler, turning once.

MAKE AHEAD

Complete steps 1 and 2. Cover and refrigerate fish and vegetable mixtures separately overnight. When you're ready to cook, complete the recipe.

3. In a large square of cheesecloth, tie fish trimmings. Add to stoneware along with water, ensuring trimmings are submerged. Cover and cook on Low for 8 hours or on High for 4 hours. Remove trimmings and discard. Increase heat to High. Add marinated fish and cook about 15 minutes, until fish is tender. Remove and discard bay leaves.

4. To serve, place 2 crostini in each bowl and ladle soup over. Garnish with parsley.

Big-Batch Chicken Vegetable Soup

Chicken soup is the ultimate comfort food and it is good for you too! If you are concerned about the amount of fat in the drumsticks, you can use chicken breasts instead.

TIPS

When you're going to be freezing meal-sized portions of soup, ladle hot soup into airtight containers, leaving at least 1 inch (2.5 cm) headspace, and let it cool slightly. Refrigerate until completely cold, then freeze for up to 3 months.

This recipe is prepared without sautéing the vegetables in fat. If you prefer, add 1 tbsp (15 mL) vegetable oil to the saucepan and heat over medium heat, then sauté the celery, leeks and carrots before adding all the other ingredients. But keep in mind that doing this will affect the nutrient analysis, since you are adding fat to the recipe.

	Nutrients per serving	
Calories		68
Fat		1 g
Carbohydrates		8 g
Protein		6 g

8 to 10	skinless chicken drumsticks (about 2 lbs/1 kg total)	8 to 10
12	mushrooms, sliced	12
4	stalks celery, diced	4
4	leeks (white and light green parts only), chopped	4
4	carrots, diced	4
3	large tomatoes, chopped	3
1	large onion, chopped	1
1	can (5½ oz/156 mL) tomato paste	1
10 cups	Chicken Stock (page 201) or ready-to-use chicken broth	2.5 L
¼ cup	chopped fresh parsley	60 mL
	Salt and freshly ground black pepper (optional)	

1. In a large pot, combine drumsticks, mushrooms, celery, leeks, carrots, tomatoes, onion, tomato paste, chicken stock, parsley and salt and pepper to taste (if using). Bring to a boil over high heat. Reduce heat, cover and simmer for 30 minutes or until chicken is falling off the bone and vegetables are soft.

2. Remove drumsticks and debone. Discard bones and return chicken to saucepan. Bring back to a boil for a few minutes to reheat chicken.

This recipe courtesy of Candice Wilke.

Salads
and Wraps

Green Papaya Salad

Papaya contains papin, an enzyme that helps us digest protein and has anti-inflammatory properties.

TIPS

Green papaya is often sold in halves, cut open to expose the white seeds. To shred it, peel and thinly shred by hand with a coarse grater, mandoline, or with a food processor. Remove the seeds with a spoon. Since papaya is sticky, you may want to wear a glove.

If green papaya is unavailable, use a combination of cabbage and carrots.

This salad alone makes purchasing a good-size mortar and pestle worthwhile, but you can also just combine the chopped garlic, chiles, green beans and shredded papaya without pounding.

To prepare the shrimp floss, process 2 tbsp (30 mL) dried shrimp in a small food processor.

- **Mortar and pestle or small food processor**

3	cloves garlic, peeled	3
1½ tsp	chopped fresh red chile pepper	7 mL
½ cup	sliced green beans	125 mL
1	green papaya, peeled, seeded and shredded (about 2 cups/500 mL)	1
2 tbsp	fish sauce (nam pla)	30 mL
2 tbsp	freshly squeezed lime juice	30 mL
1 tbsp	palm or brown sugar	15 mL
1	tomato, cut into wedges	1
2 tbsp	chopped roasted peanuts or cashews	30 mL
1 tbsp	shrimp floss (optional)	15 mL

1. Using mortar and pestle or in food processor, finely chop garlic and chiles to form a coarse paste.
2. Add beans and pound to bruise. Add papaya and pound again to bruise papaya shreds, about 2 to 3 minutes, scraping down sides with a spoon.
3. Add fish sauce, lime juice and sugar and pound while scraping sides of bowl with a spoon, turning ingredients. Taste and adjust seasonings if necessary.
4. Stir in tomato, peanuts and shrimp floss (if using). Serve with some of the juices.

Nutrients per serving

Calories	90
Fat	3 g
Carbohydrates	16 g
Protein	3 g

Marinated Asparagus

It's easy to prepare a batch or two of marinated vegetables, so you can have them on hand to add to lunches or to make a quick side dish. Asparagus contains inulin, a type of fiber that is an ideal food for the beneficial bacteria (probiotics) that live in our intestines.

TIP

Once vegetables are marinated, they keep refrigerated for several days.

1 lb	asparagus	500 g
1	clove garlic, minced	1
½ cup	rice vinegar	125 mL
2 tbsp	granulated sugar	30 mL
	Salt and freshly ground black pepper	

1. Snap off asparagus ends. Steam for 2 minutes or until tender-crisp. Immerse in cold water. Drain and set aside to dry. Place in a shallow container.

2. Combine garlic, vinegar, sugar, salt and pepper. Pour mixture over asparagus.

3. Cover and refrigerate for 1 hour. Remove asparagus from vinegar and serve at room temperature.

VARIATION

Carrots, green beans and broccoli florets are excellent marinated in the same method used for asparagus.

Nutrients per serving	
Calories	61
Fat	0 g
Carbohydrates	14 g
Protein	3 g

Hot Sweet Potato Salad

Makes 6 servings

It's worth the effort to make your own ras el hanout, which adds a bundle of phytochemicals to a salad that is already rich in beta carotene, thanks to the sweet potatoes. But you can always visit your local spice market to find a readymade spice blend.

4	sweet potatoes, quartered	4
3 tbsp	olive oil	45 mL
1	leek (white and light green parts only), sliced	1
1	onion, chopped	1
½ cup	Vegetable Stock (page 200) or ready-to-use vegetable broth	125 mL
1 tbsp	blackstrap molasses or liquid honey	15 mL
2 tsp	Ras el Hanout (see recipe, opposite) or store-bought curry powder	10 mL
½ tsp	ground nutmeg	2 mL
½ tsp	salt	2 mL

1. In a large saucepan, cover sweet potatoes with water. Bring to a boil over high heat. Reduce heat and simmer for 20 minutes or until tender. Drain, let cool and remove skins. Cut into large dice and transfer to a large serving bowl. Cover tightly.

2. Meanwhile, in a large skillet, heat oil over medium heat. Add leek and onion. Sauté for 7 minutes or until soft. Stir in vegetable stock and molasses. Increase heat and bring to a boil. Reduce heat and simmer, stirring occasionally, for 10 to 12 minutes or until liquid is slightly reduced.

3. Toss leek mixture with sweet potatoes. Add Ras el Hanout, nutmeg and salt. Taste and add more seasonings, if required. Serve warm or at room temperature.

VARIATION
Add ¼ cup (60 mL) of any of the following: nuts or seeds, flaked coconut or raisins.

Nutrients per serving	
Calories	141
Fat	6 g
Carbohydrates	19 g
Protein	1 g

In Morocco, every stall in the attarine (spice street in the market) has its own ras el hanout. The literal meaning is "top of the shop" and it is the very best the spice merchant has to offer. This is a secret blend of upwards of 25, sometimes 100 different spices, herbs and aphrodisiacs that people search out until they find the one they love best.

TIPS

A mortar and pestle works best to crush and grind the toasted spices, but if necessary, use a spice grinder or small food processor.

Store and label spice in a small clean jar with lid in the refrigerator or cool dark place for up to 2 months.

Ras el Hanout

- **Mortar and pestle (see tip, at left)**

1	2-inch (5 cm) cinnamon stick	1
1 tbsp	whole allspice berries	15 mL
1 tbsp	whole coriander seeds	15 mL
1 tbsp	whole fennel seeds	15 mL
2 tsp	whole cardamom seeds	10 mL
2 tsp	whole cumin seeds	10 mL
2 tsp	whole fenugreek seeds	10 mL
2 tsp	whole black peppercorns	10 mL
3	whole cloves	3
1	whole star anise	1
1 tbsp	sea salt	15 mL
1 tbsp	ground turmeric	15 mL
1 tsp	ground ginger	5 mL

1. Break cinnamon into small pieces. In a small spice wok or dry cast-iron skillet, combine cinnamon, allspice, coriander, fennel, cardamom, cumin, fenugreek, peppercorns, cloves and star anise. Toast over medium-high heat for 4 to 5 minutes or until the seeds begin to pop and their fragrance is released. Let cool.

2. With mortar and pestle, pound toasted spices until coarse or finely ground. Add salt, turmeric and ginger to ground spices and mix well.

VARIATION

Just before adding to a dish, add 1 minced garlic clove and $\frac{1}{4}$ tsp (1 mL) finely shredded fresh gingerroot for every 1 to 2 tbsp (15 to 25 mL) ras el hanout blend.

Nutrients per 1 tsp (5 mL)	
Calories	6
Fat	0 g
Carbohydrates	1 g
Protein	0 g

Autumn Harvest Salad

Makes 4 servings

An abundance of delicious root vegetables makes for a nutrient-packed salad. Using a food processor to shred the vegetables makes it quick and easy too!

TIP

Shaving or shredding the root vegetables makes them easy to combine and digest.

Nutrients per serving	
Calories	228
Fat	18 g
Carbohydrates	17 g
Protein	5 g

1 cup	shredded carrot	250 mL
½ cup	shredded turnip	125 mL
½ cup	shredded beet	125 mL
1	apple, diced	1
2	green onions, thinly sliced on the diagonal	2
2 tbsp	fresh thyme leaves	30 mL
1 tbsp	chopped fresh sage	15 mL
⅓ cup	Harvest Dressing (see recipe, below)	75 mL
¼ cup	coarsely chopped cashews	60 mL
3 tbsp	sesame seeds	45 mL

1. In a large salad bowl, combine carrot, turnip, beet, apple, green onions, thyme and sage. Toss well to combine. Drizzle Harvest Dressing over top and toss well. Scatter cashew nuts and sesame seeds over top and serve immediately.

Makes about ⅓ cup (75 mL)

TIP

Any finely shredded herb or leaf vegetable is called "chiffonade."

Nutrients per 1 tbsp (15 mL)	
Calories	76
Fat	8 g
Carbohydrates	1 g
Protein	1 g

Harvest Dressing

1	whole head garlic, roasted (or 1 clove garlic, finely chopped)	1
3 tbsp	olive oil	45 mL
1 tbsp	tamari or soy sauce	15 mL
1 tbsp	freshly squeezed lemon juice	15 mL
2 tbsp	chiffonade basil (see tip, at left)	30 mL
	Salt (optional)	

1. In a jar with lid or small bowl, combine garlic, oil, tamari, lemon juice and basil. If using roasted garlic, squeeze soft cloves into the container and mash with a fork. Shake or whisk ingredients to mix well. Taste and adjust seasonings, adding salt, if needed.

Carrot and Ginger Salad

Makes 4 servings

This salad is brightly colored and full of flavor. As a bonus, carrots are an excellent source of beta carotene, which becomes vitamin A in the body.

TIPS

For added convenience, shredded carrots can be purchased at the grocery store.

To peel gingerroot without a vegetable peeler, use the edge of a large spoon to scrape the skin off.

Gingerroot can be grated ahead of time and frozen in 1 tbsp (15 mL) portions, ready for use. Or you can purchase frozen grated ginger.

- **Food processor**

1 lb	carrots, cut into 3-inch (7.5 cm) lengths	500 g
2 tbsp	extra virgin olive oil	30 mL
1 tbsp	freshly grated gingerroot	15 mL
1 tbsp	poppy seeds	15 mL
	Salt and freshly ground black pepper	

1. In food processor fitted with shredding blade, shred carrots. Transfer to a large salad bowl. Add oil, ginger, poppy seeds, and salt and pepper to taste. Cover and refrigerate to allow flavors to meld, about 30 minutes. Serve at room temperature.

Nutrients per serving	
Calories	122
Fat	9 g
Carbohydrates	12 g
Protein	2 g

Quinoa Beet Potato Salad

Quinoa contains a significant amount of the antioxidant mineral manganese, and beets contain the phytochemical betalain, so this salad is an inflammation-fighting powerhouse. Quinoa also provides a complete protein, so you can eat this salad as a main course.

TIPS

The beet stains the other ingredients, but the taste is worth the pink food.

To cook quinoa, in a saucepan over medium-high heat, bring 2 cups (500 mL) vegetable stock or water and ½ tsp (2 mL) salt to a boil. Add 1 cup (250 mL) rinsed quinoa. Cover and reduce heat to medium-low. Simmer for 12 to 15 minutes or until liquid is absorbed and grains are translucent and tender. Let stand, covered, for 5 minutes. Fluff with a fork. Makes about 3½ cups (875 mL).

1½ lbs	small potatoes	750 g
1	large carrot, shredded	1
1	beet, shredded	1
¼	fennel bulb, shredded	¼
2 cups	cold or cooled cooked quinoa (see tip, at left)	500 mL
½ cup	finely chopped red onion	125 mL
¼ cup	chopped fresh parsley	60 mL
2 tbsp	chopped fresh tarragon	30 mL
½ cup	Tofu Mayonnaise (page 196 or store-bought)	125 mL
	Sea salt and freshly ground black pepper	

1. In a large saucepan, cover potatoes with water and bring to a boil over high heat. Cover, reduce heat to medium-low and simmer for 20 minutes or until potatoes are almost tender and show some resistance when pierced with the tip of a knife. Drain and rinse under cold water. Let stand, and when cool enough to handle, cut into ½-inch (1 cm) cubes.

2. Meanwhile, in a bowl, combine carrot, beet, fennel, quinoa, onion, parsley and tarragon. Add potatoes and mayonnaise. Stir to mix well. Season to taste with salt and pepper.

Nutrients per serving	
Calories	175
Fat	3 g
Carbohydrates	34 g
Protein	6 g

Lemon-Dill White Bean Salad

Dill is an unsung hero in the herb world. It may help prevent free radical damage in our bodies, and may help control the growth of bacteria. Here, it also adds a fresh flavor to this zesty salad.

Nutrients per serving	
Calories	171
Fat	5 g
Carbohydrates	25 g
Protein	9 g

1	can (19 oz/540 mL) white kidney beans, drained and rinsed	1
¼ cup	chopped red onion	60 mL
¼ cup	finely chopped red bell pepper	60 mL
2 to 3 tbsp	Lemon Vinaigrette (see recipe, below)	30 to 45 mL
	Freshly ground black pepper	

1. In a medium bowl, stir together beans, onion and red pepper.
2. Add dressing and pepper to taste. Cover and refrigerate for several hours or overnight.

VARIATION

Try this with red kidney beans instead of white and a green pepper instead of red, or a mix of all.

Makes about ½ cup (125 mL)

This very useful vinaigrette is one to keep on hand in the refrigerator. Enjoy it with cooked vegetables such as asparagus, green beans or broccoli or drizzled over fish fillets before baking or grilling.

Nutrients per 1 tbsp (15 mL)	
Calories	78
Fat	9 g
Carbohydrates	1 g
Protein	0 g

Lemon Vinaigrette

⅓ cup	extra virgin olive oil	75 mL
3 tbsp	freshly squeezed lemon juice	45 mL
2 tbsp	chopped fresh dill	30 mL
	Salt and freshly ground black pepper	

1. In a container with a tight-fitting lid, combine oil, lemon juice and dill. Cover and shake well to blend. Season with salt and pepper to taste.
2. Store in the refrigerator for up to 2 weeks.

Soba Noodle Salad with Edamame

A great salad is all about creating a pleasing combination of taste, texture and color. We feast with our eyes! Nori, an edible seaweed, is high in iodine, which can be a problem for some people, but it's easy enough to leave it out.

TIPS

Salads that include noodles absorb a lot of dressing as they stand. Taste and add more dressing before serving, if needed.

Edamame are young, tender soybeans available shelled and frozen in the pod. They have a pleasing crunch and are good for you, too!

8 oz	soba noodles	250 g
	Kosher or sea salt	
8 oz	frozen edamame in the pod	250 g
4 oz	snow peas, trimmed	125 g
2	radishes, julienned	2
2	green onions, thinly sliced on the diagonal	2
Pinch	hot pepper flakes	Pinch
½ to ⅔ cup	Miso Dressing (see recipe, opposite)	125 to 150 mL
1	sheet toasted nori (optional)	1
1 tbsp	toasted white sesame seeds (optional)	15 mL
1 tbsp	toasted black sesame seeds (optional)	15 mL

1. In a large saucepan of boiling salted water, cook noodles until tender, 6 to 8 minutes, or prepare noodles according to package instructions. Drain and rinse under cold water. (You should have 4 cups/1 L cooked soba noodles.) Set aside.

2. Cook edamame in ½ cup (125 mL) lightly salted water, covered, according to package instructions, about 4 minutes. Gently squeeze beans from pod. (You should have about ¾ cup/175 mL.)

3. Blanch snow peas for 30 seconds. Drain and rinse under cold water. Cut into fine slivers.

4. In a large bowl, combine noodles, edamame, snow peas, radishes, green onions and hot pepper flakes. Toss with dressing.

5. If using nori, use kitchen scissors to cut it lengthwise into thirds and then into fine strips. Sprinkle on top of salad. Garnish with white and black sesame seeds (if using).

Nutrients per serving	
Calories	231
Fat	10 g
Carbohydrates	28 g
Protein	8 g

Drizzling this dressing over a salad adds an extra hit of protein thanks to the miso, which also provides other important antioxidant nutrients, such as zinc and manganese. The ginger and garlic add even more flavor.

TIP

A hand-held immersion blender does a great job of blending small quantities of dressings, sauces and even soups.

Miso Dressing

- **Food processor or blender**

²⁄₃ cup	unseasoned rice vinegar	150 mL
¼ cup	yellow or white miso	60 mL
2 tbsp	chopped gingerroot	30 mL
2 tbsp	granulated sugar	30 mL
1 tbsp	chopped garlic	15 mL
	Salt and freshly ground black pepper	
1 cup	vegetable oil	250 mL
1 tbsp	sesame oil (optional)	15 mL

1. In food processor, combine vinegar, miso, ginger, sugar, garlic and salt and pepper to taste. Slowly drizzle in vegetable oil and sesame oil, if using, through the feed tube. Add water, 1 tbsp (15 mL) at a time, to make sauce a light, creamy consistency. Taste and adjust seasoning.

Nutrients per 1 tbsp (15 mL)	
Calories	79
Fat	8 g
Carbohydrates	2 g
Protein	0 g

Tabbouleh

This intriguing, healthy, delicious salad is packed with parsley, which is, in turn, packed with antioxidant nutrients, including vitamin C. However, parsley also contains a significant amount of vitamin K, so if you are taking blood thinners, check with your dietitian before eating this salad.

TIPS

This recipe uses a minimum quantity of oil, because I like my tabbouleh tart. If you prefer a sweeter taste, add 2 tbsp (30 mL) more oil.

Leftover tabbouleh can be kept in the refrigerator, covered, for up to 3 days. Be sure to bring it back up to room temperature before serving.

2 cups	packed chopped fresh parsley	500 mL
1	onion, finely chopped	1
1	tomato, finely chopped	1
½ cup	bulgur wheat	125 mL
6 tbsp	freshly squeezed lemon juice	90 mL
¼ cup	olive oil	60 mL
	Salt and freshly ground black pepper	

1. In a bowl, combine parsley, onion and tomato. Mix well. Set aside.

2. In a saucepan, boil bulgur wheat in plenty of water for 6 to 8 minutes, until tender. Drain and refresh with cold water. Drain again completely and add cooked bulgur to the vegetables in the bowl. Mix well.

3. Sprinkle lemon juice and olive oil over the salad. Add salt and pepper to taste. Toss to mix thoroughly. Transfer to a serving plate. The salad can be served immediately, although it'll be better if it waits up to 2 hours, covered and unrefrigerated.

Nutrients per serving	
Calories	118
Fat	10 g
Carbohydrates	9 g
Protein	2 g

Quinoa and Corn Salad with Cumin Lime Dressing

Makes 6 servings

The type of fiber in corn promotes the growth of healthy bacteria in the intestine. You can use frozen corn in this recipe if it's too difficult for you to cut the kernels off the cobs.

TIPS

When you buy quinoa, it has been rinsed and air-dried to remove the naturally occurring bitter saponins, a resin-like coating. Still, rinse it again before use to remove any powdery residue that may remain.

Look for other interesting and healthful oils, such as avocado, pumpkin seed or almond oil, in specialty food shops and use instead of olive oil.

Instead of pumpkin seeds, try almonds, walnuts or pine nuts.

Cook extra cobs of corn, cut off the kernels and use in soups and salads.

1 cup	quinoa, rinsed	250 mL
	Salt	
¼ cup	olive oil	60 mL
1 tsp	grated lime zest	5 mL
2 tbsp	freshly squeezed lime juice	30 mL
1½ tsp	ground cumin	7 mL
½ tsp	hot pepper sauce, or to taste	2 mL
	Freshly ground black pepper	
3	green onions, thinly sliced	3
2	tomatoes, seeded and diced	2
½	seedless cucumber, diced	½
2 cups	cooked fresh corn kernels (about 3 cobs)	500 mL
2	Hass avocados, peeled and diced	2
½ cup	coarsely chopped fresh cilantro	125 mL
⅓ cup	raw green pumpkin seeds (optional)	75 mL

1. In a medium saucepan, bring 2 cups (500 mL) water to a boil over high heat. Add quinoa and ½ tsp (2 mL) salt. Cover, reduce heat to medium-low and simmer for 15 minutes or until quinoa is tender and water is absorbed. Uncover and fluff with a fork. Let cool.

2. In a small bowl, combine oil, lime zest and juice, cumin, hot pepper sauce and salt and pepper to taste.

3. In a serving bowl, combine quinoa, green onions, tomatoes, cucumber and corn. Pour in half the dressing and toss to coat. (Can be prepared up to 4 hours ahead; cover and refrigerate.)

4. Shortly before serving, add avocados, cilantro and pumpkin seeds (if using). Drizzle with remaining dressing and toss lightly.

Nutrients per serving	
Calories	229
Fat	20 g
Carbohydrates	14 g
Protein	3 g

Kasha and Beet Salad with Celery and Feta

In this hearty salad, beets, parsley and feta are the perfect balance for assertive buckwheat. Buckwheat is not actually a grain, so it contains none of the proteins associated with gluten intolerance. Feta cheese, which can be found in regular and lower-fat versions, can be quite high in sodium, so you may choose to rinse it in cold water before sprinkling it on the salad.

TIP

Place the celery and green onions in the feed tube together so that the celery provides support to the less rigid onions.

- **Food processor**

2 cups	Chicken Stock (page 201), Vegetable Stock (page 200) or ready-to-use chicken or vegetable broth	500 mL
2	cloves garlic, minced	2
1 cup	kasha or buckwheat groats (see tip, at right)	250 mL
3	beets, cooked, peeled and cut to fit feed tube of food processor	3
4	stalks celery, cut to fit feed tube of food processor	4
6	green onions, white part only	6
3 oz	crumbled feta cheese or vegan alternative	90 g

Dressing

1 cup	fresh flat-leaf (Italian) parsley leaves	250 mL
1/4 cup	red wine vinegar	60 mL
1 tsp	Dijon mustard	5 mL
1/2 tsp	salt	2 mL
1/2 tsp	freshly ground black pepper	2 mL
1/4 cup	extra virgin olive oil	60 mL

1. In a saucepan over medium-high heat, bring chicken stock and garlic to a boil. Gradually add kasha, stirring constantly to prevent clumping. Reduce heat to low. Cover and simmer until all the liquid is absorbed and kasha is tender, about 10 minutes. Remove from heat. Fluff up with a fork, transfer to a serving bowl and let cool slightly.

Nutrients per serving	
Calories	129
Fat	9 g
Carbohydrates	10 g
Protein	4 g

TIP

Buckwheat groats that are already toasted are known as kasha. If you prefer a milder buckwheat flavor, use groats rather than kasha in this dish. Just place them in a dry skillet over medium-high heat and cook, stirring constantly, until they are nicely fragrant, about 4 minutes. In the process, they will darken from a light shade of sand to one with a hint of brown. Groats you toast yourself have a milder flavor than store-bought kasha.

2. *Dressing:* Meanwhile, in food processor fitted with a metal blade, pulse parsley, vinegar, mustard, salt and pepper until parsley is chopped and mixture is blended, about 5 times, stopping and scraping down sides of the bowl once or twice. With motor running, add olive oil through feed tube, stopping and scraping down sides of the bowl as necessary. Pour over kasha.

3. Replace metal blade with slicing blade and slice beets, celery and green onions (see tip, page 232). Add to kasha along with the dressing and toss well. Chill until ready to serve. Just before serving, sprinkle feta over top.

Everyday Tuna and Red Rice Salad

The unrefined rice in this tasty and nutritious salad contains fiber and important antioxidant minerals, and contributes a nutty, earthy taste.

TIPS

Bhutanese red and Kalijira brown rice are available at specialty stores or Asian grocery stores.

To cook the rice for this recipe: In a heavy saucepan with a tight-fitting lid, bring 1½ cups (375 mL) water to a rapid boil. Stir in ¾ cup (175 mL) rice and return to a boil. Reduce heat to low. Cover and simmer until liquid is absorbed and rice is tender, about 25 minutes. (If liquid remains, remove lid and return to element for a few minutes until it evaporates.)

- **Food processor with mini bowl attachment**

¼ cup	fresh flat-leaf (Italian) parsley leaves	60 mL
1	shallot, quartered	1
1	clove garlic, coarsely chopped	1
1 tbsp	white wine vinegar or freshly squeezed lemon juice	15 mL
1 tsp	Dijon mustard	5 mL
½ tsp	salt	2 mL
	Freshly ground black pepper	
¼ cup	extra virgin olive oil	60 mL
1	can (6 oz/170 g) tuna, drained	1
1 cup	cooked sliced green beans, cooled (optional)	250 mL
½	red bell pepper, finely chopped	½
¼ cup	sliced pitted black olives (or 1 tbsp/15 mL diced capers)	60 mL
4	green onions, white part only, thinly sliced (or ¼ cup/60 mL finely chopped red onion)	4
1	oil-packed sun-dried tomato, drained and finely chopped (or ½ cup/125 mL quartered cherry or grape tomatoes)	1
¾ cup	Bhutanese red or Kalijira brown rice, cooked (see tips, at left)	175 mL
	Lettuce leaves or hearts of romaine (optional)	

1. In mini bowl fitted with metal blade, pulse parsley, shallot, garlic, vinegar, mustard, salt, and pepper to taste, to chop and blend, about 5 times. With motor running, add olive oil through feed tube, stopping and scraping down sides of the bowl as necessary. Set aside.

2. In a bowl, combine tuna, green beans (if using), bell pepper, olives, green onions and sun-dried tomato. Toss until blended. Add dressing and toss well.

3. To serve, spoon warm rice onto plates and top with tuna mixture. Or, if using lettuce, line a platter with leafy lettuce or hearts of romaine. Spoon rice onto lettuce and top with tuna mixture.

Nutrients per serving	
Calories	250
Fat	17 g
Carbohydrates	14 g
Protein	13 g

Tuna Avocado Salad

Many of the nutrients in avocados are in the dark green flesh near the skin.

TIPS

To prepare an avocado, first cut around the avocado lengthwise, cutting through to the pit. Twist one half to separate the avocado into two halves. To easily pop out the pit, use a sharp knife to pierce the pit; turn the knife and twist. Cut avocado flesh inside the skin in a crisscross pattern; remove avocado pieces with a large spoon. Avocados brown easily, so once cut, dip the pieces in lemon juice.

1	can (6 oz/170 g) water-packed tuna, drained	1
1	avocado, peeled, pitted and cut into bite-size pieces	1
1	small tomato, diced	1
½	small red onion, finely chopped	½
¼ cup	frozen corn kernels, thawed	60 mL
2 tbsp	chopped fresh parsley	30 mL
2 tbsp	olive oil	30 mL
1 tsp	freshly squeezed lemon juice	5 mL
	Freshly ground black pepper (optional)	
	Hot pepper sauce (optional)	

1. In a small bowl, combine tuna, avocado, tomato, red onion, corn, parsley, olive oil, lemon juice, pepper (if using) and hot pepper sauce (if using).

This recipe courtesy of Cindy McKenna.

Nutrients per serving			
Calories	201	Carbohydrates	9 g
Fat	15 g	Protein	10 g

Tuna Lettuce Pockets

Choose tuna that is canned in water, broth or olive oil.

Nutrients per serving	
Calories	102
Fat	4 g
Carbohydrates	4 g
Protein	11 g

1	can (6 oz/170 g) tuna, drained and crumbled	1
1	carrot, finely shredded	1
2 tbsp	mayonnaise	30 mL
1½ tbsp	Italian dressing	22 mL
4	large leaves iceberg lettuce (or 8 small)	4

1. Combine tuna, carrot, mayonnaise and dressing.
2. Cut the center ribs from the lettuce leaves and place 2 to 3 tbsp (30 to 45 mL) of the tuna mixture in the center of each leaf. Fold leaf around filling to form an edible cup. Serve 1 or 2 pockets per person, depending on size of pockets.

Spicy Chicken Salad

Roast a chicken and use it to make this salad. Otherwise, use the deli-roasted chicken, but be aware that it can be much higher in sodium than homemade.

TIP

Concerned about the amount of sodium in a deli-roasted chicken? Roast your own chicken. In fact, roast 2 or 3 chickens. Freeze the meat in individual portions, then thaw what you need and use it to make this salad.

- **Food processor**

1	3-lb (1.5 kg) deli-roasted chicken, skin and bones removed, cut into bite-size pieces	1
8 oz	elbow macaroni, cooked, rinsed and drained	250 g
1	red bell pepper, seeded and quartered	1
2	jalapeño peppers, seeded	2
3	shallots, quartered	3
3	stalks celery, cut into 3-inch (7.5 cm) lengths	3
2 tbsp	liquid honey	30 mL
1 tbsp	Dijon mustard	15 mL
1 tsp	grated lemon zest	5 mL
1 tbsp	freshly squeezed lemon juice	15 mL
2 cups	salad greens	500 mL
	Salt and freshly ground black pepper	

1. In a large salad bowl, combine chicken and pasta. Set aside.

2. In food processor fitted with metal blade, pulse bell pepper, jalapeños and shallots, about 10 times. Transfer to salad bowl.

3. Replace metal blade with slicing blade and slice celery. Add to salad bowl. Add honey, mustard and lemon zest and juice to salad bowl. Stir to coat fully.

4. Place greens on a large platter. Arrange chicken mixture on top. Season with salt and pepper to taste.

Nutrients per serving	
Calories	521
Fat	9 g
Carbohydrates	33 g
Protein	75 g

Citrus Chicken Salad

Makes 4 servings

This salad is tangy and fresh with citrus flavors. Studies show that people who consume adequate amounts of vitamin C — abundant in oranges — have healthier cartilage. As a bonus, tarragon contains phytochemicals that are associated with better heart health and better blood sugar control.

- **Food processor**

1 tbsp	mayonnaise	15 mL
1 tbsp	liquid honey	15 mL
1 tsp	Dijon mustard	5 mL
2 cups	orange segments	500 mL
½	head napa cabbage, cut into wedges to fit feed tube of food processor	½
3	carrots, cut into 3-inch (7.5 cm) lengths	3
2	stalks celery, cut into 3-inch (7.5 cm) lengths	2
3	green onions (green part only), cut in half	3
3 tbsp	fresh tarragon leaves	45 mL
3 cups	shredded cooked chicken	750 mL
	Salt and freshly ground black pepper	

1. In a salad bowl, whisk together mayonnaise, honey and mustard. Add orange segments. Set aside.
2. In food processor fitted with shredding blade, shred cabbage. Add to salad bowl.
3. Replace shredding blade with slicing blade and slice carrots and celery. Add to salad bowl.
4. Replace slicing blade with metal blade and pulse green onions and tarragon, about 5 times. Add to salad with chicken and toss to coat. Season with salt and pepper to taste.

Nutrients per serving	
Calories	262
Fat	4 g
Carbohydrates	32 g
Protein	27 g

Rainbow Lettuce Wraps

Makes about 2 cups (500 mL) filling		

These wraps make a great alternative to a sandwich in a lunch box or substitute for a hamburger at a barbecue.

TIPS

You could also use cooled cooked cabbage leaves as the wraps.

Butter lettuce is a type of head lettuce that has, as the name implies, a smooth, buttery texture. Varieties of butter lettuce include Boston and Bibb.

Stirring ground meat can be difficult when you have sore shoulders or hands. Instead, brown the turkey in a low-oil fryer, such as an ActiFry.

1 lb	lean ground turkey or chicken	500 g
1 tbsp	grated gingerroot	15 mL
2 tsp	canola oil	10 mL
¾ cup	finely chopped red bell pepper	175 mL
¾ cup	finely chopped yellow bell pepper	175 mL
½ cup	finely chopped onion	125 mL
2	cloves garlic, minced	2
1	can (8 oz/227 mL) sliced water chestnuts, drained and chopped	1
¼ cup	hoisin sauce	60 mL
¾ tsp	Chinese five-spice powder	3 mL
¼ to ½ tsp	hot pepper flakes	1 to 2 mL
½ cup	shredded carrot	125 mL
1	head butter lettuce, leaves separated	1

1. In a large nonstick skillet, over medium heat, brown turkey and ginger, breaking up turkey with a spoon, for 5 to 6 minutes or until no longer pink. Transfer to a bowl and set aside.

2. In the same skillet, heat oil over medium heat. Sauté red pepper, yellow pepper and onion for 4 to 5 minutes or until vegetables are softened. Add garlic and sauté for 30 seconds. Return turkey to skillet and stir in water chestnuts, hoisin sauce, ¼ cup (60 mL) water, five-spice powder and hot pepper flakes to taste; cook, stirring often, for 3 to 4 minutes or until heated through. Transfer to a serving bowl.

3. Arrange carrot and lettuce leaves on a large platter and set out with the turkey mixture. Top each lettuce leaf with 2 tbsp (30 mL) of the turkey mixture, then carrot. Wrap lettuce to enclose filling.

VARIATION

Ground beef, pork or vegetarian ground round can be used in place of turkey.

This recipe courtesy of dietitian Heather McColl.

Nutrients per 2 wraps	
Calories	69
Fat	3 g
Carbohydrates	5 g
Protein	6 g

Vegetarian Mains

Roasted Vegetable Lasagna

Makes 6 servings

Lasagna with no noodles! This combination of vegetables supplies all the protein you need. Eggplant is a great source of nutrients and contains lots of soluble fiber, so this meal will keep you full for a long time.

TIP

Choose seasonal greens for this year-round dish — spinach and dandelion greens in spring, or cabbage, Swiss chard and kale in winter.

- Preheat oven to 375°F (190°C)
- 2 rimmed baking sheets, lightly oiled
- 11- by 7-inch (28 by 18 cm) baking pan, lightly oiled

1	large eggplant, trimmed and cut lengthwise into 1/4-inch (0.5 cm) slices	1
2	red bell peppers, halved lengthwise	2
5 tbsp	olive oil, divided	75 mL
1 tbsp	balsamic vinegar	15 mL
1	large onion, chopped	1
2 cups	sliced mushrooms	500 mL
2	cloves garlic, minced	2
2 tbsp	chopped fresh mixed herbs (such as oregano, thyme and basil)	30 mL
1	can (19 oz/540 mL) crushed tomatoes	1
1	can (14 to 19 oz/398 to 540 mL) lima beans, drained and rinsed	1
3 cups	shredded greens (see tip, at left)	750 mL

1. Arrange eggplant slices on one baking sheet and brush with 1 tbsp (15 mL) of the oil. Arrange red pepper halves, cut side down, on the other baking sheet and brush with 1 tbsp (15 mL) of the oil. Bake in preheated oven for 15 minutes or until the tip of a knife easily pierces the eggplant and the skin of the red peppers is dark and blistered. Do not overcook the eggplant. Let cool completely. Slip skin off red peppers and slice into wide strips. In a bowl, toss pepper strips with 1 tbsp (15 mL) of the oil and the vinegar and set aside.

Nutrients per serving	
Calories	289
Fat	14 g
Carbohydrates	34 g
Protein	10 g

TIP

To wash or not wash mushrooms? You can wipe them with a damp cloth, if you wish. However, I feel it's important to wash all produce that comes into my kitchen. I quickly rinse mushrooms under cold water and immediately wrap in a clean, dry kitchen towel or paper towels to absorb excess moisture.

2. In a skillet, heat remaining oil over medium heat. Add onion and mushrooms and cook, stirring frequently, for 6 to 8 minutes or until slightly softened. Add garlic and cook, stirring frequently, for 2 minutes or until onion and garlic are soft. Add herbs and tomatoes. Reduce heat to medium-low and simmer, stirring occasionally, for 10 minutes. Add lima beans and greens and cook for 1 to 5 minutes or until greens are wilted or, in the case of winter greens, tender when pierced with the tip of a knife.

3. Line prepared baking pan with one-third of the eggplant slices. Lay half the red pepper over the eggplant. Spread with one-third of the tomato sauce. Layer another one-third of the eggplant slices and the remaining red pepper slices and spread another one-third of the sauce over. Top with remaining eggplant slices and spread with remaining tomato sauce. Lasagna may be covered and stored in the refrigerator overnight. Bring back to room temperature before baking. Bake in preheated oven for 40 minutes or until sauce is bubbly.

Split Yellow Peas with Zucchini

Makes 6 servings

Since this tasty, easy-to-prepare dish freezes well, make a double batch and freeze in small portions. It's great for a quick lunch or supper. The split peas provide all the protein you need. Start the meal with vegetable soup and finish with fruit.

TIPS

When adding dry spices, it is important to sauté them for 3 to 4 minutes to remove the "raw taste" of the spices. The spices will neither soften nor be recognizably fragrant. If anything, they may turn slightly darker.

To freeze, transfer to an airtight container and freeze for up to 3 months. Reheat in microwave or on stovetop over low heat.

1 cup	yellow split peas (channa dal)	250 mL
2 tbsp	vegetable oil	30 mL
1½ tbsp	minced gingerroot	22 mL
2 tsp	minced green chile pepper (preferably serrano)	10 mL
1 cup	finely chopped onion	250 mL
3 cups	chopped zucchini (½-inch/1 cm pieces)	750 mL
1 tsp	coriander powder	5 mL
1 tsp	salt, or to taste	5 mL
½ tsp	ground turmeric	2 mL
½ tsp	cayenne pepper	2 mL
1	can (14 oz/398 mL) tomatoes, including juice, chopped	1

1. Clean and pick through dal for any small stones and grit. Rinse several times in cold water until water is fairly clear. Soak in 2 cups (500 mL) water for 20 to 30 minutes.

2. In a saucepan, heat oil over medium-high heat. Add ginger and chiles and sauté for 1 minute. Add onion and sauté until soft and translucent, 6 to 7 minutes.

3. Add zucchini and mix well. Cover and cook for 5 minutes. Add coriander, salt, turmeric and cayenne. Mix well and cook, stirring, 3 to 4 minutes (see tip, at left).

4. Add tomatoes with juice and dal with soaking liquid, plus enough additional water to cover. Stir to mix well. Cover, reduce heat to low and simmer, stirring every 10 minutes, until dal is soft and a little liquid remains, resulting in a thin gravy (sauce), 20 to 25 minutes.

Nutrients per serving	
Calories	193
Fat	5 g
Carbohydrates	28 g
Protein	9 g

Red Lentil Curry with Coconut and Cilantro

Easy to make, these red lentils have a luxurious coconut finish and a lovely bright yellow color. If you are trying to reduce your caloric intake, make this recipe with light coconut milk. Choose fortified coconut milk to increase your intake of calcium and vitamin D.

TIPS

Traditionally, Indian lentil dishes such as this one are served very loose and almost soupy. You can adjust the texture to your taste by adding more water or simmering longer to thicken in step 2.

Leftovers will thicken considerably upon cooling. If reheating in the microwave or a saucepan, add boiling water before heating to return to desired consistency.

2 tbsp	vegetable oil	30 mL
1	small onion, finely chopped	1
2	cloves garlic, minced	2
1 tbsp	minced gingerroot	15 mL
	Salt	
1 tsp	ground coriander	5 mL
1 tsp	ground cumin	5 mL
¼ tsp	ground turmeric	1 mL
1 cup	dried red lentils (masoor dal), rinsed	250 mL
1	can (14 oz/400 mL) coconut milk	1
1 cup	water	250 mL
¼ cup	torn fresh cilantro leaves	60 mL
	Garam masala	

1. In a saucepan, heat oil over medium heat. Add onion and cook, stirring, until softened and starting to brown, about 5 minutes. Add garlic, ginger, 1 tsp (5 mL) salt, coriander, cumin and turmeric; cook, stirring, until softened and fragrant, about 2 minutes.

2. Stir in lentils until coated with spices. Stir in coconut milk and water; bring to a boil, scraping up bits stuck to pan and stirring to prevent lumps. Reduce heat to low, partially cover and simmer, stirring often, until lentils are very soft and mixture is thick, about 15 minutes.

3. Remove from heat, cover and let stand for 5 minutes. Season to taste with salt. Stir in all but a few leaves of cilantro. Serve sprinkled with remaining cilantro and garam masala.

VARIATION

To add some heat to this dish, add 1 or 2 hot red or green chile peppers, minced, with the garlic.

Nutrients per serving	
Calories	288
Fat	19 g
Carbohydrates	22 g
Protein	10 g

Red Lentils with Garlic and Cilantro

The spices and herbs in this recipe add much more than great flavor: they also contribute phytochemicals that will help ward off inflammation and heart disease. Add some Gujarati Sambhar Masala (see recipe, opposite) with the cilantro for even more anti-arthritis action.

- • **Immersion blender or upright blender**

2 cups	dried red lentils (masoor dal)	500 mL
¾ tsp	ground turmeric	3 mL
2 tsp	salt, or to taste	10 mL
1½ cups	chopped tomatoes	375 mL
3 tbsp	minced gingerroot	45 mL
4 tsp	minced green chile pepper (preferably serrano)	20 mL
2 cups	fresh cilantro leaves, chopped	500 mL
2 tbsp	vegetable oil	30 mL
12 to 14	cloves garlic, sliced	12 to 14
2	sprigs fresh curry leaves, stripped (20 to 25)	2

1. Clean and pick through dal for any small stones and grit. Rinse several times in cold water until water is fairly clear. Soak in 8 cups (2 L) water in a saucepan for 10 minutes. Bring dal to a boil over medium-high heat. Skim any froth off the top. Reduce heat to medium-low. Stir in turmeric and simmer, partially covered, until dal is soft, about 20 minutes. Stir in salt.

2. Using an immersion blender or in a blender, in batches if necessary, purée mixture. Return to saucepan if necessary. Return to a gentle boil over medium heat.

3. Add tomatoes, ginger, chiles and cilantro. Cover, reduce heat to medium-low and simmer for 10 minutes.

4. In a small saucepan, heat oil over medium heat. Add garlic and sauté for 1 minute. Add curry leaves and cook until garlic is golden, 2 to 3 minutes. Pour mixture into dal. Cover and remove from heat. Allow to infuse for 5 minutes before serving with rice.

Nutrients per serving	
Calories	216
Fat	5 g
Carbohydrates	32 g
Protein	14 g

This mixture is a concentrate used for flavoring otherwise bland dishes such as dals. It can also be folded into cooked, slightly smashed potatoes with great success. Fenugreek has anti-arthritis effects, and is being tested in some supplements.

Gujarati Sambhar Masala

2 tbsp	vegetable oil	30 mL
1 tbsp	salt	15 mL
2 tsp	cayenne pepper	10 mL
1 tsp	pounded and semi-crushed dark mustard seeds	5 mL
1 tsp	pounded and semi-crushed fenugreek seeds (methi)	5 mL
½ tsp	asafetida (hing)	2 mL

1. In a bowl, combine oil, salt, cayenne, mustard seeds, fenugreek and asafetida. Store in an airtight container at room temperature indefinitely.

Nutrients per 1 tsp (5 mL)	
Calories	31
Fat	3 g
Carbohydrates	1 g
Protein	0 g

Rajasthani Mixed Dal

If you are new to eating dried beans and peas, you may find that they give you gas. This can be greatly reduced if you soak them overnight, changing the water a few times.

TIPS

Ghee — clarified butter — can be purchased at specialty grocery stores.

If curry leaves have dried naturally in the refrigerator over several weeks, they are most likely still aromatic. The dried ones sold in Indian markets have no aroma or flavor, and I would advise against those.

1 cup	split white lentils (urad dal)	250 mL
½ cup	yellow mung beans (mung dal)	125 mL
¼ cup	split yellow peas (channa dal)	60 mL
½ tsp	ground turmeric	2 mL
1½ tsp	salt	7 mL
2 tbsp	ghee	30 mL
1 tsp	cumin seeds	5 mL
¼ tsp	asafetida (hing)	1 mL
4	bay leaves	4
3	whole cloves	3
3	green cardamom pods, crushed	3
1	sprig fresh curry leaves, stripped (12 to 15 leaves) (optional)	1
1½ cups	chopped tomatoes	375 mL
2 tbsp	minced green chile pepper (preferably serrano)	30 mL
1 tbsp	minced gingerroot	15 mL
1 tsp	cayenne pepper	5 mL
1 cup	loosely packed fresh cilantro leaves	250 mL

1. Clean and pick through urad, mung and channa dals for any small stones and grit. Rinse several times in cold water until water is fairly clear. Soak in 7 cups (1.75 L) water in a saucepan for 1 hour.

2. Bring dals to a boil over medium-high heat. Stir in turmeric and boil gently, partially covered, until dals are soft but not mushy and water does not appear to be separated (see tip, opposite), about 30 minutes. Stir in salt. Set aside.

Nutrients per serving	
Calories	195
Fat	5 g
Carbohydrates	28 g
Protein	11 g

TIP

With some exceptions, in India, dal is usually cooked with plenty of water, which is seldom drained. A layer of water will be present on top of the cooked dal. Instead of draining this off, when the dal is soft, it is mashed or blended with the remaining water, allowing the starch in the dal to break down and act as a thickener. The mashed dal is usually the consistency of cream soup. (This technique is uncommon in Western cooking, where lentils and beans are cooked until soft, then drained, retaining their shape.)

3. In another saucepan, heat ghee over medium heat. Add cumin, asafetida, bay leaves, cloves, cardamom and curry leaves (if using) and sauté for 20 seconds. Add tomatoes, chiles, ginger and cayenne and sauté for 2 minutes.

4. Pour dal into tomato mixture and mix well. If there is excess water, cook, uncovered, over medium-low heat until water looks absorbed but without drying dal too much. (It should be thick but liquidy enough to pour over rice.) Adjust consistency with a little additional warm water if too thick. Sprinkle cilantro over dal before serving.

Buttery Mung Dal

A cup (250 mL) of mung beans contains almost 60% of the fiber you need for the whole day. The fiber in most beans is soluble, which helps control blood sugar and cholesterol levels while also helping you feel full longer.

TIPS

The starch in this particular dal makes it creamy when pressed through a sieve, which you could do if you don't have an immersion blender.

Choose canola oil, avocado oil, olive oil or grapeseed oil to sauté the garlic. Overheating the oil can destroy some of its health benefits, so keep the heat at medium or below.

- **Immersion blender or upright blender (optional)**

1½ cups	yellow mung beans (yellow mung dal)	375 mL
¼ tsp	ground turmeric	1 mL
1½ tsp	salt, or to taste	7 mL
1½ tsp	ground coriander	7 mL
¾ tsp	ground cumin	3 mL
½ tsp	cayenne pepper	2 mL
½ tsp	garam masala	2 mL
1½ tbsp	vegetable oil	22 mL
3 tbsp	coarsely chopped garlic	45 mL
1½ tsp	mango powder (amchur) (optional)	7 mL
¾ tsp	freshly ground black pepper	3 mL

1. Clean and pick through beans for any small stones and grit. Rinse several times in cold water until water is fairly clear. Soak in 4 cups (1 L) water in a large saucepan for 10 minutes.

2. Bring to a boil over medium heat, skimming froth off surface. Stir in turmeric and adjust heat to maintain a gentle boil. Cook, partially covered, until dal is very soft, about 20 minutes. Stir in salt.

3. Remove from heat. Using an immersion blender, blend until creamy and smooth. Alternatively, transfer to blender or press through a sieve (see tip, at left). Texture should be very thick, like lightly whipped cream.

4. Return mixture to very low heat. Pile coriander, cumin, cayenne pepper and garam masala in the center of the dal. Do not stir to mix.

5. In a small saucepan, heat oil over medium heat. Sauté garlic until golden, 3 to 4 minutes. Pour over spices. Remove from heat.

6. Gently transfer dal to a serving bowl, trying not to disturb the spice and garlic mixture. Sprinkle mango powder (if using) and pepper over entire surface of dish. Serve with Indian bread.

Nutrients per serving	
Calories	164
Fat	3 g
Carbohydrates	26 g
Protein	10 g

Herbed Nut and Bean Patties

Makes 6 patties

These tasty patties are a great substitute for burgers. If you're trying to avoid wheat, wrap them in lettuce leaves or use gluten-free hamburger buns.

TIP

While the patties hold together quite nicely for baking, they are still soft and fragile, definitely not suited to grilling on a barbecue.

VARIATION

For a meatless main course loaf, pack the mixture into a lightly oiled 9- by 5-inch (23 by 12. 5 cm) loaf pan and bake in a 375°F (190°C) oven for 20 minutes or until mixture is set and begins to come away from sides of the pan. Let stand for 10 minutes before serving. Slice and top with barbecue sauce. Serve hot or cold.

- **Preheat oven to 375°F (190°C)**
- **Food processor**
- **Baking sheet, lightly oiled**

1	can (19 oz/540 mL) chickpeas, drained and rinsed	1
1	small onion, cut into quarters	1
2	cloves garlic	2
1	carrot, cut into chunks	1
1	small apple, quartered	1
1	slice candied ginger (or $\frac{1}{2}$-inch/1 cm piece gingerroot)	1
$\frac{1}{2}$ cup	spelt flakes	125 mL
$\frac{1}{4}$ cup	natural almonds	60 mL
$\frac{1}{4}$ cup	sunflower seeds	60 mL
2 tbsp	ground flax seeds (flaxseed meal)	30 mL
4	fresh parsley sprigs, stems trimmed	4
$1\frac{1}{2}$ to 3 tsp	Cajun spice blend	7 to 15 mL
1 tbsp	fresh thyme leaves	15 mL
1 tsp	salt	5 mL
2 tbsp	olive oil	30 mL
1	large egg	1
$\frac{1}{2}$ cup	barbecue sauce (optional)	125 mL
6	hamburger buns (optional)	6

1. In a food processor, combine chickpeas, onion, garlic, carrot, apple and ginger. Pulse until chopped. Add spelt, almonds, sunflower seeds, flax seeds, parsley, Cajun spice to taste, thyme and salt. Process until finely chopped. With motor running, add oil and egg through the feed tube. Process until well mixed and holding together.

2. Spoon about one-sixth of the mixture directly onto prepared baking sheet, and pat into a compact patty, about 4 inches (10 cm) in diameter. Repeat until 6 patties are formed. Bake in preheated oven for 15 minutes. Top each patty with barbecue sauce (if using) and place in hamburger buns (if using).

Nutrients per patty	
Calories	260
Fat	14 g
Carbohydrates	27 g
Protein	9 g

Zucchini with Yellow Mung Beans

This recipe uses a great mix of spices that promote good health. The beans add protein and fiber, as well as antioxidant minerals and phytochemicals. Choose canola oil for its omega-3 fatty acids.

TIP

Many people find that eating beans gives them gas. Try introducing them into your diet gradually. Some people use Beano or a similar product that contains the enzyme needed to digest the complex carbohydrate in beans and other foods that causes gas.

1 cup	yellow mung beans (yellow mung dal)	250 mL
2 tbsp	vegetable oil	30 mL
1 tsp	mustard seeds	5 mL
1 tsp	cumin seeds	5 mL
1/2 tsp	fenugreek seeds (methi)	2 mL
1/2 cup	sliced green onions (2 to 3)	125 mL
2 tsp	minced garlic	10 mL
2 tsp	minced gingerroot	10 mL
2 cups	chopped tomatoes	500 mL
4 tsp	sambar powder	20 mL
1 tsp	ground coriander	5 mL
1/2 tsp	ground turmeric	2 mL
3	zucchini (about 1 1/2 lbs/750 g), sliced 1/4 inch (0.5 cm) thick	3
1 tsp	salt, or to taste	5 mL
	Juice of 1 lime or 1/2 lemon	
1/2 cup	fresh cilantro leaves, chopped, divided	125 mL
1 tsp	garam masala	5 mL

1. Clean and pick through beans for any small stones and grit. Rinse several times in cold water until water is fairly clear. Soak in 4 cups (1 L) water in a large saucepan for 10 minutes.

2. Meanwhile, heat oil in a large saucepan over high heat until a couple of mustard seeds thrown in start to sputter. Add remaining mustard seeds and cover immediately. When seeds stop popping after a few seconds, reduce heat to medium. Add cumin and fenugreek seeds. Sauté for 20 to 30 seconds. Do not allow seeds to burn.

Nutrients per serving	
Calories	157
Fat	5 g
Carbohydrates	22 g
Protein	9 g

TIPS

To peel gingerroot without a vegetable peeler, use the edge of a large spoon to scrape the skin off.

Gingerroot can be grated ahead of time and frozen in 1 tbsp (15 mL) portions, ready for use.

3. Stir in green onions, garlic and ginger. Sauté for 1 minute. Add tomatoes, sambar powder, coriander and turmeric. Mix well and sauté until tomatoes are soft, about 5 minutes.

4. Drain dal and add to onion mixture. Sauté for 3 to 4 minutes. Pour in 2 cups (500 mL) water. Cover and bring to a boil. Reduce heat to low and simmer, stirring occasionally, for 15 minutes.

5. Stir in zucchini and salt. Cover and cook, stirring occasionally, until vegetables and dal are soft, 15 to 20 minutes. Dal should be completely mushy and thickened.

6. Remove from heat. Stir in lime juice and all but 2 tbsp (30 mL) of the cilantro. Sprinkle with garam masala and cover for 5 minutes before serving. Garnish with remaining cilantro and serve with an Indian bread or rice.

Three-Bean Chili

This hearty chili makes a filling meal. It's sure to be a family favorite, so make a double batch and freeze the leftovers for another meal. Serve with a salad on the side and some fruit for dessert.

TIPS

Because can sizes vary, we provide a range of amounts for beans in our recipes. If you're using 19-oz (540 mL) cans, add a bit of chili powder to taste.

Use diced tomatoes with or without seasonings.

This dish can be frozen for up to 2 months in an airtight container.

VARIATION

For a more substantial version of this chili, add 6 oz (175 g) soy ground meat alternative. In a skillet, heat 1 tbsp (15 mL) of olive oil over medium-high heat. Add meat alternative and reduce heat to medium. Cook, stirring frequently, for 5 minutes or until heated through. Add to chili along with the vinegar.

1 tbsp	vegetable oil	15 mL
1	large onion, coarsely chopped	1
1	red bell pepper, cut into 1-inch (2.5 cm) cubes	1
2	cloves garlic, minced	2
1½ tbsp	chili powder	22 mL
1½ tsp	ground cumin	7 mL
½ tsp	dried oregano	2 mL
½ tsp	ground cinnamon	2 mL
½ tsp	ground allspice	2 mL
¼ tsp	hot pepper flakes	1 mL
2 cups	Vegetable Stock (page 200) or ready-to-use vegetable broth	500 mL
½ cup	tomato paste	125 mL
1	can (14 to 19 oz/398 to 540 mL) black beans, drained and rinsed (see tip, at left)	1
1	can (14 to 19 oz/398 to 540 mL) red kidney beans, drained and rinsed	1
1	can (14 to 19 oz/398 to 540 mL) navy or white kidney beans, drained and rinsed	1
1	can (28 oz/796 mL) diced tomatoes, with juices	1
1 tbsp	red wine vinegar	15 mL

1. In a large pot, heat oil over medium heat for 30 seconds. Add onion and red pepper and cook, stirring, for 3 minutes or until softened. Add garlic and cook, stirring, for 1 minute. Add chili powder, cumin, oregano, cinnamon, allspice and hot pepper flakes and cook, stirring, for 1 minute.

2. Add vegetable stock and increase heat to medium-high. Bring to a simmer and cook for 5 minutes or until pepper is very soft. Add tomato paste and stir well. Add black, red kidney and navy beans, tomatoes and vinegar. Return to a boil. Reduce heat to low, cover and simmer for 35 minutes or until thickened.

Nutrients per serving	
Calories	235
Fat	3 g
Carbohydrates	40 g
Protein	12 g

Baked Beans and Rice Casserole

Makes 6 servings

Post this recipe on your pantry door and keep all the ingredients on hand for a hot home-cooked meal in a jiffy.

TIP

After increasing the oven temperature, watch carefully. You want the topping to brown but not burn.

VARIATION

Replace soy bacon with veggie franks. Use 2 franks and cut into ½-inch (1 cm) thick slices, then cut each slice in half.

- **Preheat oven to 375°F (190°C)**
- **8-cup (2 L) casserole dish, greased**

2	strips soy bacon	2
2	cans (each 14 to 16 oz/398 to 480 mL) vegetarian baked beans	2
½ tsp	chili powder	2 mL
½ tsp	hot pepper sauce, or to taste	2 mL
¼ tsp	hot pepper flakes, or to taste	1 mL
2 cups	cooked jasmine or white rice	500 mL
½ cup	dry bread crumbs	125 mL
2 tbsp	soy margarine, melted	30 mL

1. In a small nonstick skillet, cook soy bacon according to package directions until crisp. Let cool for 3 minutes. Break into small pieces that resemble bacon bits.

2. In prepared dish, combine bacon pieces, baked beans, chili powder, hot pepper sauce and hot pepper flakes. Stir in cooked rice. Sprinkle with bread crumbs and drizzle margarine over top.

3. Bake in preheated oven for 25 minutes or until hot and bubbling. Increase oven temperature to 500°F (260°C). Cook for 2 to 3 minutes or until topping is browned. Let stand for 3 to 5 minutes before serving.

Nutrients per serving	
Calories	346
Fat	10 g
Carbohydrates	54 g
Protein	12 g

Quinoa à la Med

Mediterranean-style quinoa makes a great addition to a summertime family meal. You could use frozen artichokes instead of marinated; just steam them first and use a bit more dressing.

TIPS

Store a batch of this multi-purpose dressing in the refrigerator so it's ready when you need it. It can be stored for up to 5 days.

Squeeze fresh lemons with an electric juicer and freeze the juice in ice cube trays. Defrost as many ice cubes as you need to make the dressing.

1 cup	quinoa, rinsed	250 mL
2 cups	bite-size broccoli florets, blanched and drained	500 mL
1 cup	diced tomatoes	250 mL
2/3 cup	diced drained oil-marinated artichoke hearts, patted dry	150 mL
2/3 cup	finely chopped roasted red bell peppers	150 mL
1/4 cup	finely chopped kalamata olives	60 mL
1 cup	rinsed drained canned chickpeas	250 mL

Dressing

2 tbsp	Dijon mustard	30 mL
2 tbsp	red wine vinegar	30 mL
1 tbsp	freshly squeezed lemon juice	15 mL
2 tbsp	canola oil	30 mL
3/4 tsp	freshly ground black pepper	3 mL
1/4 tsp	salt	1 mL

1. In a medium saucepan, combine quinoa and 2 cups (500 mL) water; bring to a boil over high heat. Reduce heat to low, cover and simmer for 15 to 20 minutes or until liquid is absorbed and quinoa is tender. Let stand for 5 minutes. Transfer to a large bowl and fluff with a fork. Let cool.

2. Gently stir broccoli, tomatoes, artichokes, roasted peppers, olives and chickpeas into quinoa.

3. *Dressing:* In a small bowl, whisk together mustard and vinegar. Whisk in lemon juice, oil, 2 tbsp (30 mL) water, pepper and salt. Pour over salad and stir to combine.

VARIATION

Add chopped roasted mushrooms to the salad.

This recipe courtesy of dietitian Lisa Diamond.

Nutrients per serving	
Calories	238
Fat	9 g
Carbohydrates	33 g
Protein	7 g

Mediterranean Kasha Casserole with Sun-Dried Tomatoes

Kasha, or roasted buckwheat groats, is gluten-free because, despite its name, buckwheat is actually a fruit that acts like a grain in cooking. You can use fresh basil and oregano instead of dried if you have some on hand; simply use three times the amount.

TIPS

Use whole-grain kasha to prevent sticking.

To soften sun-dried tomatoes, pour boiling water over them and soak 15 minutes or until soft. Drain and chop.

You can either leave the cheese out or substitute one of your choice.

MAKE AHEAD

Prepare up to 2 days in advance. Reheat gently.

Nutrients per serving	
Calories	143
Fat	3 g
Carbohydrates	28 g
Protein	5 g

3 cups	Vegetable Stock (page 200) or ready-to-use vegetable broth	750 mL
1 cup	whole-grain kasha	250 mL
2 tsp	vegetable oil	10 mL
2 tsp	minced garlic	10 mL
1 cup	chopped onions	250 mL
1½ cups	diced unpeeled eggplant	375 mL
1½ cups	diced unpeeled zucchini	375 mL
2 cups	chopped mushrooms	500 mL
1 cup	diced plum (Roma) tomatoes	250 mL
1 cup	tomato pasta sauce	250 mL
1 tsp	dried basil	5 mL
½ tsp	dried oregano	2 mL
½ cup	chopped softened sun-dried tomatoes (see tip, at left)	125 mL
⅓ cup	sliced black olives	75 mL
2 oz	feta cheese, crumbled (optional)	60 g

1. In a saucepan, bring vegetable stock and kasha to a boil; reduce heat to low, cover and cook until liquid is absorbed, about 10 to 12 minutes.

2. Meanwhile, in a large nonstick saucepan sprayed with vegetable spray, heat oil over medium-high heat. Add garlic and onions; cook for 2 minutes. Stir in eggplant and zucchini; cook for 5 minutes, stirring often. Stir in mushrooms, tomatoes, tomato sauce, basil and oregano; cook for 4 minutes, stirring occasionally. Remove from heat; stir in sun-dried tomatoes and olives.

3. Combine kasha with vegetable mixture. Serve sprinkled with feta cheese, if desired.

Slow Cooker Squash Couscous

This delicious one-pot meal simmers away in the slow cooker while you go on with your day.

TIPS

Butternut squash can be difficult to peel. To make the task easier, first cut the squash in half crosswise, to create two flat surfaces. Place each squash half on its flat surface and use a sharp utility knife to remove the tough peel. Or skip the peeling and buy prechopped fresh squash or frozen chopped squash.

This dish is naturally quite sweet, so you may want to reduce the sugar to taste, or even eliminate it.

VARIATIONS

Add a 4-inch (10 cm) cinnamon stick to the squash mixture in step 1. Discard before serving.

Use dried cranberries or chopped dates instead of raisins.

Nutrients per serving	
Calories	230
Fat	4 g
Carbohydrates	44 g
Protein	8 g

- **Minimum 5-quart slow cooker**

1	butternut squash (about 1½ lbs/750 g)	1
3 cups	cooked or rinsed drained canned chickpeas	750 mL
2 cups	chopped yellow summer squash or zucchini	500 mL
½ cup	thinly sliced onion	125 mL
½ cup	raisins	125 mL
2 tbsp	granulated sugar	30 mL
2 tsp	ground ginger	10 mL
½ tsp	ground turmeric	2 mL
½ tsp	freshly ground black pepper	2 mL
4 cups	Vegetable Stock (page 200) or reduced-sodium ready-to-use vegetable broth	1 L
2 tbsp	non-hydrogenated margarine	30 mL
1 cup	couscous	250 mL
¼ cup	coarsely chopped fresh parsley	60 mL

1. Peel butternut squash and cut the flesh into 1-inch (2.5 cm) cubes; you should have 4 to 5 cups (1 to 1.25 L) cubed squash.

2. In slow cooker stoneware, combine butternut squash, chickpeas, summer squash, onion, raisins, sugar, ginger, turmeric, pepper, vegetable stock and margarine. Cover and cook on Low for 4 to 5 hours or until vegetables are tender.

3. Uncover, increase heat to High and cook for 15 minutes or until liquid is reduced slightly. Using a slotted spoon, remove vegetable mixture to a large bowl. Cover and keep warm.

4. Place couscous in a large bowl and pour in 1 cup (250 mL) of the hot broth from the slow cooker. Cover with plastic wrap and let stand for 5 to 10 minutes or until couscous is plumped. Fluff with a fork.

5. Spoon vegetable mixture over couscous and ladle the remaining broth over top. Sprinkle with parsley.

This recipe courtesy of dietitian Cheryl Fisher.

Curried Vegetables with Tofu

Tofu is a concentrated source of nutrients, is high in protein and contains most of the beneficial nutrients found in soybeans. For the vegetable oil, choose canola oil: its mild taste will let the other flavors shine through.

TIPS

Fried bean curd can be found in natural food stores or Asian markets. It comes prepackaged in cubes or triangles. Because of its light and airy consistency, it absorbs flavors very nicely.

Because can sizes vary, we provide a range of amounts for chickpeas in our recipes. If you're using a 19-oz (540 mL) can, add a bit of curry powder to taste.

VARIATION

For a slightly deeper flavor, add ½ tsp (2 mL) turmeric along with the ginger. If you like a bit of heat, add 3 or 4 drops of hot sesame oil.

2 tsp	vegetable oil	10 mL
1	sweet onion (such as Vidalia), coarsely chopped	1
1	red bell pepper, cut into 1- by ½-inch (2.5 by 1 cm) strips	1
2 tsp	curry powder	10 mL
½ tsp	ground ginger	2 mL
2 cups	broccoli florets	500 mL
2 cups	cauliflower florets	500 mL
1 cup	Vegetable Stock (page 200) or ready-to-use vegetable broth	250 mL
2 or 3	carrots, cut into ¼-inch (0.5 cm) thick slices (about 1 cup/250 mL)	2 or 3
1	can (14 to 19 oz/398 to 540 mL) chickpeas, drained and rinsed	1
10 oz	firm tofu, cut into 1-inch (2.5 cm) cubes or fried bean curd (see tip, at left)	300 g
½ cup	vanilla-flavored soy milk	125 mL
3 tbsp	unsweetened shredded coconut	45 mL
2 tsp	granulated natural cane sugar	10 mL
	Salt and freshly ground black pepper	

1. In a large nonstick skillet, heat oil over medium heat for 30 seconds. Add onion and cook, stirring, for 3 minutes or until softened. Add red pepper, curry powder and ginger and cook, stirring, for 1 minute. Add broccoli, cauliflower, vegetable stock and carrots and cook, stirring, for 4 to 5 minutes or until heated through. Reduce heat to low, cover and simmer for 10 minutes or until vegetables are soft.

2. Stir in chickpeas and tofu. Increase heat to medium and cook until the mixture begins to bubble. Reduce heat to low, cover and simmer for 10 minutes or until flavors are blended.

3. Stir in soy milk, coconut, sugar and salt and pepper to taste. Simmer, uncovered, for 5 minutes.

VARIATION

Sprinkle the top of each portion with 2 tbsp (30 mL) finely chopped peanuts.

Nutrients per serving	
Calories	203
Fat	7 g
Carbohydrates	26 g
Protein	10 g

Tofu Vegetable Pilaf

Fluffy basmati rice forms the base of this Indian-inspired pilaf. If you choose brown basmati rice for its greater fiber content, keep in mind that you will have to increase the cooking time by 20 to 25 minutes.

TIPS

Be sure to remove the cinnamon sticks and cardamom pods before serving. The cardamom pods can become camouflaged by the peas, so look carefully. To make removing the spices easier, wrap them in a square of cheesecloth tied with kitchen string.

The carbohydrate in this recipe may seem high, but remember that both vegetables and grains are provided in this one dish.

Serve topped with chopped fresh cilantro and chopped roasted peanuts, with plain yogurt on the side.

2 tbsp	canola oil	30 mL
2	4-inch (10 cm) cinnamon sticks	2
4	cardamom pods	4
1 tsp	cumin seeds	5 mL
1½ cups	finely chopped onions	375 mL
1½ cups	diced potatoes	375 mL
1 cup	fresh or frozen green peas (thawed and drained if frozen)	250 mL
1 cup	diced carrots	250 mL
1 cup	cubed firm tofu	250 mL
3 tbsp	grated gingerroot	45 mL
½ tsp	ground turmeric	2 mL
1 cup	basmati rice	250 mL
½ tsp	salt	2 mL

1. In a large pot, heat oil over medium heat. Sauté cinnamon sticks, cardamom pods and cumin seeds for 1 minute or until fragrant. Add onions, potatoes, peas, carrots, tofu, ginger and turmeric; sauté for 3 to 4 minutes or until onions are softened.

2. Add rice, salt and 3 cups (750 mL) water; bring to a boil. Reduce heat to low, cover and simmer, stirring occasionally, for 15 minutes or until rice is tender and fluffy. (If rice starts to stick, stir in 1 to 2 tbsp/15 to 30 mL more water.) Discard cinnamon sticks and cardamom pods. Fluff rice with a fork.

This recipe courtesy of dietitian Shefali Raja.

Nutrients per serving	
Calories	426
Fat	12 g
Carbohydrates	64 g
Protein	16 g

Spinach Pasta

Makes 6 servings

Pasta tastes so much fresher when it's homemade, and your guests will be so impressed. As a bonus, fresh pasta cooks more quickly than dried pasta. To lower the saturated fat content of this dish, use a lower-fat Parmesan cheese.

TIP

If you don't want to make your own pasta, you can purchase fresh spinach pasta at specialty grocery stores. Or use zucchini cut into "zoodles."

- **Food processor**

3	extra-large eggs	3
5 oz	frozen chopped spinach, thawed and squeezed dry	150 g
½ tsp	salt	2 mL
2 cups	all-purpose flour	500 mL
1	clove garlic, minced	1
⅓ cup	freshly grated Parmesan cheese	75 mL
3 tbsp	extra virgin olive oil	45 mL

1. In food processor, purée eggs, spinach and salt. Add flour and pulse until a ball of dough forms.

2. On a floured board, knead dough until very smooth and elastic; cover and let rest for 10 minutes. Using a pasta machine, or on a floured board, with a floured rolling pin, roll out to desired thickness, adding flour as necessary to keep dough from sticking. Cut into noodles.

3. Cook in rapidly boiling salted water for 1 to 5 minutes, or until al dente (timing will depend on thickness). Drain and toss with garlic, Parmesan and oil.

Nutrients per serving	
Calories	296
Fat	11 g
Carbohydrates	37 g
Protein	11 g

Buckwheat Pasta with Fontina, Potatoes and Cabbage

Pizzoccheri is a flat ribbon pasta made with 80% buckwheat flour and 20% wheat flour. Buckwheat is an energizing and nutritious seed that is a very good source of manganese, copper and dietary fiber.

- **Preheat oven to 450°F (230°C)**
- **12-cup (3 L) casserole dish, buttered**

1 tsp	coarse salt	5 mL
2 to 3	potatoes, peeled and cut into small chunks	2 to 3
8 oz	savoy cabbage, halved, cored and cut into strips	250 g
1 lb	pizzoccheri (available at Italian grocery stores) or fettuccine	500 g
3 tbsp	butter	45 mL
6	cloves garlic, thinly sliced	6
12	fresh sage leaves, torn into pieces	12
Pinch	salt	Pinch
Pinch	freshly ground black pepper	Pinch
1 cup	grated Parmigiano-Reggiano cheese	250 mL
10 oz	Italian fontina or Taleggio cheese, diced	300 g

1. Bring a large pot of water to a boil. Stir in coarse salt and potatoes. Reduce heat to medium-high; cook for 3 minutes or until potatoes are softened but not cooked through. Stir in cabbage and pasta; increase heat to high and cook for 8 minutes or until pasta is not quite tender but firm. Drain, reserving 1 cup (250 mL) of cooking liquid; return pasta and vegetables to pot. Set aside.

2. In a skillet, melt butter over medium-low heat. Add garlic, sage, salt and pepper; cook for 3 minutes or until garlic is softened but not browned. Pour mixture over pasta and vegetables, along with all but a heaping tablespoon (15 mL) of the Parmigiano-Reggiano; toss together gently. Put one-third of mixture into prepared casserole dish; top with one third of diced fontina. Repeat layers twice. Sprinkle with reserved tablespoon (15 mL) Parmigiano-Reggiano. Pour ¼ cup (60 mL) of reserved cooking liquid over top to moisten slightly.

3. Bake in top half of oven for 7 minutes or until cheese is melted. Let stand for 5 minutes before serving.

Nutrients per serving	
Calories	618
Fat	22 g
Carbohydrates	72 g
Protein	28 g

Udon Noodles with Tofu and Gingered Peanut Sauce

Udon noodles can be made from buckwheat, corn flour or wheat flour, so check the ingredient list carefully if you are trying to avoid wheat. Or simply choose soba noodles, which are made from buckwheat.

TIP

This dish is intended to be served slightly warmer than room temperature; if a piping hot dish is preferred, cook the noodles after the tofu and greens have been cooked in the peanut sauce.

8 oz	udon or soba noodles	250 g
8 oz	firm tofu, drained and cut into ½-inch (1 cm) cubes	250 g
2	cloves garlic, crushed	2
1 tbsp	grated gingerroot	15 mL
1 or 2	dried cayenne peppers, crushed	1 or 2
½ cup	tamari or soy sauce	125 mL
2 tbsp	organic cane sugar or packed brown sugar	30 mL
⅓ cup	coarsely ground peanuts or natural peanut butter	75 mL
⅓ cup	warm water	75 mL
4 tbsp	olive oil, divided	60 mL
1	onion, chopped	1
2 cups	broccoli florets	500 mL
2 cups	shredded kale or spinach	500 mL

1. In a large pot of boiling salted water, cook noodles for 6 to 8 minutes or according to package directions, until al dente. Drain and rinse with cool water. Set aside.

2. Meanwhile, in a bowl, combine tofu, garlic, ginger, cayenne pepper to taste, tamari and sugar. Set aside. In another bowl, combine peanuts and warm water. Set aside.

3. In a wok or large, deep saucepan, heat 2 tbsp (30 mL) of the oil over medium-high heat. Add onion and stir-fry for 3 minutes. Using a slotted spoon, lift tofu from marinade, reserving marinade, and add to wok. Stir-fry for 2 to 3 minutes, until lightly colored. Scrape tofu and onions into marinade, stir in peanuts with water and set aside.

4. Add remaining oil to wok and heat. Add broccoli and stir-fry for 3 minutes or until tender-crisp. Stir in tofu mixture and kale. Simmer, stirring frequently, for 1 or 2 minutes, until kale is tender. Serve over cooked udon noodles.

Nutrients per serving

Calories	546
Fat	24 g
Carbohydrates	62 g
Protein	24 g

Chickpea Tofu Burgers with Coriander Mayonnaise

Makes 4 servings

The combination of chickpeas and tofu gives a rich texture to these unusual burgers. Choose eggs that are high in omega-3 fatty acids.

TIPS

Serve in pita breads or on rolls, with lettuce, tomatoes and onions.

Tofu is found in the vegetable section of your grocery store. If desired, it can be replaced with 5% ricotta cheese.

Tahini is a sesame paste, usually found in the international section of your grocery store. If unavailable, try peanut butter.

MAKE AHEAD

Prepare patties and sauce up to 1 day in advance. Bake just before serving.

- Preheat oven to 425°F (220°C)
- Food processor
- Baking sheet sprayed with vegetable spray

1 cup	rinsed drained canned chickpeas	250 mL
8 oz	firm tofu	250 g
⅓ cup	dry bread crumbs	75 mL
2 tbsp	tahini	30 mL
1½ tbsp	freshly squeezed lemon juice	22 mL
1 tsp	minced garlic	5 mL
1	large egg	1
¼ tsp	freshly ground black pepper	1 mL
¼ tsp	salt	1 mL
⅓ cup	chopped fresh cilantro	75 mL
¼ cup	chopped green onions	60 mL
¼ cup	chopped red bell peppers	60 mL
Sauce		
¼ cup	2% plain yogurt	60 mL
¼ cup	light sour cream	60 mL
¼ cup	chopped fresh cilantro	60 mL
1 tbsp	light mayonnaise	15 mL
½ tsp	minced garlic	2 mL

1. In food processor, combine chickpeas, tofu, bread crumbs, tahini, lemon juice, garlic, egg, pepper and salt; process until smooth. Add cilantro, green onions and red peppers; pulse on and off until well-mixed. With wet hands, scoop up ¼ cup (60 mL) of mixture and form into a patty. Put on prepared baking sheet. Repeat procedure for remaining patties. Bake 20 minutes, turning burgers at halfway point.

2. *Sauce:* Meanwhile, in a small bowl, stir together yogurt, sour cream, cilantro, mayonnaise and garlic; set aside.

3. Serve burgers hot with sauce on side.

Nutrients per serving	
Calories	226
Fat	10 g
Carbohydrates	21 g
Protein	15 g

Fish
and Seafood

Cod Provençal

This delicious fish dish bursts with the sunny flavors of the Mediterranean. White fish is not particularly high in omega-3 fatty acids, but the olives and olive oil add some healthy fats.

TIPS

Don't skimp on the olive oil — it's what gives this dish its distinct character and flavor.

Buy pitted Kalamata olives to make preparing this dish a breeze.

- **Preheat oven to 425°F (220°C)**
- **8-inch (20 cm) square baking dish**

1¼ lbs	skinless cod or halibut fillets, cut into 4 pieces	625 g
	Salt and freshly ground black pepper	
2	tomatoes, seeded and diced	2
2	green onions, sliced	2
1	clove garlic, finely chopped	1
¼ cup	kalamata olives, rinsed and cut into slivers	60 mL
2 tbsp	chopped fresh parsley or basil	30 mL
1 tbsp	capers, rinsed	15 mL
Pinch	hot pepper flakes (optional)	Pinch
2 tbsp	olive oil	30 mL

1. Arrange cod in a single layer in baking dish. Season with salt and pepper.

2. In a bowl, combine tomatoes, green onions, garlic, olives, parsley, capers and hot pepper flakes (if using). Season to taste with salt and pepper. Spoon tomato mixture over fish fillets; drizzle with oil.

3. Bake in preheated oven for 15 to 20 minutes or until fish flakes when tested with a fork. Serve in warmed wide shallow bowls and spoon pan juices over top.

Nutrients per serving	
Calories	222
Fat	10 g
Carbohydrates	5 g
Protein	29 g

Cumin-Crusted Halibut Steaks

Makes 4 servings

Cumin seeds contain many phytochemicals that help promote good health and digestion. They make a tasty replacement for bread crumbs.

TIPS

Sea bass, halibut, grouper or any dense white fish are all excellent cooked in this interesting crust.

It is preferable to use toasted cumin seeds, as they have more flavor than ground cumin.

- **Preheat oven to 450°F (230°C)**
- **Coffee or spice grinder**

1 tbsp	cumin seeds	15 mL
½ tsp	salt	2 mL
¼ tsp	freshly ground black pepper	1 mL
1 lb	skinless halibut or other fish steaks	500 g
2 tsp	olive oil	10 mL
	Chopped fresh parsley (optional)	

1. In a nonstick skillet over medium heat, toast cumin seeds, stirring, for 2 minutes or until golden. Place seeds, salt and pepper in a coffee or spice grinder. Pulse until finely ground. Rub mixture into both sides of fish.

2. Heat olive oil in a large nonstick skillet over medium-high heat. Add fish, in batches, if necessary, and cook for 2 minutes per side or until browned.

3. Return all fish to skillet and wrap handle with foil. Bake in preheated oven for 5 minutes or until fish is opaque and flakes easily when tested with a fork. Sprinkle with parsley (if using).

Nutrients per serving	
Calories	151
Fat	5 g
Carbohydrates	1 g
Protein	24 g

Mediterranean-Style Mahi-Mahi

Using the slow cooker on a rainy summer day means you do not have to turn on the oven, and a cooler home may help you feel more comfortable.

TIPS

If you halve this recipe, use a 1½- to 3-quart slow cooker.

It is difficult to be specific about the timing, so you should begin checking for doneness after 1 hour. Be aware it may take up to 1½ hours.

- **3- to 5-quart oval slow cooker**

2 lbs	skinless mahi-mahi steaks	1 kg
1 tsp	dried oregano	5 mL
1	lemon, thinly sliced	1
1	can (28 oz/796 mL) tomatoes, with juice, coarsely chopped	1
½ cup	dry white wine	125 mL
¼ cup	extra virgin olive oil, divided	60 mL
1 tsp	salt	5 mL
	Freshly ground black pepper	
	Chopped black olives	

Gremolata

½ cup	finely chopped parsley	125 mL
3 tbsp	drained capers, minced	45 mL
2	whole anchovies, rinsed and finely chopped	2
	Freshly ground black pepper	

1. Place fish in slow cooker stoneware. Sprinkle with oregano and lay lemon slices evenly over top. In a bowl, combine tomatoes with juice, wine, 2 tbsp (30 mL) of the olive oil, salt and pepper to taste. Pour over fish. Cover and cook on High for 1 hour (see tip, at left), until fish flakes easily when pierced with a knife.

2. *Gremolata:* Meanwhile, in a bowl, combine parsley, capers, anchovies, remaining 2 tbsp (30 mL) of the olive oil and pepper to taste. Mix well and set aside in refrigerator until fish is cooked.

3. To serve, transfer fish and tomato sauce to a warm platter. Spoon gremolata evenly over and garnish with olives.

Nutrients per serving	
Calories	410
Fat	16 g
Carbohydrates	13 g
Protein	46 g

Salmon with Spinach

Salmon is one of the best sources of omega-3 fatty acids. Spinach is a great source of beta carotene and other phytochemicals, as well as a fat-like substance that protects the digestive tract from being damaged by inflammation. Spinach also provides about 1000% of the recommended daily intake of vitamin K.

- **Preheat oven to 450°F (230°C)**
- **Shallow oblong pan, greased**

1	package (10 oz/300 g) frozen chopped spinach, thawed	1
1 tbsp	grated gingerroot	15 mL
2	large mushrooms, thickly sliced	2
	Salt and freshly ground black pepper	
4	skinless salmon steaks or fillets	4

1. In a sieve, drain spinach, pressing with a spoon to remove excess liquid. Discard liquid. Spread spinach in bottom of prepared pan in a shape resembling the size of the fish. Arrange gingerroot and mushrooms evenly over spinach. Season lightly with salt and pepper. Add fish. Sprinkle lightly with salt and pepper.

2. Cover pan loosely with a tent of foil. Bake in preheated oven for 15 minutes or until fish is opaque and flakes easily when tested with a fork.

VARIATIONS

As well as salmon, any white or firm-fleshed fish will do. These are turbot, swordfish, halibut or tuna. For ease of serving fish fillets, cut them into serving-size pieces before baking.

Crusty Layered Salmon: Sprinkle toasted sesame seeds over the fish before baking to give it a crusty crunch.

Nutrients per serving	
Calories	284
Fat	12 g
Carbohydrates	3 g
Protein	36 g

Oven-Steamed Salmon with Chiles and Ginger

When preparing this light, refreshing dish, remember that cooking at high temperatures increases the formation of advanced glycation end products (AGEs), which might increase inflammation. To be on the safe side, you might want to cook at 300°F (150°C) for a longer time; just make sure to cook until the fish is opaque and flakes easily with a fork.

- Preheat oven to 400°F (200°C)

4	skinless salmon fillets (each about 6 oz/175 g)	4
1 tbsp	chopped gingerroot	15 mL
1 tbsp	chopped fresh cilantro stems	15 mL
2	cloves garlic, finely chopped	2
2 tsp	chopped fresh red chile pepper	10 mL
2 tbsp	freshly squeezed lime juice	30 mL
1 tbsp	fish sauce (nam pla)	15 mL
2 tsp	brown or granulated sugar	10 mL
2	green onions, thinly sliced	2
	Fresh cilantro leaves	

1. Arrange salmon in a single layer in a shallow baking dish.
2. In a bowl, combine ginger, cilantro stems, garlic, chile, lime juice, fish sauce and sugar. Spoon mixture over fillets. Cover dish with foil and seal edges.
3. Bake in preheated oven for 8 to 10 minutes, or until fish is opaque and flakes easily with a fork.
4. Garnish with green onions and cilantro leaves.

Nutrients per serving	
Calories	272
Fat	12 g
Carbohydrates	4 g
Protein	34 g

Poached Salmon with Lemon and Chives

Poaching is a great cooking method for people with arthritis because it uses a lower cooking temperature, thereby reducing the formation of advanced glycation end products (AGEs). If you prefer not to use wine, try fish stock or vegetable broth instead.

Nutrients per serving	
Calories	269
Fat	10 g
Carbohydrates	3 g
Protein	30 g

1 cup	dry white wine	250 mL
½ cup	water	125 mL
	Juice of 1 large lemon	
	Salt and freshly ground black pepper	
4	skinless salmon fillets (each about 5 oz/150 g)	4
⅓ cup	finely chopped fresh chives	75 mL
12	chive blossoms (optional)	12
¼ to ⅓ cup	butter, cut into cubes	60 to 75 mL

1. In a large skillet, bring wine, water, lemon juice, and salt and pepper to taste to a boil over medium-high heat. Add salmon, reduce heat and simmer for 8 to 10 minutes, or until fish is opaque and flakes easily with a fork. Transfer salmon to a warm plate.

2. Simmer liquid until reduced by two-thirds. Add chives and chive blossoms (if using), bring to a boil and boil for 1 minute. Remove from heat and swirl in butter, a few pieces at a time, until a smooth sauce forms. Pour sauce over fish.

Maple Ginger Salmon

Here's a North American twist on an Asian classic. Maple syrup has fewer calories than the same amount of honey and contains the minerals manganese and zinc.

Nutrients per serving	
Calories	319
Fat	12 g
Carbohydrates	14 g
Protein	37 g

- **Preheat oven to 350°F (180°C)**
- **Rimmed baking sheet, lined with foil**

4	skinless salmon fillets	4
¼ cup	pure maple syrup	60 mL
2 tbsp	rice vinegar	30 mL
1 tsp	finely grated gingerroot	5 mL

1. Place salmon on prepared baking sheet.

2. In a small bowl, whisk together maple syrup, vinegar and ginger. Pour over fillets.

3. Bake in preheated oven for 10 to 15 minutes or until fish is opaque and flakes easily when tested with a fork.

Salmon Stew with Corn and Quinoa

This tasty stew is a great way to increase your intake of beneficial omega-3 fatty acids. Leeks contain the antioxidant mineral manganese, as well as phytochemicals that decrease inflammation and improve blood vessel health.

TIPS

Salmon is one of the best sources of omega-3 fatty acids, which are essential to good health. Studies show that an adequate supply of omega-3s can reduce the risk of coronary artery disease, slightly lower blood pressure and strengthen the immune system, among other benefits.

To reduce your intake of saturated fat, substitute half-and-half (10%) cream for the whipping cream.

1 tbsp	olive oil	15 mL
2 tbsp	finely chopped pancetta or bacon	30 mL
3	leeks (white part only), cleaned (see tip, page 311) and thinly sliced	3
½ tsp	dried thyme	2 mL
½ tsp	cayenne pepper	2 mL
1	bay leaf	1
½ tsp	salt	2 mL
1 cup	dry white wine	250 mL
6 cups	fish stock (or 3 cups/750 mL bottled clam juice diluted with 3 cups/ 750 mL water)	1.5 L
2 cups	corn kernels	500 mL
1 cup	quinoa, rinsed	250 mL
1½ lbs	skinless salmon fillets, cut into 1-inch (2.5 cm) pieces	750 g
½ cup	heavy or whipping (35%) cream	125 mL
¼ cup	Pernod (optional)	60 mL
½ cup	finely chopped fresh chives	125 mL

1. In a Dutch oven, heat oil over medium heat for 30 seconds. Add pancetta and cook, stirring, until it begins to brown, about 3 minutes. (If you're using bacon, cook until crisp and drain off all but 1 tbsp/ 15 mL fat from pan before proceeding with recipe.)

2. Reduce heat to medium. Add leeks and cook, stirring, until softened, about 5 minutes. Add thyme, cayenne, bay leaf and salt and cook, stirring, for 1 minute. Add wine, bring to boil and boil until reduced by half, about 5 minutes. Add fish stock and corn and return to a boil. Stir in quinoa. Reduce heat to low. Cover and cook until quinoa is almost tender, about 15 minutes.

3. Add salmon and simmer until opaque and flakes easily with a fork, about 6 minutes. Stir in whipping cream and cook until heated through, about 2 minutes. Stir in Pernod (if using). Garnish with chives.

Nutrients per serving	
Calories	373
Fat	19 g
Carbohydrates	27 g
Protein	24 g

Peachy Glazed Trout

Makes 6 servings

Trout, and especially wild trout, is one of the best sources of anti-inflammatory omega-3 fatty acids. When preparing this dish, remember that cooking at high temperatures increases the formation of advanced glycation end products (AGEs), which seem to cause inflammation. To be on the safe side, you might want to cook at 300°F (150°C) for a longer time; just make sure to cook until the fish is opaque and flakes easily with a fork.

TIPS

The blanching time of the peaches will vary depending on their ripeness.

Look for the Marine Stewardship Council's blue label to ensure that your fish comes from a well-managed fishery. For more information, visit www.msc.org.

- Preheat oven to 400°F (200°C)
- 13- by 9-inch (33 by 23 cm) glass baking dish, greased

3	peaches	3
1	clove garlic, minced	1
2 tsp	grated gingerroot	10 mL
2 tbsp	lightly packed brown sugar	30 mL
½ tsp	freshly ground black pepper	2 mL
⅓ cup	unsweetened orange juice	75 mL
1 tbsp	reduced-sodium soy sauce	15 mL
1 tbsp	Dijon mustard	15 mL
6	skinless trout fillets (about 1½ lbs/750 g total)	6

1. Using a paring knife, make a small X at the bottom of each peach. In a medium saucepan of simmering water, blanch peaches for 2 to 3 minutes or until skins begin to peel back. Using a slotted spoon, transfer peaches to ice water to stop the cooking process. Let cool for 5 minutes or until cool enough to handle. Peel off and discard skin. Chop peaches.

2. In a medium bowl, combine peaches, garlic, ginger, brown sugar, pepper, orange juice, soy sauce and mustard.

3. Pat trout fillets dry with paper towels. Place in prepared baking dish and pour sauce evenly over fish.

4. Bake in preheated oven, basting occasionally with sauce, for 12 to 15 minutes or until fish is opaque and flakes easily when tested with a fork.

VARIATIONS

Use nectarines or plums, adjusting the blanching time to suit the ripeness of the fruit.

Use salmon or arctic char instead of trout and increase the cooking time as necessary.

This recipe courtesy of Compass Group Canada.

Nutrients per serving	
Calories	203
Fat	6 g
Carbohydrates	11 g
Protein	25 g

Thai Fish en Papillote

Aromatic Thai ingredients add hot, sweet, salty and tangy flavors as the fish steams in individual parcels. Choose salmon over white fish to increase the omega-3 fats. Serve with brown rice on the side and a fruit for dessert. When preparing this dish, remember that cooking at high temperatures can increase the formation of advanced glycation end products (AGEs), which seem to increase inflammation. To be on the safe side, you might want to cook at 300°F (200°C) for a longer time; just make sure to cook until the fish is opaque and flakes easily with a fork.

- Preheat oven to 425°F (220°C)
- 4 sheets parchment paper, each about 16 by 12 inches (40 by 30 cm)

4	skinless salmon or white fish fillets (about 1 lb/500 g total)	4
1 tbsp	grated gingerroot	15 mL
¼ cup	light coconut milk	60 mL
2 tsp	fish sauce (nam pla)	10 mL
1 tsp	hot chili-garlic sauce	5 mL
	Grated zest and juice of 1 lime	
1	red bell pepper, julienned	1
1	green mango (see tip, at right), julienned	1
2 tbsp	fresh cilantro leaves	30 mL
1	lime, cut into 4 wedges	1

1. Place 1 piece of fish on each sheet of parchment paper. Fold all four sides of the paper to form creases about 4 inches (10 cm) from the edge, but do not close. (This will prevent liquids from spilling off the paper.)

2. In a small bowl, combine ginger, coconut milk, fish sauce, chili-garlic sauce, lime zest and lime juice. Drizzle evenly over fish. Divide red pepper and green mango evenly on top of fish. Bring the two long sides of the parchment paper together on top of the fish and fold over repeatedly to close the center, then fold the sides together, tucking the ends under the packet to hold them in place.

Nutrients per serving	
Calories	269
Fat	14 g
Carbohydrates	13 g
Protein	23 g

TIPS

Mature green mangos have a flavor and texture similar to those of a crisp, tart green apple. Choose one that has an unblemished skin and firm flesh.

Opening the packets at the table makes a dramatic presentation, as guests are enchanted by the aromas.

You can also use frozen fish fillets. Increase the baking time to 15 to 18 minutes.

Although botanically a fruit, coconut contains ample amounts of saturated fat and should be used in moderation. Compare the labels of regular and light versions of coconut milk; many light versions contain significantly less fat.

3. Place packets on a baking sheet. Bake in preheated oven for 10 to 12 minutes or until fish flakes easily when tested with a fork.

4. Transfer packets to serving plates. Cut paper open with a sharp knife or scissors and add cilantro and a lime wedge to each packet.

This recipe courtesy of dietitian Christina Blais.

Tomato and Fish Stew

Makes 6 servings

This colorful stew is great for casual entertaining. Bay leaves contain many antioxidant nutrients, including vitamins C and A, manganese, zinc and various phytochemicals, which will be released into the stew as it cooks.

TIP

Most supermarkets sell chopped fresh vegetables. If there are none ready, just ask the clerk in the produce department to prepare what you need.

2 tbsp	olive oil	30 mL
4	cloves garlic, minced	4
1	large onion, chopped	1
1	red or green bell pepper, chopped	1
1	can (28 oz/796 mL) whole tomatoes, with juice	1
1	bottle (8 oz/237 mL) clam juice	1
½ tsp	dried thyme	2 mL
¼ tsp	freshly ground black pepper	1 mL
¼ tsp	hot pepper flakes	1 mL
2	bay leaves	2
12	mussels	12
1⅓ lbs	skinless haddock or cod fillets	700 g
¼ cup	chopped fresh parsley	60 mL
2 tbsp	chopped green onion	30 mL

1. In large heavy saucepan, heat oil over medium heat. Cook garlic, onion and red pepper for 3 to 5 minutes or until softened.

2. Add tomatoes with their juice, breaking up tomatoes with the back of a spoon. Stir in clam juice, thyme, black pepper, hot pepper flakes and bay leaves. Bring to a boil; reduce heat to medium-low. Simmer, uncovered, stirring occasionally, for 12 to 15 minutes or until slightly thickened. Discard bay leaves.

3. Scrub mussels, removing any beards. Discard any mussels that do not close when lightly tapped on the counter. Add mussels to the tomato mixture.

4. Cut fish into 2-inch (5 cm) pieces. Add to tomato mixture; cook, covered, for 5 minutes or until fish flakes easily with a fork, and mussels open. Do not stir, but baste fish occasionally with tomato mixture. Discard any mussels that don't open. Serve immediately sprinkled with parsley and green onions.

Nutrients per serving	
Calories	120
Fat	6 g
Carbohydrates	12 g
Protein	6 g

Deep South Oyster Stew

Like other shellfish, oysters are low in saturated fat and cholesterol. They are an excellent source of zinc and protein. The bacon and cream add saturated fat, so make sure the rest of your food choices are low in saturated fat on the day you prepare this meal.

TIP

If you halve this recipe, use a 1½- to 3-quart slow cooker.

MAKE AHEAD

Complete steps 1 and 2. Cover and refrigerate bacon and vegetable mixtures separately for up to 2 days. When you're ready to cook, continue with the recipe.

- **3½- to 5-quart slow cooker**

4 oz	bacon, diced	125 g
2	onions, finely chopped	2
4	stalks celery, diced	4
2	cloves garlic, minced	2
2	bay leaves	2
1 tsp	salt	5 mL
1 tsp	cracked black peppercorns	5 mL
¼ cup	dry sherry	60 mL
4 cups	Chicken Stock (page 201) or Vegetable Stock (page 200) or ready-to-use chicken or vegetable broth	1 L
1	potato, peeled and diced	1
1 tbsp	freshly squeezed lemon juice	15 mL
¼ tsp	cayenne pepper	1 mL
4 cups	finely chopped stemmed spinach	1 L
2 cups	chopped shucked oysters, with liquor	500 mL
½ cup	heavy or whipping (35%) cream	125 mL
	Hot pepper sauce	

1. In a skillet, cook bacon over medium-high heat until brown and crisp. Using a slotted spoon, transfer to paper towel to drain. Cover and refrigerate until ready to use. Reduce heat to medium.

2. Add onions and celery to pan and cook, stirring, until softened, about 5 minutes. Add garlic, bay leaves, salt and peppercorns and cook, stirring, for 1 minute. Add sherry and bring to a boil. Boil for 1 minute.

3. Transfer to slow cooker stoneware. Stir in chicken stock and potato. Cover and cook on Low for 6 hours or on High for 3 hours. Remove and discard bay leaves.

4. In a small bowl, combine lemon juice and cayenne, stirring until dissolved. Add to stoneware. Add spinach, in batches, stirring until each batch is incorporated. Stir in oysters and whipping cream. Cover and cook on High for 20 minutes, until spinach is cooked and mixture is heated through. Pass hot pepper sauce at the table.

Nutrients per serving	
Calories	337
Fat	22 g
Carbohydrates	20 g
Protein	18 g

Golden Shrimp with Cilantro and Lime

Makes 8 servings

Here's a simple, delicious way to add seafood to your diet. For a balanced meal, serve vegetable soup to start, a salad on the side and a fruit crisp for dessert.

- **Mortar and pestle**

8	cloves garlic	8
2 tsp	salt	10 mL
3 lbs	shrimp, peeled and deveined	1.5 kg
1	bay leaf	1
½ cup	freshly squeezed lime juice, divided	125 mL
2¼ tsp	ground turmeric, divided	11 mL
1 tsp	cayenne pepper	5 mL
½ cup	fresh cilantro leaves, divided	125 mL

1. Mash garlic and salt to a paste with mortar and pestle and rub into shrimp. Set aside for 15 minutes.

2. In a large saucepan over medium-high heat, combine 8 cups (2 L) water, bay leaf, 1 tbsp (15 mL) of the lime juice and 2 tsp (10 mL) of the turmeric. Bring to a boil. When water is boiling, stir in shrimp and cook just until opaque, 2 to 3 minutes. Do not overcook. Drain and transfer shrimp to a bowl.

3. Stir together remaining turmeric, cayenne pepper and remaining lime juice. Pour over warm shrimp. Toss until well combined.

4. Chop half of the cilantro leaves and add to cooled shrimp. Add remaining whole leaves and toss. Adjust seasonings and refrigerate for at least 3 hours before serving.

Nutrients per serving	
Calories	132
Fat	2 g
Carbohydrates	4 g
Protein	24 g

Rice with Shrimp and Lemon

Makes 6 servings

Arborio rice is a short-grain white rice used to make creamy rice dishes such as risotto. It contains only 2 grams of fiber per 1-cup (250 mL) serving, so serve this dish with a high-fiber salad or dessert.

6 cups	Chicken Stock (page 201) or ready-to-use chicken broth (approx.)	1.5 L
¼ cup	extra virgin olive oil	60 mL
2 tbsp	butter	30 mL
1	onion, finely chopped	1
2	cloves garlic, minced	2
2 cups	Arborio rice	500 mL
½ cup	dry white wine	125 mL
12 oz	small shrimp, peeled and deveined	375 g
	Finely grated zest and juice of 1 large lemon	
2 tbsp	chopped fresh flat-leaf (Italian) parsley	30 mL
1 tbsp	butter	15 mL
	Salt and freshly ground black pepper	

1. In a large saucepan, bring chicken stock to a boil. Reduce heat to a slow simmer and keep the stock at this steady, slightly bubbling state throughout the rest of the cooking.

2. In a heavy-bottomed saucepan, heat olive oil and 2 tbsp (30 mL) butter over medium-high heat. Add onion and cook for 2 minutes or until translucent. Stir in garlic; cook for 2 minutes longer. Add rice all at once; cook, stirring, for 2 minutes or until grains are well coated with butter and oil. Pour in wine; cook, stirring for 1 minute or until wine is absorbed. Stir in shrimp and grated lemon zest; cook, stirring, for 3 minutes.

3. Using a ladle, start to add simmering stock ½ cup (125 mL) at a time. As each ladle of stock is added, stir the rice to keep it from sticking to the bottom and sides of saucepan; do not add more until last addition is absorbed. If the stock is absorbed too quickly, reduce the heat to maintain a slow, steady simmer. Repeat this process, ladling in the hot stock and stirring, for 15 minutes. As you near the end of the cooking time, reduce the amount of stock to ¼ cup (60 mL) at a time.

4. Continue to cook, adding more stock as necessary, until the rice is tender but with a firm heart and overall creaminess. It should not be soupy or runny looking. A minute before completion, stir in lemon juice, parsley and 1 tbsp (15 mL) butter. Season to taste with salt and pepper. Serve immediately.

Nutrients per serving

Calories	358
Fat	18 g
Carbohydrates	29 g
Protein	17 g

Chicken and Shrimp Pad Thai

Thailand's famous whole-meal noodle dish has been around for more than 200 years, but fits right into our modern lifestyle because it's quick to make, low in fat and full of flavor. Use light-tasting canola oil to add omega-3 fatty acids.

TIPS

If you have tamarind paste on hand, use it instead of ketchup.

To break rice noodles a bit before soaking, put them into a big bag so they won't scatter all over your kitchen.

Think you don't like tofu? Try purchasing it at a specialty Asian grocery store.

8 oz	rice noodles (fettuccine width)	250 g
3 tbsp	ketchup	45 mL
3 tbsp	freshly squeezed lime juice	45 mL
2 tbsp	fish sauce (nam pla)	30 mL
1 tbsp	rice vinegar	15 mL
1 tsp	hot chili paste (or ½ tsp/2 mL hot pepper flakes)	5 mL
8 oz	boneless skinless chicken breasts	250 g
2 tsp	cornstarch	10 mL
2 tbsp	vegetable oil	30 mL
1 tsp	sesame oil	5 mL
3	cloves garlic, minced	3
8 oz	medium shrimp, peeled and deveined (with tails on)	250 g
½ cup	firm tofu, cut into ½-inch (1 cm) cubes	125 mL
1	large egg	1
1 cup	bean sprouts	250 mL
4	green onions, cut into 1-inch (2.5 cm) pieces	4
½ cup	chopped fresh cilantro	125 mL
2 tbsp	coarsely chopped dry-roasted peanuts	30 mL
	Lime wedges	
	Red bell pepper slices	

1. In large bowl, soak noodles in warm water for about 10 minutes or until softened but still firm. Drain well.

2. In small bowl, combine ketchup, lime juice, fish sauce, vinegar and chili paste; set aside. Cut chicken into thin strips; toss with cornstarch and set aside.

Nutrients per serving	
Calories	698
Fat	20 g
Carbohydrates	83 g
Protein	43 g

TIP

Don't substitute anything else for fish sauce. When buying it in Asian grocery stores, look for the brand with a squid on the label and store in refrigerator after opening.

3. In large wok or skillet, heat vegetable and sesame oils over medium-high heat; stir-fry garlic and chicken for 3 minutes. Add shrimp and tofu; stir-fry for 2 to 3 minutes or until shrimp are pink. Push to side of wok. Break egg into center of wok; let set slightly before combining with chicken mixture.

4. Reduce heat to medium. Add noodles and ketchup mixture; bring to boil. Add bean sprouts, onions, half of the cilantro and half of the peanuts. Transfer to large warm platter; sprinkle with remaining peanuts and cilantro. Garnish with lime wedges and red pepper around edges.

Malaysian Curry Noodles and Seafood

These noodles are seafood-laced and doubly enriched by coconut and cashews. Cashews contain heart-healthy oils and many antioxidant nutrients, including copper and magnesium. Copper also helps the body eliminate free radicals that can cause inflammation in the joints.

TIP

Bags of mixed seafood are available in the frozen section of supermarkets and specialty fish shops. These are handy if you want a variety of seafood. You can substitute one type of your favorite seafood if you prefer.

VARIATION

Substitute 1 lb (500 g) boneless skinless chicken breast, thinly sliced, for the seafood and add in step 3 before the noodles. Simmer for 1 minute, then add noodles, cooking until chicken is no longer pink inside.

Nutrients per serving	
Calories	315
Fat	23 g
Carbohydrates	24 g
Protein	6 g

1 lb	frozen mixed seafood, thawed, drained and patted dry	500 g
½ tsp	ground turmeric	2 mL
1 tbsp	vegetable oil	15 mL
3	cloves garlic, minced	3
2 or 3	hot red or green chile peppers, minced	2 or 3
1 tbsp	minced gingerroot	15 mL
2 tsp	ground coriander	10 mL
1 tsp	salt	5 mL
⅓ cup	cashew butter or natural peanut butter	75 mL
1	can (14 oz/400 mL) coconut milk	1
1 cup	water	250 mL
4 oz	rice vermicelli	125 g
3 tbsp	freshly squeezed lemon juice	45 mL
1 cup	bean sprouts	250 mL
	Chopped fresh mint	
	Thinly sliced cucumber	
	Chopped roasted salted cashews (optional)	

1. In a bowl, combine seafood and turmeric; toss to coat evenly. Set aside at room temperature.

2. In a wok or large, deep skillet, heat oil over medium heat. Add garlic, chile peppers, ginger, coriander and salt; cook, stirring, until softened and fragrant, about 2 minutes. Stir in cashew butter until blended. Add coconut milk and water; bring to a simmer, scraping up bits stuck to pan and stirring until cashew butter is blended.

3. Stir in noodles and return to a boil, stirring gently just until noodles are immersed. Stir in seafood mixture and lemon juice; reduce heat and simmer, stirring gently often, just until seafood starts to firm up and noodles are softened, about 5 minutes. Gently stir in bean sprouts just until wilted. Divide among warmed serving bowls and serve sprinkled with mint and garnished with cucumber slices and cashews (if using).

Meat and Poultry

Slow-Cooked Chili Flank Steak or Brisket

Make sure to trim the meat before adding it to the slow cooker, to cut down on the amount of saturated fat. Serve with a salad and some brown rice or barley.

- **Minimum 4-quart slow cooker**

2 lbs	flank steak or beef brisket	1 kg
½ tsp	freshly ground black pepper	2 mL
1 tbsp	vegetable oil	15 mL
3	stalks celery, with leaves, stalks cut into chunks and leaves chopped	3
2	cloves garlic, minced	2
1	onion, cut into chunks	1
1 cup	reduced-sodium ready-to-use beef broth	250 mL
1	can (19 oz/540 mL) chili-flavored or regular stewed tomatoes, with juice (about 2⅓ cups/575 mL)	1
1	large carrot, cut into chunks	1
1	bay leaf	1
½ tsp	dried thyme	2 mL
2 tsp	chili powder	10 mL

1. Cut beef into large pieces that will comfortably fit in your slow cooker. Season with pepper.

2. In a large skillet, heat oil over medium-high heat. Cook beef for 3 to 4 minutes per side or until browned on all sides. Transfer beef to slow cooker stoneware.

3. In the fat remaining in the skillet, sauté celery (including leaves), garlic and onion until lightly browned, about 5 minutes. Add to slow cooker.

4. Add broth to skillet and scrape up any brown bits from the bottom. Pour liquid into slow cooker.

5. To the slow cooker, add tomatoes and juice, carrot, bay leaf, thyme and chili powder; stir to combine. Cover and cook on Low for 6 to 8 hours or until beef is fork-tender. Discard bay leaf.

6. Slice beef across the grain and arrange on a platter. Skim fat from sauce, pour sauce over meat and serve.

This recipe courtesy of Eileen Campbell.

Nutrients per serving	
Calories	256
Fat	12 g
Carbohydrates	8 g
Protein	26 g

Veal Stewed with Artichoke Hearts

This decadent stew delivers more than just great taste: it's packed with antioxidants and phytochemicals. If you prefer not to use wine, replace it with ½ cup (125 mL) chicken or vegetable broth.

3 lbs	veal cubes for stew	1.5 kg
¼ cup	all-purpose flour	60 mL
¼ cup	olive oil	60 mL
1	large onion, chopped	1
1	stalk celery, chopped	1
3	cloves garlic, minced	3
½ cup	dry white wine	125 mL
1 tbsp	grated lemon zest	15 mL
1	bay leaf	1
1 tsp	dried rosemary, crumbled	5 mL
1 tsp	ground thyme	5 mL
¼ tsp	ground ginger	1 mL
2 cups	Chicken Stock (page 201) or ready-to-use chicken broth	500 mL
	Salt and freshly ground black pepper	
1	can (14 oz/398 mL) artichoke hearts, drained and quartered	1
1 cup	canned diced tomatoes	250 mL
2 tbsp	chopped fresh flat-leaf (Italian) parsley	30 mL

1. Dredge veal in flour. In a large, heavy saucepan or Dutch oven, heat oil over medium-high heat. Sauté veal, in batches if necessary, until browned on all sides; remove to a plate.

2. Add onion, celery and garlic to the pan and sauté until softened. Add wine, lemon zest, bay leaf, rosemary, thyme and ginger; boil for 3 minutes.

3. Return veal to the pan and add chicken stock and salt and pepper to taste; reduce heat, cover and simmer until tender, about 45 minutes.

4. Add artichoke hearts, tomatoes and parsley; cover and simmer for 30 minutes. Discard bay leaf.

Nutrients per serving	
Calories	422
Fat	16 g
Carbohydrates	14 g
Protein	49 g

Cardamom-Scented Lamb

This classic Sindhi dish is lightly spiced and has a soupy consistency. Choose olive oil or canola oil for the vegetable oil.

TIPS

The spinach is used for flavor and as a thickener. It will be barely visible.

Cardamom may play a role in supporting heart health and in reducing inflammation.

2 tbsp	vegetable oil	30 mL
¼ cup	cardamom seeds, crushed	60 mL
2 lbs	boneless lamb, cut into bite-size pieces	1 kg
1 lb	spinach, chopped (about 4 cups/1 L)	500 g
1 cup	chopped tomatoes	250 mL
2 tsp	ground coriander	10 mL
1½ tsp	salt, or to taste	7 mL
½ tsp	freshly ground black pepper	2 mL
1½ tbsp	all-purpose flour	22 mL

1. In a large saucepan, heat oil over medium-high heat. Stir in cardamom seeds and sauté until fragrant, about 1 minute.

2. Add lamb and spinach. Reduce heat to medium. Cover and cook until spinach loses all moisture, 4 to 5 minutes. Uncover and brown lamb for 8 to 10 minutes.

3. Add tomatoes and cook until moisture is evaporated, 10 minutes longer.

4. Sprinkle with coriander, salt and pepper. Mix well and brown for 2 minutes longer.

5. Pour in 2 cups (500 mL) water. Bring to a boil over medium-high heat. Reduce heat to low. Cover and simmer until lamb is tender, 45 minutes to 1 hour.

6. Stir flour with 4 tbsp (60 mL) water to make a smooth paste. Gradually pour over lamb, stirring continuously. When thickened, remove from heat. Serve with Indian bread.

Nutrients per serving	
Calories	357
Fat	28 g
Carbohydrates	6 g
Protein	20 g

Chicken Puttanesca

Capers contain an abundance of phytochemicals that seem to survive the commercial processing. Rinse the capers under running water to reduce the amount of sodium in the recipe.

VARIATION

Puttanesca Sauce: Follow recipe but omit the chicken. Enjoy as is with pasta, or serve with spicy sausages, or over firm white fish, such as cod or halibut.

2 tbsp	extra virgin olive oil	30 mL
1	chicken (2 to 2½ lbs/1 to 1.25 kg), cut into serving-size pieces	1
	Salt and freshly ground black pepper	
2	onions, halved lengthwise and thinly sliced	2
12	cloves garlic, thinly sliced	12
2	cans (each 28 oz/796 mL) tomatoes, with juice	2
½ cup	sliced oil-packed sun-dried tomatoes	125 mL
¼ cup	coarsely chopped drained capers	60 mL
2	anchovy fillets, rinsed and chopped	2
2 tbsp	chopped fresh basil (or 2 tsp/10 mL dried)	30 mL
2 tbsp	chopped fresh oregano (or 2 tsp/10 mL dried)	30 mL
1 tsp	hot pepper flakes	5 mL
½ cup	pitted niçoise olives	125 mL
¼ cup	chopped fresh flat-leaf (Italian) parsley	60 mL

1. In a large heavy skillet, heat oil over medium-high heat. Season chicken pieces lightly with salt and pepper. Add to skillet and brown well on all sides, 3 to 4 minutes per side. Remove chicken and set aside.

2. Add onions to the skillet. Reduce heat to medium and sauté until onions are soft and beginning to brown, 5 to 7 minutes. Add garlic and sauté for 1 to 2 minutes.

3. Strain tomatoes, reserving the juice, and chop tomatoes roughly. Add tomatoes to the pan with sun-dried tomatoes, capers, anchovies, basil, oregano and hot pepper flakes. Bring sauce to a simmer, stirring occasionally.

4. Return browned chicken to the pan and coat with sauce. Cover pan, reduce heat and simmer until juices run clear when chicken is pierced, 30 to 40 minutes. Add some of the reserved tomato juices if sauce is too thick. Stir in olives and parsley. Taste and adjust seasoning.

Nutrients per serving	
Calories	513
Fat	17 g
Carbohydrates	34 g
Protein	54 g

Lamb and White Bean Ragoût

Makes 6 servings

The sweet potatoes in this yummy stew add antioxidant vitamin A, and the herbs and red wine contribute an assortment of phytochemicals.

TIP

If you are avoiding gluten, thicken this sauce with arrowroot starch or cornstarch.

1 cup	dried navy beans	250 mL
2 lbs	boneless lamb shoulder	1 kg
1 cup	dry red wine	250 mL
3	sprigs fresh rosemary	3
1	bay leaf	1
	Salt and freshly ground black pepper	
4 tbsp	olive oil, divided	60 mL
1	onion, chopped	1
2	cloves garlic, finely chopped	2
2 tbsp	all-purpose flour	30 mL
5 cups	Chicken Stock (page 201) or ready-to-use chicken broth	1.25 L
1 tbsp	coarsely chopped fresh thyme	15 mL
1 tbsp	Worcestershire sauce	15 mL
2 tsp	finely chopped fresh rosemary	10 mL
1	sweet potato, cut into ½-inch (1 cm) cubes	1
¼ cup	coarsely chopped fresh flat-leaf (Italian) parsley	60 mL

1. Rinse and pick over dried beans. Soak in 4 cups (1 L) cold water in the refrigerator overnight.

2. Meanwhile, trim lamb and cut into cubes, about 1 inch (2.5 cm). In a large bowl or heavy-duty plastic bag, combine lamb, wine and rosemary sprigs. Cover and marinate in the refrigerator for 4 hours or overnight.

3. The next day, rinse and drain beans. In a saucepan, combine beans with 6 cups (1.5 L) cold water and bay leaf. Bring to a boil. Reduce heat, partially cover and simmer until beans are tender to the bite, 40 to 45 minutes. Remove from heat and add ½ tsp (2 mL) salt. Set aside for 5 minutes. Drain and set aside.

4. Drain lamb, reserving marinade, and pat dry. Discard rosemary sprigs from marinade. In a large heavy pot, heat 2 tbsp (30 mL) of the oil over medium-high heat. Lightly season lamb with salt and pepper. Sear lamb, in batches, on all sides until nicely browned. Do not crowd the pot. Transfer lamb to a bowl and set aside. Pour off and discard excess fat.

Nutrients per serving	
Calories	676
Fat	42 g
Carbohydrates	32 g
Protein	35 g

TIP

For speed and convenience, replace the dried beans with 1 can (14 to 19 oz/398 to 540 mL) navy beans, rinsed and drained.

5. In the same pot, heat remaining oil over medium heat. Add onion and garlic and sauté until softened and lightly browned, 4 to 6 minutes. Stir in flour and cook, stirring, 2 to 3 minutes. Stir in reserved marinade, scraping up all the browned bits on the bottom of the pot and whisk until smooth. Add chicken stock, thyme, Worcestershire sauce, chopped rosemary and browned lamb with any collected juices. Bring gently to a boil. Reduce heat to low and simmer, covered, until lamb is tender, 1 to 1½ hours. Add beans and sweet potato and cook until sweet potato is tender, 10 to 15 minutes. Remove from heat. Stir in parsley. Taste and adjust seasoning.

Chicken Tuscan Hunter-Style

Makes 6 servings

Trim any large pieces of fat off the chicken thighs to make this dish as lean as possible. After chopping the garlic, let it stand for a few minutes before cooking it; this maximizes the amount of available phytochemicals.

¼ cup	olive oil	60 mL
4	cloves garlic, finely chopped	4
1	sprig fresh rosemary, leaves only, finely chopped	1
12	fresh sage leaves, finely chopped	12
4½ lbs	chicken thighs, skin removed	2.25 kg
½ tsp	salt	2 mL
¼ tsp	freshly ground black pepper	1 mL
1 cup	dry red wine	250 mL
2 tbsp	tomato paste	30 mL
1½ cups	Chicken Stock (page 201) or ready-to-use chicken broth	375 mL

1. In a large skillet, heat olive oil over medium heat. Add garlic, rosemary and sage; cook for 1 or 2 minutes. Add chicken, in batches if necessary, and sear on both sides; continue cooking until chicken is golden brown, about 15 minutes.

2. Season chicken with salt and pepper. Splash in the red wine. Bring to a gentle boil and cook for about 5 minutes.

3. Blend the tomato paste into the stock and pour over chicken. Cover and let simmer 30 to 35 minutes or until chicken is cooked through and sauce is thickened. Serve immediately.

Nutrients per serving	
Calories	531
Fat	23 g
Carbohydrates	3 g
Protein	68 g

Coq au Vin

Makes 6 servings

For a delicious, comforting dish in true bistro-style, it's hard to beat a chicken stew that includes onions, mushrooms, bacon and generous quantities of rich sauce. Remove the skin from the chicken before cooking to reduce the amount of fat in each portion. If you choose Canadian (back) bacon, you'll get the bacon taste without the extra saturated fat.

- **6-quart (6 L) Dutch oven or wide shallow pot with lid**
- **Parchment paper (optional)**

2 tbsp	butter	30 mL
3 oz	bacon or lean salt pork, cut into ½-inch (1 cm) strips	90 g
3 lbs	chicken, cut into serving-size pieces	1.5 kg
1	carrot, finely chopped	1
1	onion, finely chopped	1
1	stalk celery, finely chopped	1
2	cloves garlic, finely chopped	2
1 tbsp	tomato paste	15 mL
3 cups	dry red wine	750 mL
	Salt and freshly ground black pepper	
½ to 1 cup	Chicken Stock (page 201) or ready-to-use chicken broth	125 to 250 mL
1 tsp	finely chopped fresh thyme	5 mL
1	bay leaf	1
	Sautéed Mushrooms (see recipe, page 290)	
	Caramelized Pearl Onions (see recipe, page 290)	
2 tbsp	finely chopped fresh flat-leaf (Italian) parsley	30 mL

1. In large Dutch oven, melt butter over medium heat. Add bacon and sauté until lightly browned. Remove with a slotted spoon and set aside to drain on paper towel.

2. Pat chicken dry. Add to pot and brown well on all sides. (You may need to do this in batches. Do not crowd the pan.) Transfer chicken to a platter and set aside.

3. Add carrot, onion, celery and garlic to the pot and sauté for about 5 minutes. Add tomato paste and cook for 2 minutes. Stir in wine and deglaze pan, scraping up browned bits on the bottom. Return chicken and bacon to the pot. Season lightly with salt and pepper.

Nutrients per serving	
Calories	564
Fat	22 g
Carbohydrates	17 g
Protein	53 g

TIPS

Cut a sheet of cooking parchment just $\frac{1}{2}$ inch (1 cm) larger than the surface of your pot or casserole. Lay the parchment directly on the surface of the meat and vegetables, with edges turned up around the edge of the pot. Cover the pot. During braising time, the parchment sheet catches any evaporated moisture that drips into the casserole from the lid. Carefully lift off parchment and pour away accumulated water. Your sauce will not be diluted.

If space and time allow, we recommend long, slow cooking of stews to take place in a slow oven, around 325°F (160°C), rather than on top of the stove. In the confined space you are able to control a more even low heat and adjust the temperature to keep liquid at a steady gentle simmer.

4. Add chicken stock, as needed, just to cover the chicken, and thyme and bay leaf. Bring to a simmer. Cover, reduce heat to low and simmer the chicken on the stovetop until tender, or braise in preheated 325°F (160°C) oven. (Now is the time when you prepare the Sautéed Mushrooms and Caramelized Pearl Onions.) Test chicken for doneness after 20 minutes since the breast meat will cook more quickly. Remove chicken pieces as they are cooked (when the juices run clear when chicken is pierced) and set them aside. Continue simmering until all chicken is cooked, 5 to 10 minutes more.

5. Bring cooking liquids to a boil and skim off any fat. Taste, adjust seasoning, and continue to boil and reduce until sauce is richly flavored and thickened to your taste, 1 to 2 minutes.

6. Return chicken and bacon to the casserole and add Sautéed Mushrooms and Caramelized Pearl Onions. Gently stir all together to coat with sauce and heat briefly to blend flavors, about 5 minutes. The dish is now ready to be served. For best flavor, let cool, cover and refrigerate for a day or for up to 3 days. About 1 hour before serving, remove pot from refrigerator, bring to room temperature for about 30 minutes and reheat on stovetop over medium-low heat or in 325°F (160°C) oven. Simmer until all the contents are hot, 20 to 30 minutes. Garnish with parsley.

Sautéed Mushrooms

1 tbsp	olive oil	15 mL
1 lb	cremini mushrooms, whole if small, quartered if large	500 g
	Salt and freshly ground black pepper	

Mushrooms contain many phytochemicals that help keep the immune system in balance. But their phytochemical content decreases quickly when they are kept at room temperature, so be sure to store them in the refrigerator.

1. In a large skillet, heat oil over medium-high heat. Add mushrooms and sauté until lightly browned, 6 to 8 minutes. Season to taste with salt and pepper.

Nutrients per serving

Calories	48
Fat	3 g
Carbohydrates	6 g
Protein	2 g

Caramelized Pearl Onions

1 tbsp	olive oil	15 mL
8 oz	pearl onions, peeled	250 g
	Salt and freshly ground black pepper	

Peeling pearl onions can be a challenge. Make it easier by trimming the root ends, then blanching the onions for about 30 seconds. Submerge them in ice water to stop the cooking. Wait a few seconds, then squeeze the onion where the stem was. The skin will just slip off!

1. In a medium saucepan, heat oil over medium-high heat. Add onions and sauté for about 10 minutes, rolling the onions around so that they brown on all sides. Season to taste with salt and pepper.

Nutrients per serving

Calories	37
Fat	2 g
Carbohydrates	4 g
Protein	1 g

Chicken Piccata

A light, crispy coating keeps these chicken breasts moist and flavorful. Make sure to make the bread crumbs with whole wheat bread for the most fiber. If you choose to use panko instead, add fiber by incorporating some flax seeds, oat bran or wheat bran, or a mixture of all three, into the bread crumb mixture.

TIP

When is chicken cooked? Perfectly cooked chicken is tender and moist and the juices run clear. Recommended internal temperature is 165°F (74°C). Meat continues to cook and the internal temperature rises during the first 5 to 10 minutes when removed from the heat. If cooking a whole chicken, we recommend removing chicken from the heat when the internal temperature registered at the thickest part of the meat (without touching bone) is 160°F (71°C).

Nutrients per serving	
Calories	395
Fat	22 g
Carbohydrates	20 g
Protein	29 g

- **Preheat oven to 400°F (200°C)**
- **Baking sheet, lightly oiled**

6	boneless skinless chicken breasts	6
1 tsp	grated lemon zest	5 mL
2 tbsp	freshly squeezed lemon juice	30 mL
1½ cups	fresh bread crumbs or panko	375 mL
2 tbsp	finely chopped fresh basil (or 2 tsp/10 mL dried)	30 mL
2 tbsp	finely chopped fresh flat-leaf (Italian) parsley	30 mL
2 tsp	finely chopped fresh rosemary (or ½ tsp/2 mL dried)	10 mL
½ tsp	kosher or sea salt	2 mL
½ tsp	freshly ground black pepper	2 mL
Pinch	cayenne pepper	Pinch
¼ cup	butter	60 mL
¼ cup	olive oil	60 mL

1. Pound chicken breasts between sheets of plastic wrap or parchment to an even thickness of about ½ inch (1 cm). Drizzle with lemon juice.

2. In a bowl, combine bread crumbs, lemon zest, basil, parsley, rosemary, salt, black pepper and cayenne. Spread seasoned bread crumbs in a shallow dish.

3. In a small saucepan, melt butter and oil over low heat. Pat chicken dry. Dip chicken in melted butter and oil, one piece at a time, then coat in seasoned bread crumbs. Arrange in a single layer on prepared baking sheet. Discard any excess butter and bread crumb mixtures.

4. Bake in preheated oven until crust is crisp and golden and chicken is no longer pink inside, 12 to 15 minutes.

VARIATION

Pork or Veal Cutlets: Use the seasoned bread crumbs to coat thin cutlets of pork or veal. Bake in preheated oven as for Chicken Piccata, or sauté in a skillet over medium heat.

Cheater's Cassoulet

Makes 12 servings

You'll love this easy version of cassoulet, a rich, delicious, substantial country dish. To minimize the amount of saturated fat, choose a low-fat sausage, ask your butcher to remove as much fat as possible from the lamb and pork, and omit the pork belly. Replace the butter with canola oil or, if you still want the buttery taste, a mixture of canola oil and butter.

TIPS

If you are halving this recipe, be sure to use a small (approx. 3 quart) slow cooker.

Be sure to use sausage that is seasoned with "traditional spices." Those containing chile pepper, such as chorizo, will disrupt the flavors of the dish.

Nutrients per serving	
Calories	737
Fat	41 g
Carbohydrates	39 g
Protein	46 g

- **Minimum 6-quart slow cooker**

2 tbsp	olive oil, divided	30 mL
1 lb	pork sausage (see tip, at left), removed from casings	500 g
2 lbs	trimmed boneless pork shoulder or blade (butt), cut into 1-inch (2.5 cm) cubes and patted dry	1 kg
1 lb	trimmed lamb shoulder, cut into 1-inch (2.5 cm) cubes and patted dry	500 g
4	onions, chopped	4
6	cloves garlic, minced	6
2 tsp	dried thyme	10 mL
2	bay leaves	2
1 tsp	salt	5 mL
1 tsp	cracked black peppercorns	5 mL
1	can (5½ oz/156 mL) tomato paste	1
1½ cups	dry white wine	375 mL
3 cups	Chicken Stock (page 201) or ready-to-use chicken broth	750 mL
8 oz	pork belly, thinly sliced	250 g
4 cups	cooked white beans (such as navy or great Northern), drained and rinsed	1 L

Topping

2 cups	fresh bread crumbs	500 mL
½ cup	finely chopped fresh parsley	125 mL
2	cloves garlic, minced	2
	Freshly ground black pepper	
¼ cup	melted butter	60 mL

1. In a skillet, heat 1 tbsp (15 mL) of the oil over medium-high heat. Add sausage and cook, stirring, until no hint of pink remains, about 5 minutes. Transfer to slow cooker stoneware.

2. Add pork shoulder to skillet, in batches, and cook, stirring, until browned, about 4 minutes per batch. Transfer to slow cooker stoneware.

TIPS

Many butchers sell cut-up pork stewing meat, which is fine to use in this recipe.

If you prefer, substitute 1½ cups (375 mL) chicken stock plus 2 tbsp (30 mL) lemon juice for the white wine.

MAKE AHEAD

Complete step 2. Cover and refrigerate mixture for up to 2 days. When you're ready to cook, complete the recipe.

3. Add lamb to skillet, in batches, and cook, stirring, until browned, about 4 minutes per batch. Transfer to stoneware.

4. Reduce heat to medium. Add remaining 1 tbsp (15 mL) of oil to pan. Add onions and cook, stirring, until softened, about 5 minutes. Add garlic, thyme, bay leaves, salt and peppercorns and cook, stirring, for 1 minute. Stir in tomato paste. Add wine, bring to a boil and boil for 2 minutes, scraping up brown bits from bottom of pan.

5. Transfer to slow cooker stoneware. Add chicken stock, pork belly and cooked beans. Stir well. Cover and cook on Low for 8 to 10 hours or on High for 4 to 5 hours, until hot and bubbly.

6. *Topping:* Preheat oven to 350°F (180°C). In a bowl, combine bread crumbs, parsley, garlic and pepper to taste. Mix well. Spread evenly over bean mixture. Drizzle with butter. Bake in preheated oven until top has formed a crust, about 30 minutes.

VARIATION

If you are serving this to guests, you can easily bump it up a notch if you have access to prepared duck confit (many butchers are selling it these days). Just cut it into bite-size pieces and add to the cooked cassoulet before adding the topping. Don't use more than 8 oz (250 g).

Easy Skillet Chicken and Rice

To make this dish as arthritis-friendly as possible, remove the skin from the chicken before cooking it, and choose canola or olive oil.

1 tbsp	vegetable oil	15 mL
2	chicken legs	2
	Salt and freshly ground black pepper	
²⁄₃ cup	long-grain white rice	150 mL
1	onion, chopped	1
1	clove garlic, minced	1
¼ tsp	dried oregano	1 mL
¼ tsp	dried thyme	1 mL
1	can (19 oz/540 mL) kidney beans, drained and rinsed	1
1	can (10 oz/284 mL) mushrooms, drained	1
1⅓ cups	water	325 mL
	Paprika	

1. In skillet, heat oil over medium-high heat; add chicken and brown all over, about 10 minutes, sprinkling with salt and pepper. Remove chicken and set aside. Pour off all but 1 tbsp (15 mL) drippings from pan. Add rice, onion, garlic, oregano and thyme; cook, stirring, over medium heat until rice is browned, about 3 minutes.

2. Stir in beans, mushrooms and water. Arrange chicken on top. Sprinkle with paprika. Bring to boil, cover, reduce heat to low and simmer for 30 to 40 minutes or until juices run clear when chicken is pierced and rice is tender.

Nutrients per serving	
Calories	754
Fat	21 g
Carbohydrates	68 g
Protein	73 g

Buckwheat Pilaf with Paprika-Seasoned Chicken

Smoked paprika is the secret ingredient in this flavorful chicken pilaf. The smoky and slightly nippy spice is a perfect complement to the robust flavors of buckwheat.

TIPS

Kasha is toasted buckwheat groats. Since I find the taste of kasha quite overpowering, I prefer to buy plain buckwheat groats and toast them myself, which produces a more mildly flavored result. Place the groats in a dry skillet over high heat and cook, stirring constantly, until they are nicely fragrant, about 4 minutes. In the process, they will darken from a light shade of sand to one with a hint of brown.

Toasting sliced almonds enhances their flavor. Toast them in a dry skillet over medium heat until they change to a beautiful golden color. This can happen very quickly, so stir them often.

Nutrients per serving	
Calories	329
Fat	9 g
Carbohydrates	37 g
Protein	28 g

1 tbsp	olive oil	30 mL
1	onion, finely chopped	1
½	red bell pepper, finely chopped	½
2	cloves garlic, minced	2
1 tsp	smoked paprika	5 mL
½ tsp	freshly ground black pepper	2 mL
12 oz	boneless skinless chicken breasts or thighs, cut into ½-inch (1 cm) cubes	375 g
2 cups	Chicken Stock (page 201) or reduced-sodium ready-to-use chicken broth	500 mL
1 cup	toasted buckwheat groats or kasha (see tip, at left)	250 mL
¼ cup	finely chopped fresh parsley	60 mL
¼ cup	toasted sliced almonds	60 mL

1. In a large saucepan, heat oil over medium-high heat for 30 seconds. Add onion, red pepper and garlic and cook, stirring, until vegetables are softened, about 5 minutes. Add smoked paprika, black pepper and chicken and stir until chicken is well coated with mixture. Add chicken stock and bring to a boil. Stir in buckwheat and return to a boil.

2. Reduce heat to low. Cover and simmer until liquid is absorbed and chicken is no longer pink inside, about 15 minutes. Remove from heat and set aside for 5 minutes. (If the pilaf still has a bit too much liquid for your taste, return to low heat and stir until it evaporates.) Transfer to a serving dish. Garnish with parsley and almonds and serve.

Peppery Chicken Quinoa

This great one-dish meal is not just pretty to look at, it's also very easy to make. Enjoy it when peppers are in season. Red bell peppers contain a significant amount of vitamin C, as well as many other health-promoting phytochemicals.

TIP

Harissa is a North African chili paste that is often added to couscous to give it some bite. If you don't have it, pass your favorite hot pepper sauce at the table to satisfy any heat seekers in the group.

3 cups	Chicken Stock (page 201) or reduced-sodium ready-to-use chicken broth, divided	750 mL
1 tbsp	harissa (optional)	15 mL
1 cup	quinoa, rinsed	250 mL
3 tbsp	extra virgin olive oil, divided	45 mL
½ tsp	cracked black peppercorns	2 mL
1 lb	boneless skinless chicken breasts, thinly sliced	500 g
4	cloves garlic, thinly sliced	4
3	red bell peppers, cut into thin strips	3
2 tbsp	sherry vinegar	30 mL
¼ cup	finely chopped fresh parsley	60 mL

1. In a saucepan over medium heat, bring 2 cups (500 mL) of the stock to a boil. Stir in harissa (if using). Add quinoa in a steady stream, stirring constantly, and return to a boil. Reduce heat to low. Cover and simmer until tender, about 15 minutes. Remove from heat and let stand for 5 minutes. Fluff with a fork.

2. Meanwhile, in a large skillet or wok, heat 1 tbsp (15 mL) of the olive oil over medium-high heat. Add peppercorns and stir well. Add chicken and cook, stirring, until it turns white and almost cooks through, about 5 minutes. Transfer to a plate.

3. Add remaining 2 tbsp (30 mL) of oil to pan. Add garlic and cook, stirring, just until it begins to turn golden, about 2 minutes. Add bell peppers and cook, stirring, until they begin to shimmer, about 2 minutes. Add remaining 1 cup (250 mL) of stock and sherry vinegar and cook until mixture is reduced by half, about 8 minutes. Return chicken to pan and toss until heated through. Remove from heat.

4. *To serve:* Spread cooked quinoa over a deep platter and scoop out an indentation in the middle. Fill with chicken mixture and garnish with parsley.

VARIATION

Instead of quinoa, serve this over couscous or brown or red rice. If using couscous, try spelt or barley couscous instead of whole wheat.

Nutrients per serving	
Calories	418
Fat	15 g
Carbohydrates	38 g
Protein	35 g

Chicken in Dill Sauce

Makes 8 servings

This easy meal provides an abundance of nutrients. The chicken contributes protein and is low in saturated fat. Green peas contribute soluble fiber, along with phytochemicals.

TIP

The evaporated milk mimics the smooth texture of whipping cream, but with significantly less fat and calories.

VARIATION

Use green beans instead of carrots, and corn instead of peas.

- **Preheat oven to 375°F (190°C)**
- **13- by 9-inch (33 by 23 cm) glass baking dish, greased**

4	large boneless skinless chicken breasts (each about 8 oz/250 g)	4
½ tsp	salt	2 mL
½ tsp	freshly ground black pepper	2 mL
1½ cups	chopped carrots	375 mL
1 cup	chopped celery	250 mL
1 cup	chopped onion	250 mL
2 cups	Chicken Stock (page 201) or reduced-sodium ready-to-use chicken broth	500 mL
1 cup	frozen green peas, thawed	250 mL
2½ tbsp	all-purpose flour	37 mL
½ cup	2% evaporated milk	125 mL
1 tbsp	finely chopped fresh dill	15 mL

1. Place 1 chicken breast flat on a cutting board. Place one hand on top of the chicken and, using a sharp knife and slicing parallel with the board, cut through the chicken to obtain 2 thin cutlets. Repeat with the remaining breasts.

2. Place chicken cutlets in prepared baking dish, overlapping as necessary. Sprinkle with salt and pepper. Cover with carrots, celery and onion. Pour chicken stock over top. Cover with foil.

3. Bake in preheated oven for about 30 minutes or until vegetables are soft. Remove dish from oven and stir in peas. Replace foil and bake for 10 minutes or until chicken is no longer pink inside.

4. Ladle 1 cup (250 mL) of the cooking liquid into a small bowl. While whisking, sprinkle flour over the hot liquid and whisk until there are no lumps and liquid is smooth. Gradually whisk in evaporated milk and dill. Pour sauce evenly over chicken and vegetables in baking dish. Bake, uncovered, for 5 minutes or until sauce is hot.

This recipe courtesy of dietitian Dianna Bihun.

Nutrients per serving	
Calories	185
Fat	2 g
Carbohydrates	11 g
Protein	29 g

Terrific Chicken Burgers

Cooking the burgers in a skillet rather than on the barbecue allows for greater control of the temperature. Keep the heat at medium or lower. Make sure to choose lean ground chicken or turkey. If you're avoiding wheat, try replacing the bread crumbs with quick-cooking rolled oats.

TIP

Layer these patties in toasted onion buns for an easy burger supper or accompany them with stir-fried rice and vegetables.

1	large egg	1
½ cup	fine dry bread crumbs	125 mL
⅓ cup	finely chopped green onions	75 mL
1 tsp	ground coriander	5 mL
1 tsp	grated lemon zest	5 mL
½ tsp	salt	2 mL
¼ tsp	freshly ground black pepper	1 mL
1 lb	ground chicken or turkey	500 g
1 tbsp	vegetable oil	15 mL

1. In a bowl, beat egg; stir in bread crumbs, green onions, coriander, lemon zest, salt and pepper; mix in chicken. With wet hands, shape into four ¾-inch (2 cm) thick patties.

2. In a large nonstick skillet, heat oil over medium heat; cook patties for 5 to 6 minutes on each side or until golden brown on outside and no longer pink in center.

Nutrients per burger	
Calories	268
Fat	14 g
Carbohydrates	10 g
Protein	23 g

Turkey in Cranberry Leek Sauce

Makes 6 servings

Turkey is not just for special occasions, as this easy dish proves. Turkey is a great source of lean protein. For a complete, nutritious meal, serve with another vegetable and a barley or buckwheat pilaf on the side, and some fruit for dessert.

TIPS

If you're concerned about your consumption of fat, remove the skin from the turkey breast and skip step 1. Place the skinless breast in the stoneware and proceed with step 2.

Save your hands — buy leeks that are already washed and cut up.

MAKE AHEAD

This dish can be partially prepared before it is cooked. Heat oil and complete step 2. Cover and refrigerate overnight or for up to 2 days. When you're ready to cook, complete steps 1 and 3.

- **Minimum 5-quart slow cooker**

1 tbsp	olive oil	15 mL
1	skin-on bone-in turkey breast (about 1½ lbs/750 g)	1
2	leeks (white part only with just a bit of green), cleaned (see tip, page 311) and thinly sliced	2
2	cloves garlic, minced	2
2 tsp	dried thyme	10 mL
½ tsp	cracked black peppercorns	2 mL
1 tbsp	all-purpose flour	15 mL
1 cup	Chicken Stock (page 201), turkey stock or ready-to-use chicken broth	250 mL
	Salt (optional)	
½ cup	dried cranberries	125 mL
2 tbsp	finely chopped fresh parsley	30 mL

1. In a skillet, heat oil over medium-high heat for 30 seconds. Add turkey breast, skin side down, and cook until nicely browned, about 4 minutes. Transfer, skin side up, to slow cooker stoneware.

2. Reduce heat to medium. Add leeks and cook, stirring, until softened, about 5 minutes. Add garlic, thyme and peppercorns and cook, stirring, for 1 minute. Add flour and cook, stirring, for 1 minute. Add chicken stock and cook, stirring, until mixture begins to thicken, about 2 minutes. Season with salt (if using). Stir in cranberries.

3. Transfer sauce to slow cooker stoneware, covering turkey with sauce. Cover and cook on Low for 5½ to 6 hours or on High for 2½ to 3 hours, until an instant-read thermometer inserted into center of breast registers 165°F (74°C). To serve, transfer to a platter and garnish with parsley.

Nutrients per serving	
Calories	218
Fat	9 g
Carbohydrates	13 g
Protein	22 g

Smoked Turkey Chili

Makes 10 servings

If you're craving the stick-to-the-ribs satisfaction of a zesty chili but feel the need for something a little different, try this. The black-eyed peas are lighter than traditional red or pinto beans, and the smoked turkey adds intriguing depth. Choose a lower-fat cheese. If you cannot find a great-tasting reduced-fat Monterey Jack or Cheddar, try part-skim mozzarella.

TIPS

If you halve this recipe, use a 2- to 3-quart slow cooker.

For this quantity, soak, cook and drain 2 cups (500 mL) dried black-eyed peas or use 2 cans (14 to 19 oz/398 to 540 mL), drained and rinsed.

- **Minimum 5-quart slow cooker**
- **Blender**

2 tbsp	vegetable or olive oil	30 mL
2	onions, finely chopped	2
4	stalks celery, diced	4
4	cloves garlic, minced	4
2 tsp	ground cumin	10 mL
2 tsp	dried oregano	10 mL
1 tsp	ground allspice	5 mL
1 tsp	cracked black peppercorns	5 mL
½ tsp	grated lime zest	2 mL
1	2-inch (5 cm) cinnamon stick	1
1	can (28 oz/796 mL) tomatoes, with juice, coarsely chopped	1
1 cup	Chicken Stock (page 201), turkey stock or ready-to-use chicken broth	250 mL
4 cups	drained cooked black-eyed peas (see tip, at left)	1 L
3	dried ancho, New Mexico or guajillo chiles	3
2 cups	boiling water	500 mL
1 to 2	jalapeño peppers (see tip, opposite), seeded and diced	1 to 2
½ cup	coarsely chopped fresh cilantro leaves and stems	125 mL
2 tbsp	freshly squeezed lime juice	30 mL
1 tbsp	Mexican chili powder	15 mL
2 lbs	smoked turkey, shredded or cut into cubes	1 kg
2	poblano or green or red bell peppers, finely chopped	2
1 cup	shredded Monterey Jack or Cheddar cheese	250 mL
	Finely chopped red or green onion (optional)	
	Sour cream (optional)	

Nutrients per serving

Calories	310
Fat	10 g
Carbohydrates	31 g
Protein	27 g

TIPS

Use any combination of poblano peppers and red or green bell peppers. If using only sweet peppers, you may want to add an extra jalapeño pepper.

If you prefer a creamier finish, increase the quantity of cheese or be sure to add a dollop of sour cream.

MAKE AHEAD

Complete step 1. Cover and refrigerate mixture for up to 2 days. When you're ready to cook, complete the recipe.

1. In a skillet, heat oil over medium heat. Add onions and celery and cook, stirring, until softened, about 5 minutes. Add garlic, cumin, oregano, allspice, peppercorns, lime zest and cinnamon stick and cook, stirring, for 1 minute. Add tomatoes with juice and chicken stock and bring to a boil.

2. Transfer to slow cooker stoneware. Stir in black-eyed peas. Cover and cook on Low for 6 to 8 hours or on High for 3 to 4 hours, until hot and bubbly.

3. About an hour before recipe has finished cooking, in a heatproof bowl, soak dried chile peppers in boiling water for 30 minutes, weighing down with a cup to ensure they are submerged. Drain, discard stems and chop coarsely.

4. In blender, combine rehydrated chiles, jalapeño, cilantro, lime juice, chili powder and $1/2$ cup (125 mL) liquid from the chili. Purée. Add to stoneware along with smoked turkey and poblano peppers. Cover and cook on High for 20 minutes, until peppers are tender. Stir in cheese and cook on High until melted. Garnish with red onion and/or sour cream, if desired.

VARIATION

Smoked Chicken Chili: Substitute an equal quantity of smoked chicken for the turkey.

Turkey Mushroom Meatloaf

Move over, meatloaves made with ground beef. This tasty meatloaf is packed with great flavor and is sure to become a favorite. Consider doubling the recipe and stash the second cooked meatloaf in the freezer to have on hand for another meal.

TIPS

To wash or not wash mushrooms? You can wipe them with a damp cloth, if you wish. However, I feel it's important to wash all produce that comes into my kitchen. I quickly rinse mushrooms under cold water and immediately wrap in a clean, dry kitchen towel or paper towels to absorb excess moisture.

To make 1½ cups (375 mL) fresh bread crumbs, process 3 slices white sandwich bread in a food processor until finely crumbled.

Cook the meatloaf in a muffin pan and freeze each mini loaf individually for an easy-to-defrost lunch or supper.

- Preheat oven to 350°F (180°C)
- 9- by 5-inch (23 by 12.5 cm) loaf pan, greased

1 tbsp	olive oil	15 mL
1 cup	finely chopped mushrooms	250 mL
1 cup	diced peeled apple	250 mL
1	onion, finely chopped	1
½ cup	finely chopped celery	125 mL
2 tsp	dried sage	10 mL
1 tsp	dried thyme	5 mL
1 tsp	salt	5 mL
½ tsp	freshly ground black pepper	2 mL
2 tbsp	chopped fresh parsley	30 mL
2	large eggs	2
1½ lbs	ground turkey or chicken	750 g
1½ cups	soft fresh bread crumbs	375 mL

1. In a nonstick skillet, heat oil over medium heat; cook mushrooms, apple, onion, celery, sage, thyme, salt and pepper, stirring often, for 10 minutes or until vegetables are tender. Add parsley and let cool slightly.

2. In a bowl, lightly beat eggs. Stir in turkey, bread crumbs and vegetable mixture. Using a wooden spoon, gently mix until thoroughly combined.

3. Press mixture lightly into loaf pan. Bake in preheated oven for 1 to 1¼ hours or until meat thermometer registers 160°F (71°C). Let stand for 5 minutes. Drain pan juices; turn out onto a plate and cut into slices.

Nutrients per serving

Calories	413
Fat	17 g
Carbohydrates	26 g
Protein	38 g

Side Dishes

Green Beans with Cashews

The simple addition of cashews and red onions transforms ordinary green beans into a delightful companion to any main course. Cashews are rich in heart-protective monounsaturated fats and the bone-strengthening mineral magnesium.

1 lb	green beans, trimmed	500 g
2 tbsp	olive oil	30 mL
½ cup	slivered red onion	125 mL
⅓ cup	raw cashews	75 mL
¼ tsp	salt	1 mL
¼ tsp	freshly ground black pepper	1 mL
	Few sprigs fresh parsley, chopped	

1. Blanch green beans in a pot of boiling water for 5 minutes. Drain and immediately refresh in a bowl of ice-cold water. Drain and set aside.

2. In a large skillet, heat olive oil over medium-high heat for 30 seconds. Add onions, cashews, salt and pepper and stir-fry for 2 to 3 minutes, until the onions are softened. Add cooked green beans, increase heat to high, and stir-fry actively for 2 to 3 minutes, until the beans feel hot to the touch. (Take care that you don't burn any cashews in the process.) Transfer to a serving plate and garnish with chopped parsley. Serve immediately.

Nutrients per serving

Calories	519
Fat	13 g
Carbohydrates	76 g
Protein	29 g

Beans and Cabbage with Ginger

Most Thai vegetable dishes are stir-fried, with seasoning sauces added. This one includes creamy coconut milk and the added freshness of ginger and lemongrass. Ginger is rich in nutrients and has been shown to have anti-inflammatory effects.

TIP

When selecting fresh gingerroot, make sure it is firm, smooth and free of mold.

2 tbsp	vegetable oil	30 mL
2 tbsp	coarsely chopped gingerroot	30 mL
1 tbsp	chopped fresh lemongrass, white part only	15 mL
1 tsp	chopped fresh red or green chile pepper	5 mL
2 cups	sliced green beans (about 8 oz/250 g), cut into 2-inch (5 cm) lengths	500 mL
2 cups	chopped cabbage	500 mL
1/2 cup	coconut milk	125 mL
2 tbsp	fish sauce (nam pla)	30 mL
2 tsp	granulated sugar	10 mL
	Fresh sweet Thai basil leaves	

1. Heat a wok or large skillet over medium-high heat and add oil. Add ginger, lemongrass and chile and stir-fry for 30 seconds. Add beans and cabbage and stir-fry for 2 minutes.

2. Add coconut milk, fish sauce and sugar and combine. Cover and cook for 3 minutes. Remove cover and cook for 1 minute, or until beans and cabbage are just tender. Serve garnished with basil.

Nutrients per serving

Calories	103
Fat	9 g
Carbohydrates	6 g
Protein	2 g

Cumin Beets

Makes 6 servings

This dish is inspired by Indian cuisine. If you have trouble peeling the beets, try canned beets in this recipe.

TIPS

For the best flavor, toast cumin seeds and grind them yourself. *To toast seeds:* Place in a dry skillet over medium heat and cook, stirring, until fragrant, about 3 minutes. Immediately transfer to a spice grinder or mortar and grind finely.

Peeling the beets before they are cooked ensures that all the delicious cooking juices end up on your plate.

If you prefer a spicy dish, add hot pepper sauce, to taste, after the beets have finished cooking.

MAKE AHEAD

Complete step 1. Cover and refrigerate for up to 2 days. When you're ready to cook, complete the recipe.

- **2-quart slow cooker**

1 tbsp	vegetable oil	15 mL
1	onion, finely chopped	1
3	cloves garlic, minced	3
1 tsp	ground cumin (see tip, at left)	5 mL
1 tsp	salt	5 mL
½ tsp	freshly ground black pepper	2 mL
2	tomatoes, peeled and coarsely chopped	2
1 cup	water	250 mL
1 lb	beets, peeled and used whole if small, or thinly sliced	500 g
	Hot pepper sauce (optional)	

1. In a skillet, heat oil over medium heat. Add onion and cook, stirring, until softened, about 3 minutes. Stir in garlic, cumin, salt and pepper and cook, stirring, for 1 minute. Add tomatoes and water and bring to a boil.

2. Place beets in slow cooker stoneware and pour tomato mixture over them. Cover and cook on Low for 8 hours or on High for 4 hours, until beets are tender. If desired, pass hot pepper sauce at the table.

Nutrients per serving	
Calories	76
Fat	3 g
Carbohydrates	12 g
Protein	2 g

Jalapeño Broccoli

This recipe uses the sweet heat of jalapeño peppers to dress up broccoli and make it fun to eat. Caution: jalapeño peppers can be quite hot. If you are sensitive to spicy foods, make sure to remove the seeds.

TIP

This salad can be served immediately or it can stand, covered, at room temperature for up to 2 hours.

1 tsp	salt	5 mL
1	head broccoli, trimmed and separated into spears	1
1 tbsp	balsamic vinegar	15 mL
2 to 3 tbsp	olive oil	30 to 45 mL
2	fresh jalapeño peppers, thinly sliced (with or without seeds, depending on desired hotness)	2
¼ cup	toasted pine nuts	60 mL
	Few sprigs fresh coriander or parsley, chopped	

1. Bring a pot of water to a boil and add salt. Add broccoli spears and boil over high heat for 3 to 5 minutes (depending on desired tenderness). Drain and transfer broccoli to bowl of ice water for 30 seconds. Drain and lay out the cooked spears decoratively on a presentation plate. Drizzle evenly with balsamic vinegar.

2. In a small frying pan, heat olive oil over medium heat for 30 seconds. Add jalapeños and stir-fry for 2 to 3 minutes until softened. Take peppers with all the oil from the pan and distribute evenly over broccoli. Garnish with pine nuts and herbs.

Nutrients per serving	
Calories	130
Fat	11 g
Carbohydrates	8 g
Protein	5 g

Braised Carrots with Capers

Makes 8 servings

This dish is simplicity itself and yet the results are startlingly fresh. Capers contain the flavonoids rutin and quercetin, which are powerful phytochemicals. Rinse capers under running water to help reduce sodium.

TIPS

Carrots are high in beta carotene, an antioxidant that our bodies turn into vitamin A. Cooking actually increases the vegetable's beta carotene and increases its sweetness.

If you are halving this recipe, be sure to use a small (1½ to 3½ quart) slow cooker.

MAKE AHEAD

Complete step 1 and refrigerate overnight. The next day, complete the recipe.

- **2- to 4-quart slow cooker**

2 tbsp	extra virgin olive oil	30 mL
12	large carrots, peeled and thinly sliced	12
12	cloves garlic, thinly sliced	12
½ tsp	salt	2 mL
½ tsp	freshly ground black pepper	2 mL
½ cup	drained capers	125 mL

1. In slow cooker stoneware, combine oil, carrots, garlic, salt and pepper. Toss to combine.

2. Cover and cook on Low for 6 hours or on High for 3 hours, until carrots are tender. Add capers and toss to combine. Serve immediately.

VARIATION

Braised Carrots with Black Olives: Substitute ½ cup (125 mL) chopped black olives (preferably kalamata), a particularly pungent Greek variety, for the capers.

Nutrients per serving	
Calories	83
Fat	4 g
Carbohydrates	12 g
Protein	2 g

Cauliflower with Capers

Makes 4 servings

Pressed for time? This simple side dish can be prepared in less than 5 minutes. It could even be made with frozen cauliflower to make it easier on sore hands.

¼ cup	mayonnaise	60 mL
2 tsp	freshly squeezed lemon juice	10 mL
1 tsp	drained small capers	5 mL
Dash	hot pepper sauce (such as Tabasco)	Dash
1	head cauliflower, broken into florets	1

1. Combine mayonnaise, lemon juice, capers and hot pepper sauce. In a large pot of lightly salted boiling water, cook cauliflower until barely tender, about 3 minutes. Drain and toss with the mayonnaise mixture.

Nutrients per serving	
Calories	95
Fat	5 g
Carbohydrates	11 g
Protein	3 g

Orange-Braised Fennel

Makes 6 servings

Crunchy, slightly sweet fennel is commonly used in Mediterranean and Italian cuisines. It is rich in vitamin C, which acts as a powerful antioxidant and immune system enhancer. It also contains the phytochemical anethole, which has shown to reduce inflammation.

TIPS

For the best flavor, toast coriander seeds and grind them yourself. To toast seeds: Place in a dry skillet over medium heat and cook, stirring, until fragrant, about 3 minutes. Immediately transfer to a spice grinder or mortar and grind finely.

If you halve this recipe, use a 2-quart slow cooker.

- **1½- to 3½-quart slow cooker**
- **Large sheet of parchment paper**

2 tbsp	olive oil	30 mL
3	bulbs fennel, trimmed, cored and thinly sliced on the vertical	3
2	cloves garlic, minced	2
1 tsp	ground coriander (see tip, at left)	5 mL
½ tsp	salt	2 mL
½ tsp	cracked black peppercorns	2 mL
	Grated zest and juice of 1 orange	

1. In a skillet, heat oil over medium-high heat. Add fennel, in batches, and cook, stirring, just until it begins to brown, about 5 minutes per batch. Transfer to slow cooker stoneware as completed. When last batch of fennel is almost browned, add garlic, coriander, salt, peppercorns and orange zest to pan and cook, stirring, for 1 minute. Transfer to slow cooker stoneware and stir in orange juice.

2. Place a large piece of parchment over the fennel, pressing it down to brush the food and extending up the sides of the stoneware so it overlaps the rim. Cover and cook on Low for 6 hours or on High for 3 hours, until fennel is tender. Lift out the parchment and discard, being careful not to spill the accumulated liquid into the stoneware.

Nutrients per serving	
Calories	78
Fat	5 g
Carbohydrates	9 g
Protein	2 g

Simple Braised Leeks

Makes 6 servings

Leeks have a mild onion flavor that is both delicate and rich. They are a wonderful accompaniment to grilled fish or roast chicken. Like garlic and onions, leeks are rich in vitamin K and vitamin A.

TIPS

If you halve this recipe, use a 1½- to 2-quart slow cooker.

Leeks can be gritty and need to be thoroughly cleaned before cooking. Peel off the tough outer layer(s) and cut off the root. Slice leeks according to recipe instructions and submerge in a basin of lukewarm water, swishing them around to remove all traces of dirt. Transfer to a colander and rinse under cold water.

- **2- to 4-quart slow cooker**

6 to 8	leeks (white part only with just a hint of green), cleaned (see tip, at left) and cut into quarters on the vertical	6 to 8
3 tbsp	melted butter or olive oil	45 mL
1 cup	Vegetable Stock (page 200) or Chicken Stock (page 201) or ready-to-use vegetable or chicken broth	250 mL
	Salt and freshly ground black pepper	
¼ cup	finely chopped fresh parsley	60 mL

1. Pat leeks dry and place in slow cooker stoneware. Add butter and toss until well coated.

2. Place a clean tea towel, folded in half (so you will have 2 layers), over top of stoneware to absorb moisture. Cover and cook on High for 1 hour. Stir well.

3. Remove tea towel and add vegetable stock. Cover and cook on Low for 5 to 6 hours or on High for 2½ to 3 hours, until leeks are very tender. Season to taste with salt and pepper. Garnish with parsley and serve.

VARIATION

Leeks Gratin: After the leeks have finished cooking, drain off the liquid and set aside. Do not garnish with parsley. Transfer leeks to an ovenproof serving dish and keep warm. Place the liquid in a saucepan, bring to a boil, and cook until reduced by at least half. (You'll want about ½ cup/125 mL of liquid.) Meanwhile, preheat broiler. In a bowl, combine ½ cup (125 mL) dry bread crumbs, ¼ cup (60 mL) finely grated Parmesan and 2 tbsp (30 mL) finely chopped parsley. Pour reduced cooking liquid over leeks and sprinkle bread crumb mixture evenly over top. Place under broiler until cheese is melted and top is browned.

Nutrients per serving	
Calories	123
Fat	7 g
Carbohydrates	13 g
Protein	1 g

New Orleans Braised Onions

Makes 10 servings

New Orleans is famous for its flavorful and hearty foods. This simple side dish pairs well with pork. As the flavonoids in onions tend to be located in the outer layers, peel off as little as possible of the edible portion when removing the paper layer.

TIPS

Onions are high in natural sugars, which long, slow simmering brings out, as does the orange juice in this recipe.

If you halve this recipe, use a 1½- to 3½-quart slow cooker, checking to make sure the whole onions will fit.

- **Minimum 5-quart slow cooker**

2 to 3	large Spanish onions	2 to 3
6 to 9	whole cloves	6 to 9
½ tsp	salt	2 mL
½ tsp	cracked black peppercorns	2 mL
Pinch	dried thyme	Pinch
	Grated zest and juice of 1 orange	
½ cup	Vegetable Stock (page 200) or ready-to-use vegetable broth	125 mL
	Finely chopped fresh parsley (optional)	
	Hot pepper sauce (optional)	

1. Stud onions with cloves. Place in slow cooker stoneware and sprinkle with salt, peppercorns, thyme and orange zest. Pour orange juice and vegetable stock over onions, cover and cook on Low for 8 hours or on High for 4 hours, until onions are tender.

2. Using a slotted spoon, transfer onions to a serving dish and keep warm in a 250°F (120°C) oven. Transfer liquid to a saucepan over medium heat. Cook until reduced by half.

3. When ready to serve, cut onions into quarters. Place on a deep platter and cover with sauce. Sprinkle with parsley, if desired, and pass the hot pepper sauce, if desired.

Nutrients per serving	
Calories	16
Fat	0 g
Carbohydrates	3 g
Protein	0 g

Curried Root Vegetables Masala

This side dish is chock-full of colorful vegetables. Eating a rainbow of different vegetables each day will help improve your daily intake of essential vitamins and minerals. In particular, this recipe is rich in vitamin A, which contributes to eye health, and complex carbohydrates, which can improve satiety and slow digestion.

TIP

Traditionally, whole spices are left in curries when serving, but they aren't meant to be eaten. Be sure to let your guests know not to eat the whole cloves in this dish.

¼ cup	vegetable oil, divided	60 mL
1	small sweet potato, cut into ½-inch (1 cm) cubes	1
1	boiling or all-purpose potato, cut into ½-inch (1 cm) cubes	1
1	large carrot, cut into ½-inch (1 cm) thick slices	1
1	beet, cut into ½-inch (1 cm) cubes	1
1	small onion, thinly sliced	1
¼ cup	minced garlic (about 8 cloves)	60 mL
1 tsp	ground cumin	5 mL
1 tsp	hot pepper flakes	5 mL
½ tsp	whole cloves	2 mL
2 tbsp	raisins	30 mL
2 cups	canned or fresh diced tomatoes, with juice	500 mL
½ cup	water	125 mL
2 tbsp	freshly squeezed lemon juice	30 mL
	Salt	

1. In a large skillet, heat half the oil over high heat. Add sweet potato, potato, carrot and beet, in batches as necessary; cook, stirring, until vegetables start to brown and soften, about 5 minutes. Using a slotted spoon, transfer to a bowl, leaving as much oil in the pan as possible and adding more oil between batches as necessary. Set vegetables aside.

2. Return pan to medium-high heat. Add onion and cook, stirring, until starting to brown, about 2 minutes. Add garlic, cumin, hot pepper flakes and cloves; cook, stirring, for 1 minute.

3. Stir in raisins, tomatoes with juice, water and lemon juice; bring to a simmer. Simmer, stirring often, until tomatoes are softened, about 2 minutes.

4. Stir in reserved vegetables and cook, stirring occasionally, until vegetables are tender and sauce is slightly thickened, about 20 minutes. Season to taste with salt.

Nutrients per serving	
Calories	260
Fat	14 g
Carbohydrates	31 g
Protein	3 g

Hot-and-Sour Vegetable Curry

This versatile curry is a marvelous way to get a boost of healthy vegetables.

TIP

Frozen vegetables can be just as nutritious as fresh. The vegetables are usually picked at their peak of ripeness, meaning they are also at their nutritional peak. During the flash-freezing process, many of the vitamins and minerals remain intact.

- **Blender**

1½ tsp	granulated sugar	7 mL
¾ cup	white vinegar	175 mL
3 tbsp	vegetable oil, divided	45 mL
1½ cups	cubed peeled sweet potato (½-inch/1 cm cubes)	375 mL
1 cup	cubed peeled potato (½-inch/1 cm cubes)	250 mL
1 cup	cubed peeled carrots (½-inch/1 cm cubes)	250 mL
1 cup	green beans, cut into 1-inch (2.5 cm) pieces	250 mL
1 cup	frozen peas, thawed	250 mL
¼ cup	coarsely chopped garlic	60 mL
2 tbsp	coarsely chopped gingerroot	30 mL
2 cups	finely chopped onions	500 mL
1½ cups	chopped tomatoes	375 mL
1 tbsp	ground cumin	15 mL
1½ tsp	cayenne pepper	7 mL
1 tsp	ground turmeric	5 mL
1 tsp	salt, or to taste	5 mL
1 cup	packed fresh cilantro, coarsely chopped, divided	250 mL

1. In a bowl, stir sugar into vinegar to dissolve. Set aside.

2. In a nonstick skillet, heat 1 tsp (5 mL) of the oil over medium heat. Add sweet potato and sauté until pieces start to brown lightly, about 2 minutes. Transfer to a bowl. Repeat process separately with potato, carrots and green beans, adding each to bowl with sweet potatoes. Toss peas into mixture and set aside.

3. In blender, blend garlic, ginger and 3 tbsp (45 mL) water into a paste. Set aside.

4. In a saucepan, heat remaining oil over medium-high heat. Add onion and sauté until golden, 6 to 8 minutes.

Nutrients per serving	
Calories	129
Fat	6 g
Carbohydrates	18 g
Protein	3 g

To peel gingerroot without a vegetable peeler, use the edge of a large spoon to scrape the skin off.

Gingerroot can be grated ahead of time and frozen in 1 tbsp (15 mL) portions, ready for use.

5. Reduce heat to medium-low. Stir in paste, tomatoes, cumin, cayenne, turmeric and salt. Mix well. Cover and cook until tomatoes are soft and can be mashed with the back of a spoon, 6 to 8 minutes.

6. Stir in vegetables and ¾ cup (175 mL) of the cilantro. Pour vinegar mixture and ½ cup (125 mL) water over top and cook until vegetables are tender, 5 to 8 minutes. Garnish with remaining cilantro before serving.

Spiced Spinach

Makes 6 servings

Spinach is packed with many beneficial vitamins and minerals. To decrease the saturated fat content of this dish, choose reduced-fat or fat-free yogurt.

TIP

Spinach leaves tend to collect sand and soil, so make sure to wash them well. Some supermarkets now sell packages of pre-washed spinach.

2 tbsp	butter	30 mL
2 tbsp	minced onion	30 mL
1 tsp	ground coriander	5 mL
1 tsp	curry powder	5 mL
Pinch	freshly ground black pepper	Pinch
Pinch	cayenne pepper	Pinch
Pinch	ground nutmeg	Pinch
2	packages (each 10 oz/300 g) spinach leaves, coarsely chopped	2
	Salt	
⅓ cup	plain yogurt	75 mL

1. In a large skillet, melt butter over medium-high heat. Sauté onion, coriander, curry powder, black pepper, cayenne and nutmeg until onion is tender and spices are aromatic.

2. Add spinach and salt to taste; sauté until spinach is wilted and dry, about 3 minutes. Remove from heat and stir in yogurt.

Nutrients per serving	
Calories	95
Fat	5 g
Carbohydrates	12 g
Protein	3 g

Veggie Kabobs

In the summer months, flavorful veggies are easy to prepare on the grill and will please a crowd of family and friends. For a complete meal, add cubes of tofu or another favorite lean protein. Keep the grill heat at medium to reduce charring.

TIPS

Zucchini, which comes in green and yellow (or golden) versions, is a type of summer squash. In this recipe, we like to use both green zucchini and yellow summer squash for appearance. If you prefer, use just green or golden zucchini in this recipe.

The longer the marinating time, the deeper the flavors.

- **Preheat grill or broiler**
- **16 bamboo or metal skewers**

⅓ cup	freshly squeezed lemon juice	75 mL
¼ cup	olive oil	60 mL
1	clove garlic, minced (about 1 tsp/5 mL)	1
2 tsp	dried oregano (or 2 tbsp/30 mL finely chopped fresh)	10 mL
	Salt and freshly ground black pepper	
2	bell peppers (any color), cut into 1-inch (2.5 cm) strips	2
2	small zucchini, cut into 1-inch (2.5 cm) thick slices	2
2 cups	grape tomatoes or cherry tomatoes (about 16)	500 mL
2 cups	whole mushrooms (about 16)	500 mL
1	large onion, cut into 8 wedges and halved crosswise, separated into single layers	1
1	yellow summer squash (such as golden zucchini), cut into 1-inch (2.5 cm) cubes	1

1. In a large bowl or sealable plastic bag, combine lemon juice, olive oil, garlic, oregano and salt and pepper to taste. Add peppers, zucchini, tomatoes, mushrooms, onion and squash and stir to evenly coat. Marinate at room temperature for 15 to 20 minutes or in the refrigerator for up to 12 hours.

2. Thread vegetables onto skewers, alternating to form an attractive pattern and leaving a bit of space between the pieces to allow air to circulate.

3. Grill or broil, turning and basting often with remaining marinade, for 8 to 10 minutes or until vegetables are browned on all sides and tender. While cooking, rotate location of the skewers on the grill or broiler to ensure even cooking.

Nutrients per serving	
Calories	103
Fat	7 g
Carbohydrates	9 g
Protein	2 g

TIP

Any leftover veggies from these kabobs make a perfect beginning for tasty pasta dishes or salads.

VARIATIONS

Vary the flavor by replacing oregano with the same quantity of thyme, basil or rosemary.

Substitute garlic salt for the fresh garlic, but adjust seasoning accordingly.

The vegetables (unskewered) can also be spread in a single layer on two greased rimmed baking sheets and baked in a preheated 400°F (200°C) oven for 30 to 35 minutes. Turn the vegetables and rotate the pans after 20 minutes.

For convenience, cook the vegetables in a nonstick grill basket, being aware that some may cook more quickly than others.

Vegetable Fried Rice

Makes 6 servings

Vegetable fried rice is a convenient way to use up those leftover vegetables. To maximize fiber content, use brown rice.

TIPS

Most supermarket chains carry canned straw mushrooms. If you can't find them, use 2 cups (500 mL) sliced mushrooms instead.

It is preferable to use a wok when making this dish, as the vegetables will cook faster and there will be more room to manipulate the ingredients.

1 cup	jasmine, white or brown rice	250 mL
3 tbsp	peanut or vegetable oil, divided	45 mL
1	large onion, finely chopped (about 2 cups/500 mL)	1
3 cups	chopped bok choy	750 mL
1 cup	sugar snap peas, trimmed and cut into 1-inch (2.5 cm) pieces	250 mL
1	red bell pepper, thinly sliced and cut into 1-inch (2.5 cm) pieces	1
1	bunch green onions (white and green parts), coarsely chopped (about 1 cup/250 mL)	1
1	can (15 oz/450 mL) straw mushrooms, drained	1
¼ cup	chopped fresh basil	60 mL
Sauce		
½ cup	reduced-sodium soy sauce	125 mL
2 tbsp	distilled white vinegar	30 mL
1	clove garlic, minced (or ¼ tsp/1 mL garlic powder)	1
1½ tsp	granulated natural cane sugar, or to taste	7 mL
	Hot sesame oil (see tip, at left)	

1. Cook rice according to package directions. Set aside.

2. In a large skillet or wok, heat 2 tbsp (30 mL) oil over medium heat for 30 seconds. Add onion and cook, stirring, for 3 minutes or until softened. Add bok choy, sugar snap peas, red pepper, green onions and mushrooms. Reduce heat to medium-low and cook, stirring occasionally, for 4 minutes or until vegetables are tender-crisp.

Nutrients per serving	
Calories	164
Fat	8 g
Carbohydrates	20 g
Protein	5 g

3. *Sauce:* Meanwhile, in a small bowl, whisk together soy sauce, vinegar, garlic, sugar and hot sesame oil to taste. Stir half into vegetables and add basil. Reduce heat to low, cover and cook for 10 minutes or until flavors are well blended. Transfer vegetables to a bowl and cover with foil to keep warm.

4. Return skillet to high heat and add remaining 1 tbsp (15 mL) oil. Heat until sizzling. Add rice and cook for 3 to 4 minutes, pushing down with a spatula to brown rice. Stir in vegetables and remaining sauce and mix well.

Mushroom Baked Rice

Makes 4 servings

Rice is absolutely foolproof when cooked in the oven — and there's less temptation to lift the lid and have a peek.

TIP

When purchasing ready-to-use broths, be sure to read the Nutrition Facts table and nutritional claims. As elevated levels of sodium can contribute to hypertension and cardiovascular disease, select broths that have no added salt or are at least low in sodium.

- **Preheat oven to 400°F (200°C)**
- **6-cup (1.5 L) casserole dish, greased**

1 tbsp	olive oil	15 mL
1 cup	sliced mushrooms (any variety)	250 mL
1 cup	long-grain white rice	250 mL
1½ cups	hot Chicken Stock (page 201) or ready-to-use chicken or beef broth	375 mL
	Freshly ground black pepper	

1. In a nonstick skillet, heat oil over medium-high heat. Add mushrooms. Sauté for 5 minutes. Stir in rice and chicken stock.

2. Transfer to prepared casserole dish. Cover and bake in preheated oven for 20 minutes or until liquid is absorbed and rice is tender. Let stand for 5 minutes before serving. Season with pepper to taste.

Nutrients per serving	
Calories	118
Fat	5 g
Carbohydrates	15 g
Protein	4 g

Golden Curried Pineapple Rice

Makes 4 servings

Pineapple adds sweetness and flavor to this dish. Your guests will beg for more!

TIPS

If your package of basmati rice specifies a different amount of water for 1 cup (250 mL) of rice, adjust the amount accordingly.

It is traditional to serve whole spices in the rice, but they are not meant to be eaten. You can discard them if you prefer.

When purchasing a pineapple, select one that is heavy for its size. Many stores also sell fresh pineapple with the skin removed — all you have to do is chop it.

1 cup	basmati rice	250 mL
	Cold water	
1 tbsp	vegetable oil	15 mL
8	fresh curry leaves	8
1	2-inch (5 cm) cinnamon stick	1
1 tsp	cumin seeds	5 mL
1 tsp	mustard seeds	5 mL
3	cloves garlic, minced	3
1/2 tsp	salt	2 mL
1/2 tsp	ground turmeric	2 mL
1 cup	chopped fresh pineapple	250 mL
1 3/4 cups	water	425 mL
1/4 tsp	garam masala	1 mL

1. In a sieve, rinse rice under cool running water until water runs fairly clear. Transfer rice to a bowl and cover with cold water. Let soak for 20 minutes. Drain well.

2. In a saucepan, heat oil over medium heat until hot but not smoking. Add curry leaves, cinnamon, cumin seeds and mustard seeds; cook, stirring, until seeds start to pop, about 1 minute. Add garlic, salt and turmeric; cook, stirring, until blended and softened, about 1 minute. Add pineapple and cook, stirring, until pineapple starts to release its juices, about 2 minutes.

3. Stir in rice until well coated with spices. Stir in 1 3/4 cups (425 mL) water and bring to a boil. Reduce heat to low, cover and simmer until rice is tender and liquid is absorbed, about 15 minutes. Remove from heat and let stand, covered, for 5 minutes. Fluff with a fork. Discard cinnamon stick, if desired. Serve sprinkled with garam masala.

Nutrients per serving	
Calories	105
Fat	4 g
Carbohydrates	16 g
Protein	2 g

Quinoa with Almonds

Quinoa is a protein- and fiber-rich whole grain that can easily replace rice or pasta. It is also an excellent source of manganese. This dish is a great accompaniment to a main course that includes a small portion of meat that is high in saturated fat.

TIPS

When you buy quinoa, it has been rinsed and air-dried to remove the naturally occurring bitter saponins, a resin-like coating. Still, rinse it again before use to remove any powdery residue that may remain.

To toast almonds: Place nuts on a baking sheet in a 350°F (180°C) oven for 6 to 8 minutes, stirring occasionally, until lightly toasted.

1 tbsp	vegetable oil	15 mL
2	carrots, peeled and chopped	2
2	stalks celery, chopped	2
1	small onion, finely chopped	1
1½ tsp	ground coriander	7 mL
1 cup	quinoa, rinsed	250 mL
1 cup	Chicken Stock (page 201) or ready-to-use chicken broth	250 mL
1 tsp	grated orange or lemon zest	5 mL
1 cup	orange juice	250 mL
½ tsp	salt	2 mL
¼ tsp	freshly ground black pepper	1 mL
¼ cup	chopped fresh cilantro or parsley	60 mL
¼ cup	toasted sliced almonds	60 mL

1. In a medium saucepan, heat oil over medium heat. Cook carrots, celery, onion and coriander, stirring, for 5 minutes or until vegetables are softened. Add quinoa, stock, orange zest and juice, salt and pepper; bring to a boil. Reduce heat to medium-low, cover and simmer for 15 minutes or until quinoa is tender and liquid is absorbed.

2. Uncover and fluff quinoa with a fork. Let stand for 5 minutes. Stir in cilantro and almonds.

Nutrients per serving	
Calories	193
Fat	10 g
Carbohydrates	23 g
Protein	6 g

Desserts

Banana Cake with Lemon Cream Frosting

This decadent cake is higher in fiber and lower in fat and sugar than any store-bought version.

TIPS

For a simple substitute for the buttermilk, stir 1½ tsp (7 mL) lemon juice into ½ cup (125 mL) milk. Let stand for 5 to 10 minutes or until thickened.

For the smoothest frosting, use extra-smooth ricotta cheese.

For the most intense walnut flavor, use walnut oil in the cake and toast the walnuts for garnishing the cake.

- Preheat oven to 350°F (180°C)
- Food processor or blender
- 13- by 9-inch (33 by 23 cm) cake pan, sprayed with baking spray

Cake

1¾ cups	whole wheat flour	425 mL
2 tsp	baking powder	10 mL
¾ tsp	baking soda	3 mL
½ cup	buttermilk	125 mL
½ cup	liquid honey	125 mL
¼ cup	walnut oil or vegetable oil	60 mL
3	ripe bananas	3
4	large egg whites	4

Lemon Cream Frosting

1 cup	5% ricotta cheese	250 mL
1½ tbsp	liquid honey	22 mL
1 tbsp	grated lemon zest	15 mL
1 tbsp	freshly squeezed lemon juice	15 mL
1½ tsp	cornstarch or arrowroot	7 mL
¼ cup	chopped walnuts	60 mL
	Lemon zest, cut into thin strips	

1. *Cake:* In a bowl, stir together flour, baking powder and baking soda; set aside.

2. In food processor, purée buttermilk, honey, oil and bananas until smooth; stir into flour mixture just until mixed.

3. In another bowl, beat egg whites until stiff peaks form; fold into batter. Pour into prepared pan.

4. Bake 20 to 30 minutes or until tester inserted in center comes out clean. Cool in pan on wire rack.

5. *Frosting:* In clean food processor, purée ricotta, honey, grated lemon zest, lemon juice and cornstarch until smooth. Transfer to a saucepan. Cook over medium heat, stirring constantly, until steaming hot. Remove from heat. Chill.

6. Spread cold frosting over cooled cake. Sprinkle with walnuts and strips of lemon zest.

Nutrients per serving	
Calories	85
Fat	2 g
Carbohydrates	14 g
Protein	2 g

Fresh Ginger Cake

This moist, spicy ginger cake is sure to become a favorite. It's high in calories, though, so save it for special occasions.

TIPS

To make grating gingerroot easier on sore hands, peel it and store it in the freezer. Then simply grate as needed — no thawing required.

Grate gingerroot until very fine to avoid any stringy fibrous bits in the cake. Add 1 tbsp (15 mL) finely chopped crystallized ginger to the batter for those who love ginger.

- **Preheat oven to 350°F (180°C)**
- **8-inch (20 cm) round cake pan, lightly greased and lined with parchment paper**

1 cup	all-purpose flour	250 mL
½ tsp	baking soda	2 mL
½ tsp	ground cinnamon	2 mL
¼ tsp	ground cloves	1 mL
¼ tsp	freshly ground black pepper	1 mL
Pinch	salt	Pinch
⅔ cup	sunflower oil	150 mL
⅔ cup	light (fancy) molasses	150 mL
½ cup	granulated sugar	125 mL
2	large eggs	2
¼ cup	grated gingerroot	60 mL
1 tbsp	confectioners' (icing) sugar	15 mL

1. In a bowl, sift together flour, baking soda, cinnamon, cloves, pepper and salt. Set aside.

2. In a large bowl, using an electric mixer on medium speed or with a whisk, beat oil, molasses and sugar until smooth. Lightly beat in eggs and ginger. On low speed or with a wooden spoon, add dry ingredients alternately with ¼ cup (60 mL) water, making 3 additions of flour mixture and 2 of water, beating until just blended. Pour batter into prepared pan, smoothing top. Bake in preheated oven until top springs back and a tester inserted in the center comes out clean, 50 to 60 minutes.

3. Let cake stand in pan for 10 minutes. Run a knife around the inside of pan to release the cake and turn out onto a cake board or plate. Remove parchment. Invert onto a wire rack and let cool. Lightly dust top with confectioners' sugar before serving.

Nutrients per serving

Calories	581
Fat	21 g
Carbohydrates	96 g
Protein	9 g

Ancient Grains
Chocolate Chip Cookies

**Makes about
2 dozen cookies**

Flax seeds are rich in omega-3 fatty acids. While whole flax seeds have a soft crunch, the nutrients in ground flax seeds are more easily absorbed.

TIPS

Stone-ground flours give a grainier texture to cookies than refined flours. Look for them at health food or natural foods stores or well-stocked supermarkets.

For the most even baking, bake one sheet at a time. If you do bake both sheets at once, place one in the upper third of the oven and one in the lower third. Switch their positions halfway through.

Because Kamut flour is used in this recipe, it is not gluten-free.

- **Preheat oven to 350°F (180°C)**
- **Baking sheets, greased or lined with parchment paper**

½ cup	lightly packed brown sugar	125 mL
⅓ cup	non-hydrogenated margarine	75 mL
¼ cup	ground flax seeds (flaxseed meal)	60 mL
¼ cup	granulated sugar	60 mL
1	large egg	1
1 tsp	vanilla extract	5 mL
¾ cup	stone-ground Kamut flour	175 mL
¾ cup	stone-ground spelt flour	175 mL
½ tsp	baking soda	2 mL
¼ tsp	salt	1 mL
1 cup	semisweet chocolate chips	250 mL

1. In a large bowl, using an electric mixer on high speed, cream brown sugar, margarine, flax seeds and granulated sugar for 1 minute. Beat in egg and vanilla until blended. Add Kamut flour, spelt flour, baking soda and salt; mix until well blended. Stir in chocolate chips.

2. Drop by tablespoonfuls (15 mL) about 2 inches (5 cm) apart on prepared baking sheets. Bake in preheated oven for 12 to 15 minutes or until bottoms are lightly browned. Let cool on pans on a wire rack for 5 minutes, then transfer to rack to cool completely.

This recipe courtesy of dietitian Shauna Lindzon.

Nutrients per cookie	
Calories	112
Fat	6 g
Carbohydrates	16 g
Protein	2 g

Date and Nut Pinwheels

There is no doubt that dates are a very nutritious fruit. They are rich in fiber and beta carotene.

2 cups	packed chopped dates	500 mL
½ cup	finely chopped raw cashews	125 mL
1 cup	sweetened flaked or shredded coconut, divided	250 mL

1. Wrap dates in plastic wrap and place on a cutting board. Mash with a rolling pin or a wooden mallet or pulse in a food processor until they form a paste and hold together.

2. Place another large piece of plastic wrap, about 16 inches (40 cm) long, on table with the short end facing you. Spoon dates lengthwise down middle in a line about 10 inches (25 cm) long. Cover with another piece of plastic wrap. Flatten with hand into as even a rectangle as possible. With rolling pin, roll into even rectangle about 13 by 8 inches (33 by 20 cm), lifting wrap and flipping over occasionally to eliminate wrinkles.

3. Turn so long end faces you. Remove upper plastic wrap. Sprinkle date surface evenly with cashews, leaving a ¼-inch (0.5 cm) border on far long edge. Top with ½ cup (125 mL) of the coconut. Starting at edge closest to you, with the help of plastic wrap, carefully form into a roll, peeling off plastic wrap as you roll and pressing to compact. Pinch edge to seal.

4. On another piece of plastic wrap, sprinkle remaining coconut. Carefully transfer roll onto coconut and roll to cover dates completely. Roll up tightly in plastic wrap, twisting ends to enclose. Refrigerate for at least 3 hours or for up to 2 days.

5. With a sharp knife, cut into approximately ½-inch (1 cm) thick slices. (Cut straight down. Do not use sawing motion.)

Nutrients per pinwheel	
Calories	71
Fat	2 g
Carbohydrates	14 g
Protein	1 g

Fall Fruit en Papillote

Makes 4 servings

This simple dish makes a dramatic presentation for guests. The fruit is served in the pockets so that diners open the parchment at the table. Thanks to the variety of fruit, this is also a tremendously healthy dessert, packed with many different vitamins and minerals.

TIP

Be careful when selecting apple juice, as not all juices are created equal. Some are nutritious, while others are simply sugar and water. Purchase juices that are labeled "100% fruit juice" and beware of the words "drink," "punch" and "cocktail."

- **Preheat oven to 350°F (180°C)**
- **4 sheets parchment paper, each 18 by 12 inches (45 by 30 cm)**
- **Baking sheet**

¼ cup	raisins	60 mL
¼ cup	chopped pecans	60 mL
¼ cup	chopped candied ginger	60 mL
4	1-inch (2.5 cm) cinnamon sticks	4
4	1-inch (2.5 cm) pieces licorice root (optional)	4
4	1-inch (2.5 cm) pieces vanilla bean	4
4	whole cloves	4
4	dried or fresh apricots, halved	4
1	pear, cut into eighths	1
1	apple, cut into eighths	1
1	peach, quartered	1
1	plum, quartered	1
½ cup	apple cider or apple juice	125 mL
1 tsp	butter	5 mL

1. Fold a sheet of parchment paper in half. Cut out the shape of one-half of a heart, with center fold as the center of the heart. When you open up the parchment paper, you'll have a heart-shaped piece. Repeat with remaining 3 sheets.

2. On one side of the fold line of one piece of parchment, spoon 1 tbsp (15 mL) each raisins, pecans and ginger. Add 1 piece each cinnamon, licorice (if using), vanilla bean and 1 clove. Add 2 each apricot halves, pear and apple slices. Add 1 each peach and plum quarter. Sprinkle 2 tbsp (30 mL) cider and top with ¼ tsp (1 mL) butter.

3. Fold the other half of the parchment heart along the fold line, over fruit. Beginning at the top of the heart, roll and fold the 2 cut ends together. Work towards the bottom until the entire cut edge is sealed. Fruit is now enclosed in one half heart-shaped pocket. Repeat with remaining 3 hearts.

Nutrients per serving	
Calories	240
Fat	9 g
Carbohydrates	41 g
Protein	2 g

Pockets may be prepared up to 4 hours ahead of time and baked just before serving.

4. Transfer pockets to baking sheet. Bake in preheated oven for 30 to 40 minutes or until apples and pears are tender. Slide each package onto individual dessert plates. Cut an "X" on top of each package with a sharp knife. Pull back the tips of the 4 corners of the "X" to make a small opening in the parchment. Serve immediately.

Baked Peaches with Almond Crust

Makes 4 servings

Different types of peaches have distinct flavors. Peaches with white flesh are usually sweeter and less acidic than yellow-fleshed peaches.

- **Preheat oven to 350°F (180°C)**
- **Baking dish**

6 tbsp	ground almonds	90 mL
2 tbsp	packed brown sugar, liquid honey or pure maple syrup	30 mL
1 tbsp	softened unsalted butter	15 mL
2	large ripe freestone peaches	2
1 tsp	softened unsalted butter	5 mL
	Chocolate ice cream and/or raspberry coulis	

1. In a small bowl, combine ground almonds, sugar and 1 tbsp (15 mL) butter, mixing with a spoon to form a paste.

2. Cut a ring around the peaches and neatly separate them in halves. Remove pits. Lightly rub 1 tsp (5 mL) butter all over the peaches to grease the surfaces. Put peach halves in baking dish, skin-side down. Heap one-quarter of the almond paste into the pit cavity of each half.

3. Bake in preheated oven for 20 minutes. Serve (half a peach per portion) immediately, garnished with a dollop of ice cream and/or a smear of raspberry coulis.

Nutrients per serving	
Calories	141
Fat	9 g
Carbohydrates	16 g
Protein	2 g

Poached Peaches with Lavender Custard

Makes 4 servings

This vegan-friendly dessert is rich in calcium, a bone-strengthening mineral that is often deficient in vegan diets.

TIPS

Just make sure to purchase soy milk or rice milk that is fortified with calcium and vitamin D.

Use only organic lavender, which has not been chemically treated.

- Blender or food processor

4	peaches, halved	4
¾ cup	apple juice	175 mL
½ cup	white wine	125 mL

Lavender Custard

½ cup	soy milk or rice milk	125 mL
1	3-inch (7.5 cm) piece vanilla bean	1
1	2-inch (5 cm) piece licorice root (optional)	1
1 tbsp	dried lavender buds (see tip, at left)	15 mL
12 oz	silken tofu	375 g

1. In a saucepan, combine peach halves, apple juice and wine. Bring to a boil over medium heat. Reduce heat and simmer for 10 minutes or until the tip of a knife meets with some resistance when inserted. Remove from heat and let peaches stand in the poaching liquid until ready to serve or overnight.

2. *Lavender Custard:* In a saucepan over medium-low heat, combine soy milk, vanilla bean, licorice (if using) and lavender. Cover, reduce heat and simmer until bubbles form around outside edge of pan. Let cool with cover on. Strain and discard vanilla, licorice and lavender. In blender, process tofu until smooth. With the motor running, add cooled soy milk through the feed tube. Blend until smooth.

3. Using a slotted spoon, lift peaches into bowls and top with custard. Custard will keep tightly covered in the refrigerator for up to 2 days.

Nutrients per serving	
Calories	163
Fat	3 g
Carbohydrates	24 g
Protein	6 g

Wine-Poached Pears

Makes 4 servings

This classic preparation for pears is an impressive way to end a special meal. Try garnishing it with low-fat Greek yogurt, which is naturally higher in protein than regular yogurt.

TIPS

Poach the pears the day ahead. They are best served well chilled.

Select pears that are not overly ripe so they will hold their shape when sliced.

2 cups	red wine or cranberry juice cocktail	500 mL
½ cup	granulated sugar	125 mL
1	cinnamon stick	1
3	whole cloves	3
2	3-inch (7.5 cm) strips orange peel	2
4	Bartlett pears, peeled, halved lengthwise and cored	4
	Whipped cream or extra-thick yogurt	
	Freshly grated nutmeg	
	Mint sprigs	

1. In a saucepan, combine wine, sugar, cinnamon stick, cloves and orange peel. Bring to a boil; stir to dissolve sugar. Add pear halves; reduce heat, cover and simmer for 15 minutes or until just tender when pierced with a knife. Remove with a slotted spoon to a dish; let cool.

2. Bring poaching liquid in saucepan to a boil over high heat; boil until reduced to ¾ cup (175 mL). Strain through a sieve to remove spices; let cool and refrigerate.

3. Place pears cut side down on work surface. Beginning near the stem end, cut each pear half into ¼-inch (0.5 cm) lengthwise slices. (Do not cut through the stem itself; slices will still be attached at stem end.) Arrange 2 pear halves on each dessert plate, pressing down gently to fan out slices. Spoon syrup over top. Garnish with a dollop of whipped cream or extra-thick yogurt and sprinkle with grated nutmeg. Garnish with mint sprigs.

Nutrients per serving	
Calories	173
Fat	1 g
Carbohydrates	47 g
Protein	1 g

Melon Balls with Warm Ginger Sauce

Makes 6 servings

Although honeydew melons and cantaloupes are increasingly available throughout the year, they are usually in season between June and August. For the most nutrients, choose fully ripened melons.

TIP

If you don't have a melon baller, use a small spoon to scoop melon flesh, or cut flesh into small cubes, or take a shortcut and buy cut-up pieces of melon.

MAKE AHEAD

Make sauce in advance and store covered in refrigerator up to 2 days; reheat before serving.

1	small ripe honeydew melon	1
2	small ripe cantaloupes	2
Sauce		
2 cups	orange juice	500 mL
2 tbsp	minced gingerroot (or $\frac{1}{2}$ tsp/2 mL ground ginger)	30 mL
1 tbsp	raspberry or red wine vinegar	15 mL
1 tsp	liquid honey	5 mL
$\frac{1}{2}$ tsp	freshly squeezed lemon juice	2 mL
	Fresh mint leaves	

1. Cut melons in half and discard seeds. With a melon baller, scoop out flesh. Divide melon balls among 6 individual dessert dishes.

2. *Sauce:* In a saucepan, combine orange juice, ginger, vinegar, honey and lemon juice. Bring to a boil; cook until reduced to $\frac{1}{2}$ cup (125 mL). Spoon warm sauce over melon balls and serve garnished with mint leaves.

Nutrients per serving	
Calories	109
Fat	1 g
Carbohydrates	26 g
Protein	2 g

Rice Pudding

Makes 4 servings

This version of a comfort food classic is made with almond milk, which can be consumed by people with milk allergies or lactose intolerance. While it has fewer calories than other non-dairy milks, it also has less protein. Choose fortified almond milk.

- **Four 1-cup (250 mL) ramekins**

1 cup	jasmine rice	250 mL
4 cups	unsweetened almond milk, divided	1 L
1	3-inch (7.5 cm) cinnamon stick	1
¼ cup	pure maple syrup	60 mL
1 tsp	vanilla extract	5 mL
	Ground cinnamon	
	Ground nutmeg	

1. In a medium saucepan over medium-high heat, stir together rice, 3 cups (750 mL) of the almond milk and cinnamon stick and, stirring often, bring to a boil.

2. Reduce heat, cover and simmer for 15 to 20 minutes to partially cook rice. Stir in maple syrup, vanilla and remaining almond milk. Simmer, stirring and ensuring mixture doesn't become too dry, for 15 to 20 minutes or until most of the milk has been absorbed and rice is tender. Do not overcook.

3. Remove and discard cinnamon stick. Divide rice mixture evenly among ramekins. Sprinkle with cinnamon and nutmeg. Serve warm or cool.

Nutrients per serving	
Calories	197
Fat	3 g
Carbohydrates	40 g
Protein	3 g

Banana Raspberry Tapioca Pudding

This easy-to-prepare treat is also good for you. Tapioca is a starch derived from the root of the shrub-like cassava plant. It is flavorless and makes an excellent thickener for puddings, jellies and soups.

- Four ³/₄-cup (175 mL) ramekins, lightly greased
- Cook's torch

2 cups	milk	500 mL
3 tbsp	granulated sugar	45 mL
2 tbsp	wheat-free instant tapioca	30 mL
1	large egg, lightly beaten	1
1	banana	1
½ cup	raspberries	125 mL
4 tsp	packed brown sugar	20 mL

1. In a medium heavy-bottomed pot, stir together milk, granulated sugar and tapioca. Let stand for 15 minutes.

2. Over medium heat, whisk in egg until blended and cook, stirring occasionally, for about 10 minutes or until boiled and thickened. Set aside and let cool.

3. Slice banana and evenly divide slices among ramekins. Evenly top with raspberries. Spoon tapioca mixture evenly over fruit, smoothing top. Cover and refrigerate overnight.

4. Sprinkle brown sugar evenly over puddings. Brown with a cook's torch until sugar has melted to form a crunchy crust.

Nutrients per serving	
Calories	182
Fat	4 g
Carbohydrates	32 g
Protein	6 g

Coconut Ice Cream

Coconut milk is high in calories and saturated fat, so save this dessert for special occasions. Light coconut milk is available and contains less saturated fat.

MAKE AHEAD
Ice cream can be packed into a freezer container and frozen for 2 weeks.

Nutrients per serving	
Calories	282
Fat	24 g
Carbohydrates	21 g
Protein	2 g

3 cups	coconut milk	750 mL
¾ cup	granulated sugar	175 mL
½ tsp	salt	2 mL
	Coconut Caramel Sauce (see recipe, below)	
	Toasted coconut or chopped pecans	

1. In a saucepan, combine coconut milk, sugar and salt. Place over medium heat and bring to a low boil, stirring until sugar dissolves.
2. Pour into a bowl and refrigerate for 2 to 3 hours, or until very cold. For faster chilling, place over a bowl of ice water and stir frequently.
3. Transfer to an ice cream maker and freeze according to manufacturer's directions or freeze in a metal container until firm, stirring 4 to 5 times during freezing process.
4. Serve topped with Coconut Caramel Sauce and toasted coconut or chopped peanuts.

This versatile sauce can be used to complement desserts, waffles and even satays.

Nutrients per 1 tbsp (15 mL)	
Calories	58
Fat	3 g
Carbohydrates	9 g
Protein	0 g

Coconut Caramel Sauce

1 cup	granulated sugar	250 mL
¼ cup	water	60 mL
1 cup	coconut milk	250 mL

1. In a saucepan, combine sugar and water. Bring to a boil over medium-high heat and cook, without stirring, for 5 to 6 minutes, or until mixture starts to caramelize. When mixture starts to color, swirl pan gently for even coloring and cook for 2 to 3 minutes, or until golden, being careful not to burn caramel. Remove pan from heat.
2. Carefully pour coconut milk into saucepan (mixture may seize in a lump). Return to medium heat and cook, stirring, until caramel has dissolved.

Pomegranate, Ginger and Clove Granita

Makes 8 servings

This fruity ice is sweet, tart and spicy all at once — perfect as a palate cleanser or a light dessert. Pomegranate is an exotic fruit with many health benefits.

TIP

If desired, scrape the mixture with a fork every hour for 3 to 5 hours while it's freezing; this will promote the formation of ice crystals.

- **13- by 9-inch (33 by 23 cm) metal baking pan**

½ cup	granulated sugar	125 mL
1 tbsp	grated gingerroot	15 mL
1 tsp	ground cloves	5 mL
4 cups	unsweetened pomegranate juice	1 L
¼ cup	pomegranate seeds	60 mL
8	fresh mint sprigs	8

1. In a large saucepan, combine sugar, ginger, cloves and pomegranate juice. Bring to a boil over high heat, stirring to dissolve sugar. Reduce heat to medium-low and simmer for 5 minutes to allow flavors to infuse juice. Strain, if desired.

2. Pour juice into baking pan. Freeze for at least 6 hours, until solid, or overnight.

3. Scrape the mixture with a fork to create a shaved ice texture. Portion into serving bowls and top with pomegranate seeds and a sprig of mint.

This recipe courtesy of dietitian Mary Sue Waisman.

Nutrients per serving	
Calories	121
Fat	0 g
Carbohydrates	30 g
Protein	0 g

Library and Archives Canada Cataloguing in Publication

Title: The complete arthritis health, diet guide & cookbook : includes 125 recipes for managing inflammation & arthritis pain / Kim Arrey, BSC, RD, with Dr. Michael R. Starr, MD, FRCPC.
Other titles: Complete arthritis health, diet guide and cookbook
Names: Arrey, Kim, author. | Starr, Michael R., author.
Description: Second edition.
Identifiers: Canadiana 20190201045 | ISBN 9780778806561 (softcover)
Subjects: LCSH: Arthritis—Popular works. | LCSH: Arthritis—Nutritional aspects—Popular works. | LCSH: Arthritis—Diet therapy—Popular works. | LCSH: Arthritis—Diet therapy—Recipes.
Classification: LCC RC933 .A637 2019 | DDC 616.7/22—dc23

Selected References

A complete list of references is available upon request.

Autenrieth C, Schneider A, Döring A, et al. Association between different domains of physical activity and markers of inflammation. *Med Sci Sports Exerc*, 2008 Sep;41(9):1706–13.

Baillet A, Zeboulon N, Gossec L et al. Efficacy of cardiorespiratory aerobic exercise in rheumatoid arthritis: Meta-analysis of randomized controlled trials. *Arthritis Care Res* (Hoboken), 2010 Jul;62(7): 984–92.

Brichford C. *Rheumatoid Arthritis: Shopping for Healthy Foods*. Available at: http://www.everydayhealth.com/rheumatoid-arthritis/rheumatoid-arthritis-healthy-foods.aspx. Accessed Sept 2011.

Campbell KL, Campbell PT, Ulrich CM, et al. No reduction in C-reactive protein following a 12-month randomized controlled trial of exercise in men and women. *Cancer Epidemiol Biomarkers Prev*, 2008 Jul;17(7):1714–18.

Canadian Association of Occupational Therapists. *Managing and Preventing Arthritis*. Available at: http://www.caot.ca/default.asp?pageid=3694. Accessed Sept 2011.

Chen YS, Yan W, Geczy CL, et al. Serum levels of soluble receptor for advanced glycation end products and of S100 proteins are associated with inflammatory, autoantibody, and classical risk markers of joint and vascular damage in rheumatoid arthritis. *Arthritis Res Ther*, 2009;11(2):R39. Epub 2009 Mar 11.

Childers NF, Margoles MS. An apparent relation of nightshades (Solanaceae) to arthritis. *J Neurol Orthop Med Surg*, 1993;12:227–31.

Clegg DO, Reda DJ, Harris CL, et al. Glucosamine, chondroitin sulfate, and the two in combination for painful knee osteoarthritis. *N Engl J Med*, 2006, Feb 23; 354(8):795–808.

Cooney JK, Law RJ, Matschke V, et al. Benefits of exercise in rheumatoid arthritis. *J Aging Res*, 2011 Feb 13;2011:681640.

Darlington LG, Ramsey NW, Mansfield JR. Placebo-controlled, blind study of dietary manipulation therapy in rheumatoid arthritis. *Lancet*, 1986 Feb 1;1(8475):236–38.

Dietitians of Canada. *Rheumatoid Arthritis: Key Practice Points*. Available at: http://www.pennutrition.com/KnowledgePathway.aspx?kpid=978&pqcatid=146. Accessed Sept 2011.

Elkan AC, Sjöberg B, Kolsrud B, et al. Gluten-free vegan diet induces decreased LDL and oxidized LDL levels and raised atheroprotective natural antibodies against phosphorylcholine in patients with rheumatoid arthritis: A randomized study. *Arthritis Res Ther*, 2008;10(2):R34. Epub 2008 Mar 18.

Elmali N, Baysal O, Harma A, et al. Effects of resveratrol in inflammatory arthritis. *Inflammation*, 2007 (Apr); 30(1–2):1–6.

Foley D, Ancoli-Israel S, Britz P, Walsh J. Sleep disturbances and chronic disease in older adults: Results of the 2003 National Sleep Foundation Sleep in America Survey. *J Psychosom Res*, 2004 May;56(5):497–502.

Ford ES. Does exercise reduce inflammation? Physical activity and C-reactive protein among U.S. adults. *Epidemiology*, 2002 Sep;13(5): 561–68.

Frostegård, J. Atherosclerosis in patients with autoimmune disorders. *Arterioscler Throm Vasc Biol*, 2005 Sep;25(9): 1776–85. Epub 2005 Jun 23.

Gillespie ND, Lenz TL. Reducing inflammation: Statins or lifestyle? *AJLM*, 2012 Jan/Feb;6(1):21–23.

Goldring MB, Otero M. Inflammation in osteoarthritis. *Curr Opin Rheumatol*, 2011 Sep;23(5):471–78.

Hafström I, Ringertz B, Spångberg A, et al. A vegan diet free of gluten improves the signs and symptoms of rheumatoid arthritis: The effects on arthritis correlate with a reduction in antibodies to food antigens. *Rheumatology* (Oxford), 2001 Oct;40(10):1175–79.

Hagen KB, Byfuglien MG, Falzon L, et al. Dietary interventions for rheumatoid arthritis. *Cochrane Database Syst Rev*, 2009 Jan 21;(1): CD006400.

Haugen MA, Kjeldsen-Kragh J, Skakkebaek N, et al. The influence of fast and vegetarian diet on parameters of nutritional status in patients with rheumatoid arthritis. *Clin Rheumatol*, 1993 Mar; 12(1):62–69.

Holst-Jensen SE, Pfeiffer-Jensen M, Monsrud M, et al. Treatment of rheumatoid arthritis with a peptide diet: A randomized, controlled trial. *Scand J Rheumatol*, 1998; 27(5):329–36.

Jessop DS, Harbuz MS. A defect in cortisol production in rheumatoid arthritis: Why are we still looking? *Rheumatology* (Oxford), 2005 Sep; 44(9): 1097–1100.

Kavanaghi R, Workman E, Nash P, et al. The effects of elemental diet and subsequent food reintroduction on rheumatoid arthritis. *Br J Rheumatol*, 1995 Mar;34(3):270–73.

Kjeldsen-Kragh J. Rheumatoid arthritis treated with vegetarian diets. *Am J Clin Nutr*, 1999 Sep;70(3 Suppl):594S-600S.

Kjeldsen-Kragh J, Haugen M, Borchgrevink CF, et al. Controlled trial of fasting and one-year vegetarian diet in rheumatoid arthritis. *Lancet*, 1991 Oct 12;338(8772): 899–902.

Mahan LK, Escott-Stump S. *Krause's Food & Nutrition Therapy*, 12th ed. St. Louis, MO: Saunders Elsevier, 2008.

McDougall J, Bruce B, Spiller G, et al. Effects of a very low-fat, vegan diet in subjects with rheumatoid arthritis. *J Altern Complement Med*, 2002 Feb;8(1):71–75.

McKellar G, Morrison E, McEntegart A, et al. A pilot study of a Mediterranean-type diet intervention in female patients with rheumatoid arthritis living in areas of social deprivation in Glasgow. *Ann Rheum Dis*, 2007 Sep; 66(9):1239–43.

Müller H, de Toledo FW, Resch KL. Fasting followed by vegetarian diet in patients with rheumatoid arthritis: A systematic review. *Scand J Rheumatol*, 2001;30(1):1-10.

Nanri A, Moore MA, Kono S. Impact of C-reactive protein on disease risk and its relation to dietary factors. *Asian Pac J Cancer Prev*, 2007 Apr–Jun; 8(2):167–77.

National Collaborating Centre for Chronic Conditions (UK). *Rheumatoid Arthritis: National Clinical Guideline for Management and Treatment in Adults*. London: Royal College of Physicians (UK), 2009 Feb.

Nenonen MT, Helve TA, Rauma AL, Hänninen OO. Uncooked, lactobacilli-rich, vegan food and rheumatoid arthritis. *Br J Rheumatol*, 1998 Mar;37(3):274–81.

Peltonen R, Nenonen M, Helve T, et al. Faecal microbial flora and disease activity in rheumatoid arthritis during a vegan diet. *Br J Rheumatol*, 1997 Jan;36(1):64–68.

Perry MG, Kirwan JR, Jessop DS, Hunt LP. Overnight variations in cortisol, interleukin 6, tumour necrosis factor alpha and other cytokines in people with rheumatoid arthritis. *Ann Rheum Dis*, 2009 Jan;68(1):63–68. Epub 2008 Mar 28.

Plaisance EP, Grandjean PW. Physical activity and high-sensitivity C-reactive protein. *Sports Med*, 2006; 36(5): 443–58.

Pronsky Z, Crowe J. Food-Medication Interactions, 16th ed. Birchrunville, PA: *Food-Medication Interactions*, 2010.

Pullerits R, Bokarewa M, Dahlberg L, Tarkowski A. Decreased levels of soluble receptor for advanced glycation end products in patients with rheumatoid arthritis indicating deficient inflammatory control. *Arthritis Res Ther*, 2005;7(4):R817–24. Epub 2005 Apr 25.

Scherer E. Tips for cooking when you have arthritis. *Discovery Health*, 2011. Available at: http://health.howstuffworks.com/diseases-conditions/arthritis/overview/cooking-with-arthritis.htm.

Scott R. Pain-free grocery shopping. *Arthritis Today*, 2009. Available at: http://www.arthritistoday.org/daily-living/do-it-easier/in-the-kitchen/shopping-tips.php.

Sköldstam L, Hagfors L, Johansson G. An experimental study of a Mediterranean diet intervention for patients with rheumatoid arthritis. *Ann Rheum Dis*, 2003 Mar;62(3):208–14.

Sköldstam L, Larsson L, Lindström FD. Effect of fasting and lactovegetarian diet on rheumatoid arthritis. *Scand J Rheumatol*, 1979; 8(4):249–55.

Uribarri J, Woodruff S, Goodman S, et al. Advanced glycation end products in foods and a practical guide to their reduction in the diet. *J Am Diet Assoc*, 2010 Jun; 110(6):911–16.

Vancouver Coastal Health. *Before, During and After Hip and Knee Replacement Surgery: A Patient's Guide*. Vancouver: Oasis, 2011.

Vander AJ, Sherman J, Luciano DS. *Human Physiology: The Mechanisms of Body Function*, 8th ed. New York: McGraw-Hill, 2011.

Verdaet D, Dendale P, De Bacquer D, et al. Association between leisure time physical activity and markers of chronic inflammation related to coronary heart disease. *Atherosclerosis*, 2004 Oct;176(2):303–10.

Best Websites

American College of Rheumatology: www.rheumatology.org

Arthritis Australia: www.arthritisaustralia.com.au

The Arthritis Society (Canada): www.arthritis.ca

Arthritis Today: www.arthritistoday.org

European League Against Rheumatism: www.eular.org

National Rheumatoid Arthritis Society (UK): www.nras.org.uk

Natural Medicines Comprehensive Database: http://naturaldatabase.therapeuticresearch.com

Office of Dietary Supplements, National Institutes of Health: http://ods.od.nih.gov

Contributing Authors

Byron Ayanoglu with contributions from Algis Kemezys
125 Best Vegetarian Recipes
Recipes from this book are found on pages 188, 230, 304, 307 and 329.

Byron Ayanoglu and Jennifer MacKenzie
Complete Curry Cookbook
Recipes from this book are found on pages 208, 243, 280, 313 and 321.

Johanna Burkhard
500 Best Comfort Food Recipes
Recipes from this book are found on pages 183, 201, 213, 231, 264, 298, 322 and 331.

Pat Crocker
The Vegan Cook's Bible
Recipes from this book are found on pages 173, 181, 190, 195, 196 (bottom), 226, 240, 261 and 330.

Pat Crocker
The Vegetarian Cook's Bible
Recipes from this book are found on pages 178, 182 (bottom), 198, 222, 224, 249 and 328.

Dietitians of Canada
Simply Great Food
Recipes from this book are found on pages 182 (top), 202, 218, 235 (top) and 282.

Maxine Effenson-Chuck and Beth Gurney
125 Best Vegan Recipes
Recipes from this book are found on pages 207, 212, 252, 253, 257, 316 and 318.

Judith Finlayson
The Complete Whole Grains Cookbook
Recipes from this book are found on pages 175, 179, 270, 295 and 296.

Judith Finlayson
The Convenience Cook
Recipes from this book are found on pages 194 and 200.

Judith Finlayson
The Healthy Slow Cooker
A recipe from this book is found on page 299.

Judith Finlayson
Slow Cooker Comfort Food
Recipes from this book are found on pages 216, 266, 275, 295, 300 and 311.

Judith Finlayson
The Vegetarian Slow Cooker
Recipes from this book are found on pages 306, 308, 310 and 312.

George Geary and Judith Finlayson
650 Best Food Processor Recipes
Recipes from this book are found on pages 191 (bottom), 203, 206, 225, 232, 234, 236 and 237.

Margaret Howard
The 250 Best 4-Ingredient Recipes
Recipes from this book are found on pages 174, 180, 211, 221, 227, 265 and 320.

Rose Murray
125 Best Casseroles and One-Pot Meals
Recipes from this book are found on pages 274 and 294.

Dr. Maitreyi Raman, Angela Sirounis and Jennifer Shrubsole
The Complete IBS Health & Diet Guide
Recipes from this book are found on pages 173, 186, 269 (bottom), 333 and 334.

Lynn Roblin, Nutrition Editor
500 Best Healthy Recipes
Recipes from this book are found on pages 255, 262, 324 and 332.

Jane Rodmell
All the Best Recipes
Recipes from this book are found on pages 189, 196 (top), 200, 228, 285, 286, 288, 291 and 325.

Andrew Schloss with Ken Bookman
2500 Recipes
Recipes from this book are found on pages 187, 191 (top), 235 (bottom), 259, 269, 283, 299 and 315.

Kathleen Sloan-McIntosh
125 Best Italian Recipes
Recipes from this book are found on pages 192, 204, 214, 260, 277 and 287.

Linda Stephen
Complete Book of Thai Cooking
Recipes from this book are found on pages 197, 209, 220, 268, 278, 305 and 335.

Suneeta Vaswani
Complete Book of Indian Cooking
Recipes from this book are found on pages 183, 240, 244, 246 and 314.

Suneeta Vaswani
Easy Indian Cooking
Recipes from this book are found on pages 184, 248, 250, 276, 284 and 327.

Mary Sue Waisman
Dietitians of Canada Cook!
Recipes from this book are found on pages 177, 238, 254, 256, 258, 271, 297, 326 and 336.

Donna Washburn and Heather Butt
Complete Gluten-Free Cookbook
A recipe from this book is found on page 176.

About the Nutrient Analyses

··

Computer-assisted nutrient analysis of the recipes was prepared by Kimberly Zammit, HBSc (the project supervisor was Len Piché, PhD, RD, Division of Food & Nutritional Sciences, Brescia University College, London, ON), using Food Processor® SQL, version 10.9, ESHA Research Inc., Salem OR (this software contains over 35,000 food items based largely on the latest USDA data and the entire Canadian Nutrient File, 2007b). The database was supplemented when necessary with data from the Canadian Nutrient File (version 2010) and documented data from other reliable sources.

The analysis was based on:

- imperial weights and measures (except for foods typically packaged and used in metric quantities);
- the smaller ingredient quantity when there was a range;
- the first ingredient listed when there was a choice of ingredients.

Calculations involving meat and poultry use lean portions without skin and with visible fat trimmed. A pinch of salt was calculated as $\frac{1}{8}$ tsp (0.5 mL). All recipes were analyzed prior to cooking. Optional ingredients and garnishes, and ingredients that are not quantified, were not included in the calculations.

Index